POCKETBOOK
of ORAL DISEASE

for Elsevier:
Commissioning Editor: Alison Taylor
Development Editor: Lynn Watt
Project Manager: Andrew Riley
Designer/Design Direction: Stewart Larking

POCKETBOOK
of ORAL DISEASE

Crispian Scully CBE
MD PhD MDS MRCS BSc FDSRCS FDSRCPS FFDRCSI FDSRCSE FRCPath
FMedSci FHEA FUCL DSc DChD DMed[HC] DrHC
Emiritus Professor, University College London, UK

Jose V Bagan MD DDS PhD
Professor of Oral Medicine, Valencia University and
Hospital General Universitario de Valencia, Valencia, Spain

Marco Carrozzo MD DSM
Professor of Oral Medicine, Newcastle University, Honorary Consultant,
Royal Victoria Infirmary Hospital, Newcastle upon Tyne, UK

Catherine M Flaitz DDS MS
Professor of Oral and Maxillofacial Pathology and Pediatric Dentistry,
The University of Texas School of Dentistry at Houston; Associate Faculty,
McGovern Center for Humanities and Ethics, The University of Texas
Medical School at Houston; and Associate Staff, Texas Children's
Hospital, Baylor College of Medicine, Texas, USA

Sergio Gandolfo MD DDS
Professor, Head of the Oral Medicine and Oral Oncology
Section, Department of Oncology,
University of Turin, Orbassano (Turin), Italy

CHURCHILL LIVINGSTONE

ELSEVIER

Edinburgh   London   New York   Oxford   Philadelphia   St Louis   Sydney   Toronto 2012

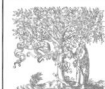

CHURCHILL
LIVINGSTONE
ELSEVIER

Figures in Chapter 7 © S. Gandolfo; C. Scully & M. Carrozzo. Originally published in Gandolfo *et al.* Oral Medicine ISBN 9780443100376, Elsevier 2006.

ISBN 978-0-702-04649-0

Reprinted 2013, 2015, 2016

British Library Cataloguing in Publication Data

A catalogue record for this book is available from the British Library

Library of Congress Cataloging in Publication Data

A catalog record for this book is available from the Library of Congress

Notices

Knowledge and best practice in this field are constantly changing. As new research and experience broaden our understanding, changes in research methods, professional practices, or medical treatment may become necessary.

Practitioners and researchers must always rely on their own experience and knowledge in evaluating and using any information, methods, compounds, or experiments described herein. In using such information or methods they should be mindful of their own safety and the safety of others, including parties for whom they have a professional responsibility.

With respect to any drug or pharmaceutical products identified, readers are advised to check the most current information provided (i) on procedures featured or (ii) by the manufacturer of each product to be administered, to verify the recommended dose or formula, the method and duration of administration, and contraindications. It is the responsibility of practitioners, relying on their own experience and knowledge of their patients, to make diagnoses, to determine dosages and the best treatment for each individual patient, and to take all appropriate safety precautions.

To the fullest extent of the law, neither the Publisher nor the authors, contributors, or editors, assume any liability for any injury and/or damage to persons or property as a matter of products liability, negligence or otherwise, or from any use or operation of any methods, products, instructions, or ideas contained in the material herein.

ELSEVIER your source for books, journals and multimedia in the health sciences

www.elsevierhealth.com

Working together to grow libraries in developing countries

www.elsevier.com | www.bookaid.org | www.sabre.org

ELSEVIER BOOK AID International Sabre Foundation

The Publisher's Policy is to use **paper manufactured from sustainable forests**

Printed in China

Last digit is the print number: 10   9   8   7   6   5   4

CONTENTS

PREFACE

This *Pocketbook of Oral Disease* is aimed at graduating dental care students and, as such, assumes knowledge of basic sciences and human diseases and offers the basics of oral diseases. The emphasis is on diagnosis and treatment in primary care settings, and the rather complex language and terminology is clarified in the glossaries of eponymous syndromes and abbreviations at the back of the book.

Since reliable epidemiological data are sparse, we have termed conditions seen by most practitioners as 'common', and those seen mainly by specialists only, as 'uncommon' or 'rare'. Graduating dentists are usually expected to know mainly about 'common' conditions and those that can be life-threatening.

The subject is presented initially by symptoms and signs, then discussing the various sites and giving synopses of the various conditions most commonly seen. Diagnosis, investigations, referral and care in primary care settings are then outlined.

This book was developed on the basis of a successful enterprise, the *Colour Guide to Oral Disease*, published with Professor Roderick Cawson, which was highly popular and went to several editions. Some of those illustrations appeared also in his *Essentials of Oral Pathology and Oral Medicine*, co-authored with Edward Odell.

This current guide has been thoroughly updated and expanded, and includes leading oral medicine clinicians as co-authors, originating from the USA (Professor Catherine Flaitz), Spain (Professor Jose Bagan) and Italy (Professor Marco Carrozzo and Professor Sergio Gandolfo), and includes some material from the book *Oral Medicine*, co-authored with these Italian colleagues.

Finally, our thanks are due to our patients and nurses, and, for various pieces of advice, to our colleagues Drs Monica Pentenero, Pedro Diz Dios and David Wiesenfeld.

C.S.
2012

Introduction

Oral medicine has been defined as being 'concerned with the oral health care of patients with chronic recurrent and medically related disorders of the mouth and with their diagnosis and non-surgical management'. Oral diseases can affect people of any background, gender or age.

Children are usually most liable to dental caries and the sequelae of odontogenic infections, and to acute viral infections, but oral diseases are generally more common in adults, especially older people or people with systemic disease. Immunocompromised individuals are especially prone to oral disease, and also to serious outcomes.

Factors predisposing to oral disease may include:

- Genetic predisposition: prominent especially in autosomal dominant conditions
- Systemic disease: including mental health issues
- Lifestyle habits: including poor oral hygiene and/or use of tobacco, alcohol, betel and recreational drugs
- Iatrogenic (doctor-induced) influences: such as the wearing of oral appliances; radiation therapy; transplantation procedures; drugs
- Nutrition: malnutrition and eating disorders.

Dangerous conditions

Many oral medicine conditions are recurrent or chronic and some are serious, with considerable associated morbidity (illness), often affecting the quality of life (QoL), and some are potentially lethal.

Conditions that are potentially dangerous or have a high mortality include disorders such as pemphigus, cancer and chronic infections such as HIV/AIDS, tuberculosis or syphilis (all of which may be lethal). Other conditions have a high morbidity (incidence of ill health), and these include temporal arteritis (cranial or giant cell arteritis), pemphigoid or Behçet syndrome (which can lead to blindness), trigeminal neuralgia and facial palsy (which may signify serious neurological diseases), and potentially malignant oral disorders such as leukoplakia, lichen planus and submucous fibrosis.

It is important to refer or biopsy a patient with any unusual lesion, especially a single lesion persisting 3 or more weeks (which could be a cancer), or if there are typically multiple persisting ulcers when a vesiculo-bullous disorder such as pemphigus is suspected (since this is potentially lethal).

Changes that might suggest malignant disease such as cancer could include any of the following persisting more than 3 weeks:

- A sore on the lip or in the mouth that does not heal
- A lump on the lip or in the mouth or throat
- A white or red patch on the gums, tongue, or lining of the mouth
- Unusual bleeding, pain, or numbness in the mouth
- A sore throat that does not go away, or a feeling that something is caught in the throat
- Difficulty or pain with chewing or swallowing
- Swelling of the jaw that causes dentures to fit poorly or become uncomfortable
- A change in the voice, and/or
- Pain in the ear
- Enlargement of a neck lymph gland.

If in any doubt – refer the patient for a second or a specialist opinion.

History

The history gives the diagnosis in the majority (possibly about 80%) of cases. Important questions to answer include, what is this chief or primary complaint (Complaining of [CO] or Chief Complaint [CC]) and what is the history (History of the Present Complaint [HPC]) – is this:

- The first episode?
- Persistent or recurrent?
- Changing in size or appearance?

and are there:

- Single or multiple lesions/symptoms?
- Specific or variable symptoms?
- Extraoral lesions?

The Relevant Medical History (RMH), Family History (FH) and Social History (SH) should be directed to elicit a relevant history in terms of a range of aspects. One way to remember all this is by the acronym **GSPOT, MED, RAGES**:

- **G**enetics: family history?
- **S**ocial history?
- **P**ets?
- **O**ccupation?
- **T**ravel history?
- **M**edical history/medications?
- **E**ating habits?
- **D**rugs and habits? (drugs of misuse; tobacco; alcohol; betel; artefactual [this means self-induced, or factitial])
- **R**espiratory features?
- **A**nogenital features?
- **G**astrointestinal features?
- **E**ye features?
- **S**kin, hair or nail features?

Additionally, other aspects are needed in relation to complaints specific to different systems, as detailed below.

History related to dental problems

The history related to dental (tooth) problems should also include at least:

- date of onset of symptoms
- swelling details, such as duration and character
- pain details, such as duration, site of maximum intensity, severity, onset, daily timing, character, radiation, aggravating and relieving factors, relationship to meals and associated phenomena
- mouth-opening restriction
- changes in the occlusion of the teeth
- hyposalivation details.

Disorders that affect the teeth may appear to be unilateral, but the other teeth should always be considered, and it is important to consider the possibility of related systemic disorders, especially those affecting:

- musculo-skeletal/connective tissue
- the neurological system (e.g. seizures)
- nutrition (eating disorders such as bulimia).

History related to mucosal problems

The history related to mucosal problems should also include at least:

- date of onset of symptoms
- lesional details, such as duration and character
- pain/discomfort details, such as duration, site of maximum intensity, severity, onset, daily timing, character, radiation, aggravating and relieving factors, relationship to meals and associated phenomena
- mouth-opening restriction.

Disorders that affect the mucosa may appear to be unilateral, but all the other oral mucosa should always be examined, and it is important to consider the possibility of related systemic disorders, especially infections, and those affecting:

- the haematopoietic system (e.g. anaemia or leukaemia)
- the gastrointestinal tract (e.g. Crohn disease)
- the skin and/or anogenital (e.g. lichen planus) or conjunctival or other mucosae (e.g. erythema multiforme)
- nutrition (disorders such as hypovitaminosis).

History related to salivary problems

The history related to salivary problems should also include at least:

- date of onset of symptoms
- swelling details such as site, duration and character, and relation to meals and whether enlarging
- quality and quantity of saliva, both observed and perceived, and details of any speech difficulties, dysphagia or taste alterations
- pain details, such as duration, daily timing, character, radiation, aggravating and relieving factors, relationship to meals and associated phenomena
- mouth-opening restriction

- history of dry eyes or dryness of other mucosa
- personal or family history of arthritis
- occupation, such as glass blowing or trumpet playing, which might introduce air into the gland (pneumoparotid).

Disorders that affect the salivary glands may appear to be unilateral, but the other glands should always be considered, and it is important to consider the possibility of related systemic disorders, especially those affecting:

- lachrymal and other exocrine glands (e.g. Sjögren syndrome)
- endocrine glands (e.g. diabetes)
- hepatobiliary system (e.g. alcoholic cirrhosis may underlie sialosis)
- connective tissues (e.g. rheumatoid arthritis or systemic lupus erythematosus).

History related to jaw problems

The history should also include:

- date of onset of symptoms
- precipitating factors (e.g. trauma)
- swelling details, such as duration and character
- pain details, such as site of maximum intensity, onset, duration, severity, daily timing, character, radiation, aggravating and relieving factors, relationship to meals and associated phenomena
- mouth-opening restriction
- history of dry eyes or dryness of other mucosa
- personal or family history of arthritis.

Disorders that affect the jaws or temporomandibular joint (TMJ) may appear to be unilateral, but the other areas should always be evaluated, and it is important to consider the possibility of related systemic disorders, especially infections and those affecting:

- bones (e.g. osteoporosis)
- joints (e.g. osteoarthritis)
- connective tissues (e.g. rheumatoid arthritis).

History related to pain and neurological problems

The history should also include at least (Box 1.1):

- date of onset of symptoms
- symptom details, such as duration and character, referred pain

> **Box 1.1** Characteristics of pain (SOCRATES)
>
> **S**ite
> **O**nset
> **C**haracter
> **R**adiation
> **A**ssociated features
> **T**ime course
> **E**xacerbating and relieving factors
> **S**everity

- pain details, such as duration, daily timing, character, radiation, aggravating and relieving factors, relationship to meals, and associated phenomena
- movement disorders
- sensory loss, including visual changes.

Disorders that affect the neurological system may appear to be unilateral, but the cranial nerves and neurological system should always be considered, and it is important to consider the possibility of related systemic disorders, especially those affecting the cardiovascular system (e.g. thromboembolism).

Examination

Careful examination is crucial and should include at the very least those extraoral areas readily inspected, such as (usually) the head and neck, and hands – with due consideration for culture.

Extraoral examination

Extraoral examination should include assessment of general features such as:

- anxiety or agitation
- appearance
- behaviour
- breathing
- communication
- conscious level
- movements

- posture
- sweating
- temperature
- wasting
- weight loss or gain

and careful inspection of the face for:

- facial symmetry
- facial colour – for pallor (e.g. fear, anaemia) or
- facial erythema (e.g. anxiety, alcoholism, polycythaemia) or rashes (e.g. infections, lupus) or other lesions (e.g. basal cell carcinoma)
- facial swellings – for soft tissue or salivary gland swellings (e.g. allergies, infections or inflammatory lesions), enlarged masseter muscles (masseteric hypertrophy) or bony enlargement
- fistulas or sinuses (which may be odontogenic in origin)
- pupil size (e.g. dilated in anxiety or cocaine abuse, constricted in opioid abuse).

Neck examination is mandatory, especially examination of cervical lymph nodes. Lesions in the neck may arise mainly from the cervical lymph nodes, but also from the thyroid gland, salivary glands and heterotopic salivary tissue, or from skin, subcutaneous tissues, muscle, nerve, blood vessels or other tissues.

Lesions arising from the skin can usually be moved with the skin and are generally readily recognizable.

Jaws

The jaws should be palpated to detect swelling or tenderness. Maxillary, mandibular or zygomatic deformities, fractures or enlargements may be more reliably confirmed by inspection from above (maxillae/zygomas) or behind (mandible).

Following trauma, all borders and sutures should be palpated for tenderness or a step deformity (at the infraorbital rim, the lateral orbital rim, the zygomatic arch and the zygomatic buttress intraorally).

The jaw joints (TMJ) should then be examined by inspecting:

- facial symmetry
- facial and intraoral discolouration and swelling (haematoma, ecchymoses, laceration)
- jaw opening and movements

and by palpating the bones, main masticatory muscles (temporalis, masseters and pterygoids), and TMJ – using fingers placed over the joints in front of the ears, to detect pain, or swelling.

Finally, the dental occlusion should be examined.

The neurological system

Cranial nerve examination may also be needed (Table 1.1), by inspecting:

- ■ facial symmetry and movement
- ■ ocular movements
- • testing trigeminal nerve
  - ■ corneal reflex (this tests Vth and VIIth cranial nerves); touching the cornea gently with sterile cotton wool should produce a blink.
  - ■ touch (tested with cotton wool or stream of air)
  - ■ vibration (tested with a tuning fork)
  - ■ proprioception (move a joint slightly with the patient's eyes closed and ask them to recognize the direction of the movement)
  - ■ pain (pin-prick testing)
  - ■ temperature (test with a warm or cold object)
- • hearing assessment
- • examining the eyes
- • testing taste sensation (gustometry) using stimuli on a cotton-tipped applicator, including:
  - ■ citric acid or hydrochloric acid (sour taste)
  - ■ caffeine or quinine hydrochloride (bitter)
  - ■ sodium chloride (salty)
  - ■ saccharose (sweet)
  - ■ monosodium glutamate (umami taste).

Electrogustometry examines taste sensitivity by means of electric excitability thresholds determined through the response to the irritation of taste buds area with electrical current of different intensity.

Trigeminal motor functions that should be tested include:

- • jaw jerk
- • palpating muscles of mastication during function:
  - ■ masseters during clenching
  - ■ temporalis during clenching
  - ■ pterygoids during jaw protrusion.

Table 1.1 Cranial nerve examination

Nerve		Test/examination/consequence of lesion
Number	**Name**	
I	Olfactory	Smell
II	Optic	Visual fields Visual acuity Pupils equal reactive to light and accommodation (PERLA) Fundoscopy
III	Oculomotor	Eye movements
IV	Trochlear	Diplopia
V	Abducens	Nystagmus
VI	Trigeminal	Sensory-fine touch, pin prick, hot and cold Masticatory muscle power Corneal reflex Jaw jerk
VII	Facial	Facial movements Corneal reflex Taste
VIII	Vestibulocochlear	Hearing Balance
IX	Glossopharyngeal	Taste
X	Vagus	Gag reflex Speech Swallow Cough
XI	Accessory	Rotate head Shrug shoulders
XII	Hypoglossal	Tongue protrusion

Assess the mental state and level of consciousness (Glasgow Coma Scale) and, if necessary:

- assess speech
  - dysarthria (oropharyngeal, neurological or muscular pathology)
  - dysphonia (respiratory pathology), or
  - dysphasia (abnormal speech content due to damage in the brain language areas)
- check for neck stiffness (meningeal inflammation)
- look for abnormal posture or gait (broad-based in cerebellar deficit, shuffling in Parkinsonism, high stepping in peripheral leg neuropathy, swinging leg in hemiparesis, etc).

Specific neurological disease may be encountered, and thus the dental surgeon should be adept in examining the cranial nerves, especially the trigeminal and the facial nerves.

Trigeminal (V) nerve
This nerve conveys sensation from the head, face and mouth, and motor supply to the muscles of mastication, mylohyoid, anterior belly of digastric, tensor veli palatini and tensor tympani.

Test: light touch sensation (with cotton wool); pain (with pin prick); corneal reflex (touch the cornea with a wisp of cotton wool); open and close jaw against resistance; jaw jerk.

Abnormal findings include facial anaesthesia (sensory loss), hypoaesthesia (sensory diminution), dysaesthesia or paraesthesia (abnormal sensations like 'pins and needles'); abnormal reflexes; weakness and wasting of masticatory muscles.

Facial (VII) nerve
The facial nerve is motor to muscles of facial expression, stylohyoid, posterior belly of digastric, and stapedius; secretomotor (parasympathetic fibres to lachrymal, submandibular and sublingual salivary, nasal and palatine glands); and taste (from anterior two-thirds of tongue via the chorda tympani).

Test: facial movements (eye shutting, smiling, etc.); Schirmer test (a special paper strip to assess lacrimation); check for hyposalivation; taste sensation (apply salty, sweet, sour and bitter substances to the tongue as above); hearing, for hyperacusis. The facial nerve can be tested by asking patients to close their eyes and lips tightly – the strength of closure can be felt by manually trying to open them; asking patients to show their teeth;

asking patients to look upwards, raising the eyebrows and creasing the forehead; and also asking patients to whistle or fill their cheeks with air with their lips tightly pursed – if the face is weak, the patient will find it difficult to hold in the air. Tapping each inflated cheek reveals the weakness.

Lesions

Abnormal findings include contralateral facial weakness with partial sparing of the upper face (bilateral innervation) in upper motor neurone (UMN) lesions (brain lesions); ipsilateral facial weakness, impaired lacrimation, salivation and taste in lower motor neurone (LMN) lesions (e.g. Bell palsy, parotid surgery, etc.).

Neurological disorders may appear to be unilateral, but the other cranial nerves should always be examined. An overall neurologic examination should be performed to evaluate for widespread disease. It is important to consider drug use and the possibility of related systemic disorders.

Intraoral examination

For mouth examination:

- Use a good light via
  - conventional dental unit light
  - special loupes or
  - otorhinolaryngology light.
- Remove any dental appliance to examine beneath.
- Examine all visible mucosa.
- Begin away from focus of complaint or location of known lesions.
- Examine the dorsum of tongue, ventrum of tongue, floor of the mouth, hard and soft palate mucosa, gingivae, labial and buccal mucosa, and teeth.
- A systematic and consistent approach to the examination is important.

Mucosal lesions are not always readily visualized and, among attempts to aid this, but not proven superior to conventional visual examination in terms of specificity or sensitivity, are:

Toluidine blue staining (also known as tolonium blue or vital staining). The patient rinses with 1% acetic acid for 20 seconds to clean the area, then with plain water for 20 seconds, then with 1% aqueous toluidine blue solution for 60 seconds, then again rinses with a 1% acetic acid for 20 seconds, and finally with water for 20 seconds. Toluidine blue stains some areas blue – these are mainly but not exclusively pathological areas.

Chemiluminescent illumination. The technique uses light refraction and relies on fluorophores that naturally occur in cells after rinsing the mouth with 1% acetic acid using excitation with a suitable wavelength. The visibility of some lesions may thus be enhanced.

Fluorescence spectroscopy. Tissues are illuminated with light and lesions change the fluorophore concentration and light scattering and absorption. Their visibility may thus be enhanced.

There are limitations in these aids, discussed in Chapter 7, but combinations of these approaches may enhance the evaluation of the tissues and assist in the decision-making.

Lesions once identified should be described using standardized nomenclature, as shown in Table 1.3 at the end of the chapter, and entered onto a diagram of the mouth. Photographs may be indicated.

The lips

The lips should be examined in a systematic fashion to ensure that all areas are included. The lips should first be inspected and examination is then facilitated if the mouth is gently closed and the lips everted.

The lips consist of skin on the external surface and mucous membrane on the inner surface within which are bundles of striated muscle, particularly the orbicularis oris muscle. The upper lip includes the philtrum, a midline depression, extending from the columella of the nose to the superior edge of the vermilion zone. The oral commissures are the angles where the upper and lower lips meet.

The epithelium of the lip vermilion, the transitional zone between the glabrous skin and the mucous membrane, is distinctive, with a prominent stratum lucidum and a thin stratum corneum: the dermal papillae are numerous, with a rich capillary supply, which produces the reddish-pink colour of the lips. Melanocytes are abundant in the basal layer of the vermilion of pigmented skin, but are infrequent in white skin. The vermilion zone contains no hair or sweat glands but does contain ectopic sebaceous glands (Fordyce spots) – yellowish pinhead-sized papules particularly seen in the upper lip and at the commissures. They also appear intraorally, mainly in the buccal mucosa. The lips feel slightly nodular because of the minor salivary glands they contain, and the labial arteries are readily palpable. The normal labial mucosa appears moist with a fairly prominent vascular arcade, and in the lower lip particularly many minor salivary glands which are often exuding mucus are visible.

Intraoral mucosae

The intraoral mucosa is divided into lining, masticatory and specialized types.

- Lining mucosa (buccal, labial and alveolar mucosa, floor of mouth, ventral surface of tongue, soft palate, lips) is non-keratinized.
- Masticatory mucosa (hard palate, gingiva) is adapted to the forces of pressure and friction and is keratinized.
- Specialized mucosa is seen where taste buds are found, on the lingual dorsum mainly.

The tongue

The specialized mucosa on the dorsum of the tongue, adapted for taste and mastication, is keratinized but pink. A healthy child's tongue is rarely coated but a mild and thin whitish coating is commonly seen in healthy individuals.

The anterior two-thirds of the tongue, called the oral tongue, is embryologically different from the posterior third, or pharyngeal tongue. The anterior (oral) tongue also bears a number of different papillae. Filiform papillae, which form an abrasive surface to control the food bolus as it is pressed against the palate, cover the entire surface of the anterior two-thirds of the tongue dorsum.

Fungiform papillae are fewer and are scattered between the filiform papillae, mainly anteriorly; they are mushroom-shaped, red structures covered by non-keratinized epithelium and with taste buds on their surface.

Circumvallate papillae are 8–12 large papillae each surrounded by a deep groove into which open ducts of the serous minor salivary glands; they are located adjacent and anterior to the sulcus terminalis – the line that separates the oral from the pharyngeal tongue. The lateral walls of the circumvallate papillae contain taste buds. Foliate papillae – 4–11 parallel ridges alternating with deep grooves in the mucosa – lie on the lateral margins posteriorly and also have taste buds.

The posterior tongue contains large amounts of lymphoid tissue – the lingual tonsil – which is part of the Waldeyer ring of lymphoid tissue that surrounds the entrance to the pharynx. The round or oval prominences of lymphoid tissue with intervening lingual crypts lined by non-keratinized epithelium lie between the epiglottis posteriorly and the circumvallate papillae anteriorly. The posterior third of the tongue is usually divided in the midline by a ligament. The posterior third of the tongue is thus embryologically and anatomically distinct from the anterior two-thirds (the oral tongue) and the two parts are joined at a V-shaped groove, the sulcus terminalis. The tongue dorsum is best inspected by protrusion The floor of the mouth and tongue ventrum are best examined by asking the patient to push the tongue first into the palate and then into each cheek in turn. This raises for inspection the floor of the mouth, an area where tumours may start (the 'coffin' or 'graveyard' area of the mouth). The tongue can be held with gauze to facilitate examination.

The posterior aspect of the floor of the mouth is the most difficult area to examine well and one where lesions are most likely to be missed. It can be inspected with the aid of a mirror but examination in the conscious patient induces retching. Use of topical anaesthetics or examination under conscious sedation or general anaesthesia (EUA) may be indicated in some cases.

Abnormalities of tongue movement (neurological or muscular disease) may be obvious from dysarthria or involuntary movements and any fibrillation or wasting noted. The voluntary tongue movements and sense of taste should be formally tested. Taste sensation can be tested with salt, sweet, sour, bitter and umami by applying solutions of salt, sugar, vinegar (acetic acid), 5% citric acid and glutamate to the tongue on a cotton swab or cotton pellet.

The palate

The palate and fauces consist of a hard and keratinized anterior and non-keratinized soft posterior palate, the tonsillar area and pillars of the fauces, and the oropharynx. The mucosa of the hard palate is firmly bound down as a mucoperiosteum (similar to the gingivae) and with no obvious vascular arcades. Rugae are present anteriorly on either side of the incisive papilla that overlies the incisive foramen.

The soft palate and fauces may show a faint vascular arcade. In the soft palate, just posterior to the junction with the hard palate, is a conglomeration of minor salivary glands, a region that is often also yellowish due to submucosal fat or pigmented due to racial pigmentation.

The palate should be inspected and movements examined when the patient says 'Aah'. Using a mirror permits inspection of the posterior tongue, tonsils and oropharynx, and can even offer a glimpse of the epiglottis and larynx.

Glossopharyngeal palsy may lead to uvula deviation to the contralateral side. It is also advisable to evaluate for vibration and mobility of the soft palate to determine if a submucous cleft palate is present.

The gingivae

The gingivae consist of a free gingival margin overlapping the cemento-enamel junction of the tooth and a strip of attached 'keratinized' gingiva bound down to the alveolar bone that supports the teeth. The attached gingiva is clearly demarcated from the non-keratinized vascular alveolar mucosa. The gingivae in health are firm, pale pink, sometimes with melanin racial pigmentation, with a stippled surface, and have sharp gingival papillae reaching up between adjacent teeth to the tooth contact point.

The dentogingival junction is a unique anatomical feature concerned with the attachment of the gingiva to the tooth. Non-keratinized gingival epithelium forms a cuff surrounding the tooth, and at its lowest point on the tooth is adherent to the enamel or cementum. This 'junctional' epithelium is unique in being bound both on its tooth and lamina propria aspects by basement membranes. Above this is a shallow sulcus or crevice (up to 2 mm deep), the gingival sulcus or crevice.

The tooth root is connected to the alveolar bone by fibres of the periodontal ligament, which run to the cementum. Bands of tissue, which may contain muscle attachments (fraena), run from the labial mucosa centrally onto the alveolar mucosa and from the buccal mucosa in the premolar region onto the alveolar mucosa.

Examine particularly for abnormalities such as gingival redness, swelling, ulceration or bleeding on gently probing the gingival margin, pocket depth and for tooth mobility.

The buccal and labial mucosa

These mucosa are non-keratinized. The labial mucosa has a vascular pattern and prominent minor salivary glands but these are not obvious in the buccal mucosa.

Fordyce spots may be conspicuous, particularly in the upper lip and near the commissures and retromolar regions in adults.

Stensen ducts (parotid papillae) can be seen opening by the crowns of the maxillary second molars.

The teeth

The teeth develop from neuroectoderm, and development (odontogenesis) of all the deciduous and some of the permanent dentition begins in the fetus. Mineralization of the primary dentition commences at about 14 weeks *in utero* and all primary teeth are mineralizing by birth. Tooth eruption occurs after crown formation when mineralization is largely complete but before the roots are fully formed (Table 1.2). The first or primary (deciduous or milk) dentition begins to erupt at age 6 months and by 3 years is complete, comprising two incisors, a canine and two molars in each of the four mouth quadrants. There are 10 deciduous (primary or milk) teeth in each jaw.

Permanent incisor and first molar teeth begin to mineralize at, or close to, the time of birth, mineralization of other permanent teeth starting later. The secondary or permanent teeth begin to erupt at about the age of 6–7 years and the deciduous teeth are slowly lost by normal root resorption. The full permanent (adult) dentition consists of 16 teeth in each jaw: two incisors, a canine, two premolars and three molars in each quadrant (Table 1.2). Normally most teeth have erupted by about 12–14 years of age. However, some deciduous (milk) teeth may still be present at the age of 12–13 years. The last molars (third molars or 'wisdom teeth'), if present, often erupt later or may impact and never appear in the mouth.

A fully developed tooth comprises a crown of insensitive enamel, surrounding sensitive dentine, and a dentine root which has a cementum rather than enamel covering. Teeth contain a vital pulp (nerve). The fibres of the periodontal ligament run from the alveolus to attach through cementum to the dentine surface and thus attach the tooth to the jaw.

The salivary glands

The major salivary glands are the parotids, submandibular and sublingual glands. Minor salivary glands are found elsewhere in the mouth – especially in the lips, ventrum of the tongue and soft palate. The major salivary glands should be inspected and palpated, noting any swelling or tenderness, and the character and volume of saliva exuding from the salivary ducts.

Early enlargement of the parotid gland is characterized by outward deflection of the lower part of the ear lobe, which is best observed by inspecting

Table 1.2 Tooth eruption times

Deciduous (primary) teeth	Upper (mth)	Lower (mth)
A Central incisors	8–13	6–10
B Lateral incisors	8–13	10–16
C Canines (cuspids)	16–23	16–23
D First molars	13–19	13–19
E Second molars	25–33	23–31
Permanent (secondary) teeth	**Upper (yr)**	**Lower (yr)**
1 Central incisors	7–8	6–7
2 Lateral incisors	8–9	7–8
3 Canines (cuspids)	11–12	9–10
4 First premolars (bicuspids)	10–11	10–12
5 Second premolars (bicuspids)	10–12	11–12
6 First molars	6–7	6–7
7 Second molars	12–13	11–13
8 Third molars	17–21	17–21

the patient from behind. This simple sign may allow distinction of parotid enlargement from simple obesity. Swelling of the parotid sometimes causes trismus. The parotid duct (Stensen duct) is most readily palpated with the jaws clenched firmly since it runs horizontally across the upper masseter where it can be gently rolled, to open at a papilla on the buccal mucosa opposite the upper molars.

The submandibular gland is best palpated bimanually with a finger of one hand in the floor of the mouth lingual to the lower molar teeth, and a finger of the other hand placed over the submandibular triangle (bimanual palpation). The submandibular duct (Wharton duct) runs anteromedially across the floor of the mouth to open at the side of the lingual fraenum.

Examine intraorally for normal salivation from these ducts, and pooling of saliva in the floor of the mouth. Any exudate obtained by massaging or milking the ducts should be noted.

Examine for signs of hyposalivation (frothy or stringy saliva, lack of saliva pooling or frank dryness). Place the surface of a dental mirror against the buccal (cheek) mucosa; the mirror should lift off easily but, if it adheres to the mucosa or draws a string of thick saliva as it is slowly moved away, then hyposalivation is present.

Anatomical features or developmental anomalies

Anatomical features or developmental anomalies that may be noticed by patients or clinicians and cause concern include:

- Bifid uvula: this is symptomless but may overlie a submucous cleft palate. That may not immediately be obvious but there may be slight nasal intonation of speech.
- Bony-hard enlargements:
  - exostoses – benign, painless and self-limiting broad-based surface bony-hard masses with normal overlying mucosa (Figures 1.1, 1.2) seen on the facial aspect of the jaw, most commonly on the maxilla. They begin to develop in early adulthood and may enlarge slowly over years. They have no malignant potential.
  - pterygoid hamulus – bilateral, palpable and bony hard lumps located posterior to the last maxillary molars. They may give rise to concern about an 'unerupted tooth'.

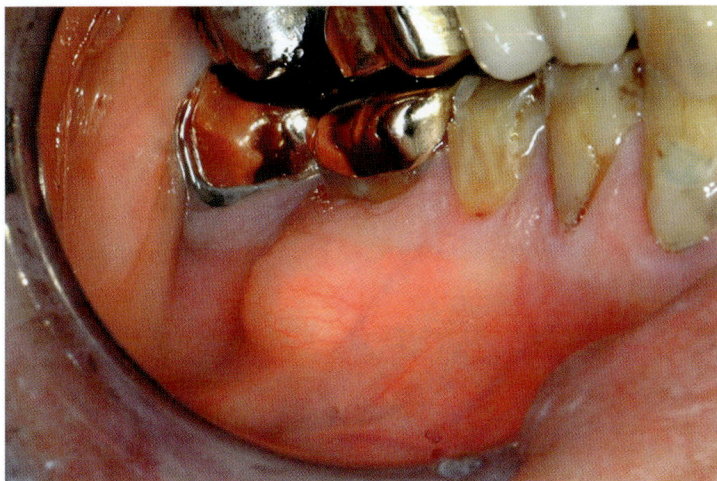

Figure 1.1 Exostosis.

Figure 1.2 Exostosis.

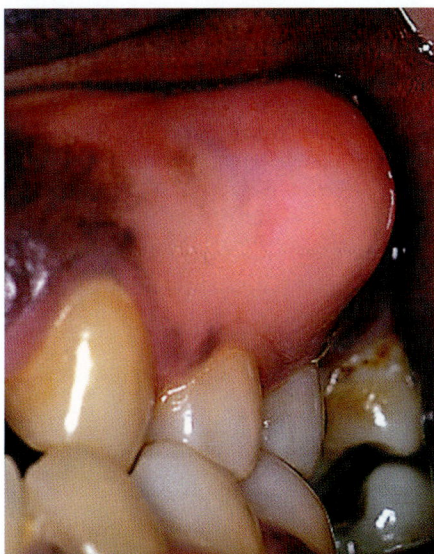

Anatomical features or developmental anomalies (continued)

- torus mandibularis – fairly common benign, painless and self-limiting broad-based surface bony-hard masses with normal overlying mucosa seen lingual to the mandibular premolars, usually bilaterally. These are variable in size and shape (Figures 1.3–1.5). They have no malignant potential.

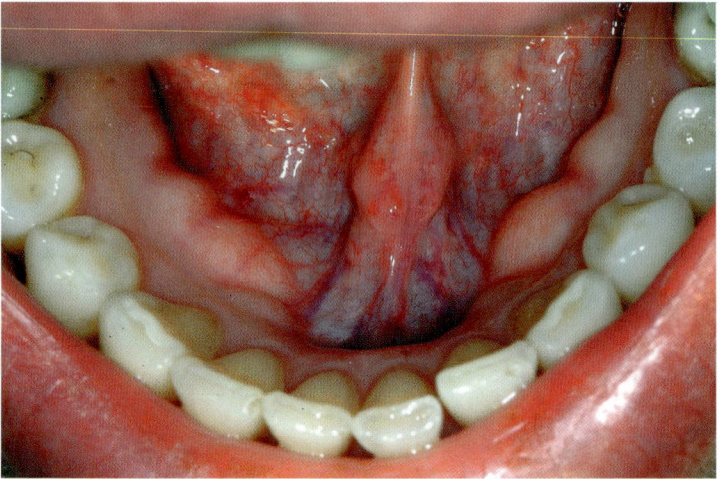

Figure 1.3 Torus mandibularis.

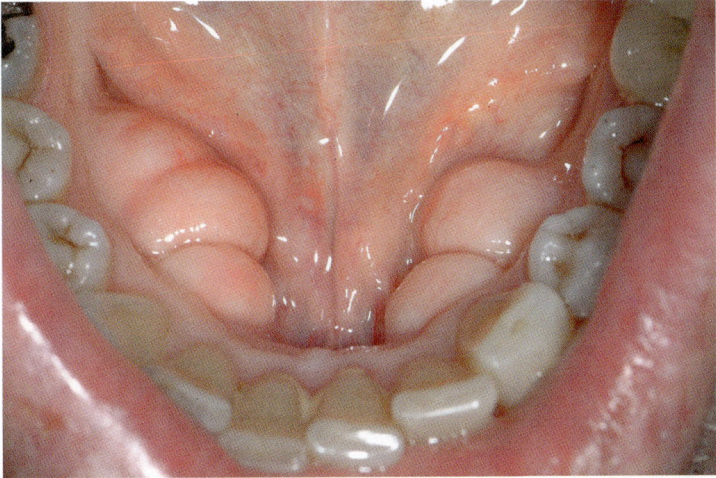

Figure 1.4 Torus mandibularis.

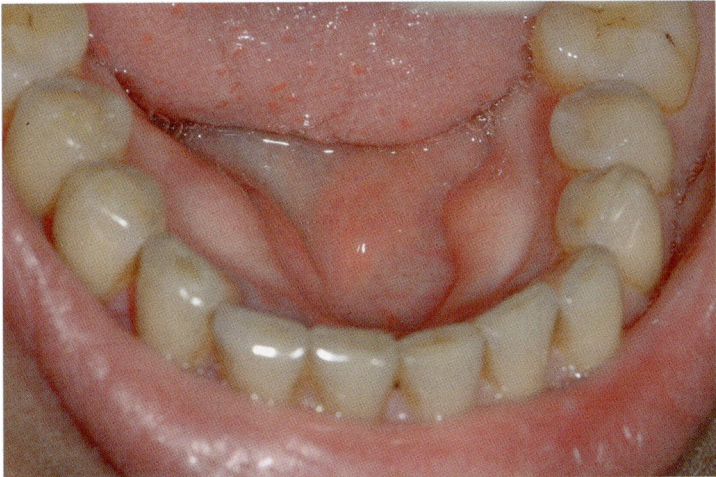

Figure 1.5 Torus mandibularis.

Anatomical features or developmental anomalies (continued)

- torus palatinus – fairly common benign, painless and self-limiting broad-based surface bony-hard masses with normal overlying mucosa seen in the centre of the hard palate. They may be smooth-surfaced or lobulated (Figures 1.6 and 1.7). They have no malignant potential.
- unerupted teeth – mainly third molars, second premolars and canines.

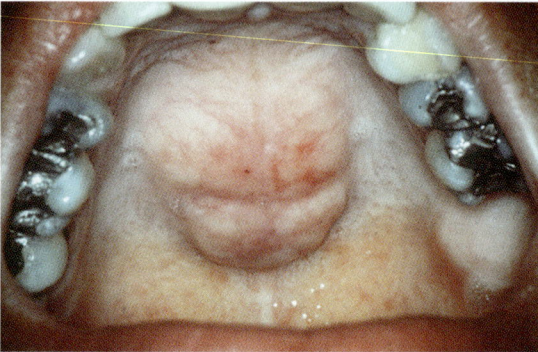

Figure 1.6 Torus palatinus.

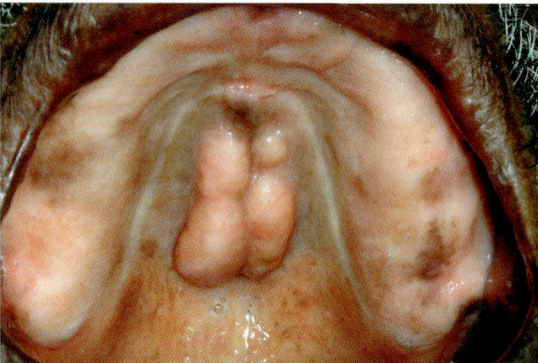

Figure 1.7 Torus palatinus.

- Fissured tongue is common (Figures 1.8, 1.9) and usually inconsequential, although erythema migrans (geographic tongue) is often associated. Fissured tongue is usually isolated and developmental but can be associated with systemic disease (Down syndrome, Melkersson–Rosenthal syndrome or Sjögren syndrome).

Figure 1.8 Fissured tongue.

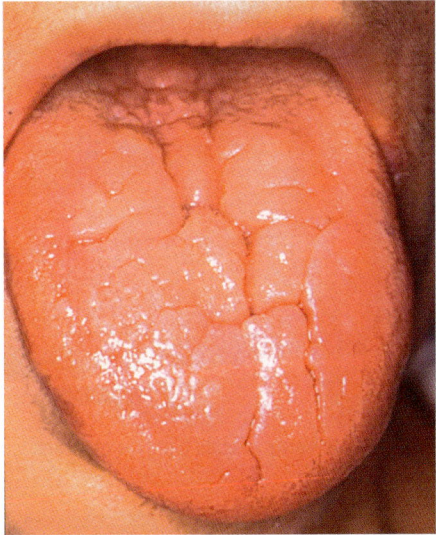

Figure 1.9 Fissured tongue.

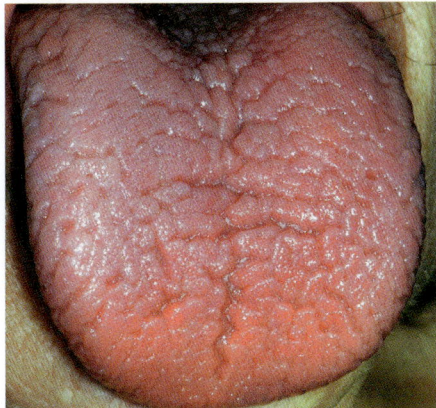

Anatomical features or developmental anomalies (continued)

- Fordyce spots: sebaceous glands seen mainly in the upper lip, commissures and retromolar regions (Figures 1.10, 1.11).

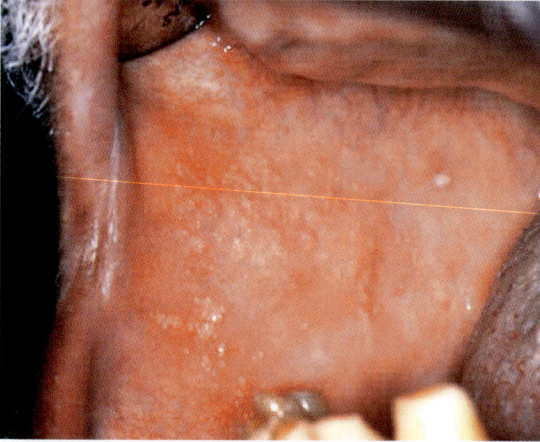

Figure 1.10 Fordyce spots (Fordyce granules).

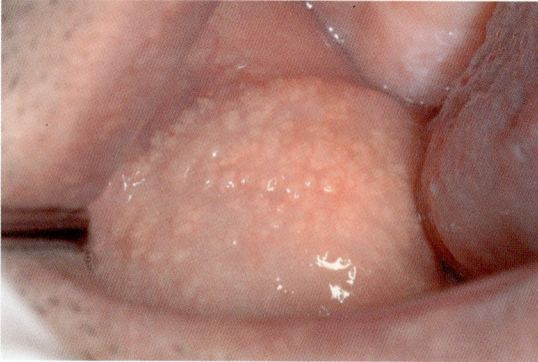

Figure 1.11 Fordyce spots (Fordyce granules).

- Leukoedema: a normal variation more prevalent in people of colour, in which there is a white-bluish tinge of the buccal mucosa that disappears when the cheek is stretched (Figures 1.12, 1.13).

Figure 1.12 Leukoedema.

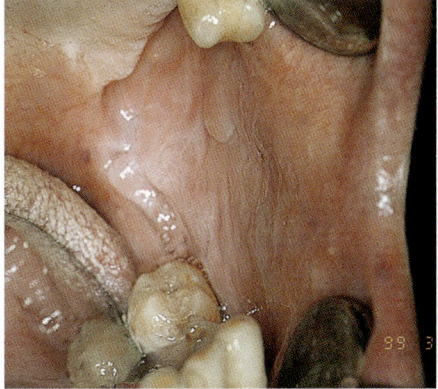

Figure 1.13 Leukoedema: same case as in figure 1.12 but after stretching mucosa.

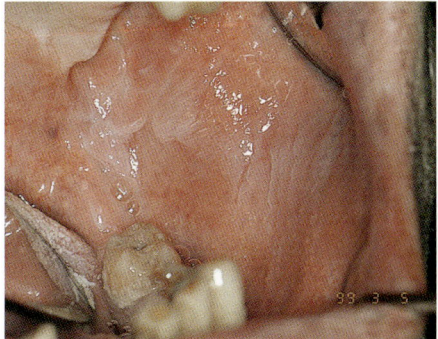

Anatomical features or developmental anomalies (continued)

- Lingual varicosities: inconsequential dilated sublingual veins seen mainly in older men (Figure 1.14).
- Lingual tonsils: rounded masses of normal lymphoid tissue covering the posterior third of the tongue, and part of Waldeyer ring of lymphoid tissue (along with the tonsils and adenoids).
- Papillae:
  - incisive – in the anterior palate (palatal to and between the central incisors); may be tender if traumatized
  - lingual
    a circumvallate – run in a V-shaped line across the posterior aspect of the anterior (oral) tongue (Figure 1.15)
    b filiform – these are the smallest lingual papillae and scattered across the anterior two-thirds of the tongue (Figure 1.16)
    c fungiform – bigger than the filiform but scattered in the same way across the anterior two-thirds of tongue (Figure 1.16)
    d foliate – bilateral but not necessarily symmetrical on the posterior borders of the tongue; occasionally become inflamed (foliate papillitis also called hypertrophy of the foliate papillae) and can mimic carcinoma (Figure 1.17).

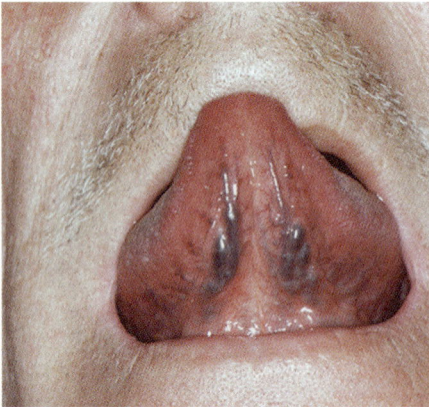

Figure 1.14 Sublingual varices.

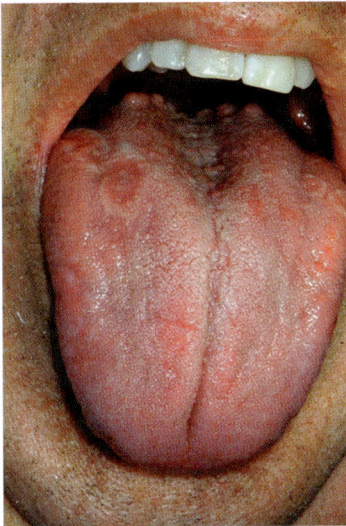

Figure 1.15 Circumvallate papillae (erythema migrans also present).

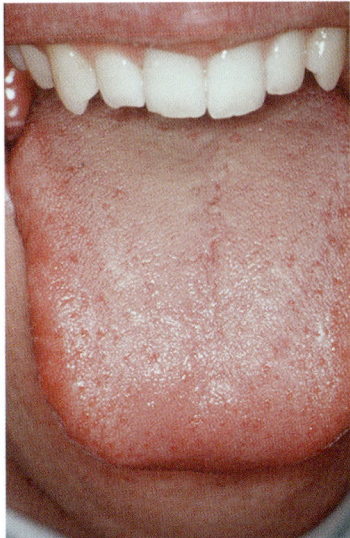

Figure 1.16 Filiform and fungiform papillae.

Figure 1.17 Foliate papillae.

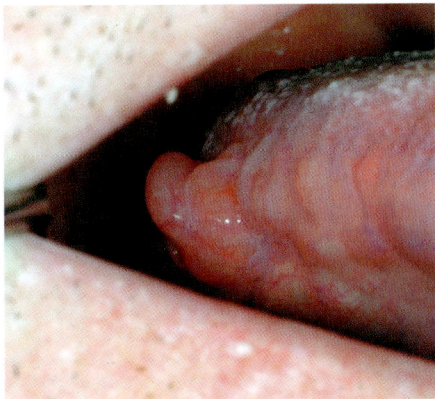

Anatomical features or developmental anomalies (continued)

- retrocuspid – usually bilateral and found on the lingual gingiva in the mandibular canine region, it resembles the incisive papilla
- salivary duct
  a parotid (orifice of Stensen duct) – bilateral and may occasionally be traumatized by biting, or by an orthodontic or other appliance
  b submandibular duct – in floor of mouth on either side of lingual fraenum.
- Racial pigmentation is the most common cause of oral pigmentation, and can be seen in many people, particularly, but not exclusively, in people of colour. Usually brown (rarely black), the pigmentation especially is seen on the gingiva, dorsal tongue or palate (Figures 1.18–1.20).
- Stafne bone cavity is most typically seen on radiographs as a unilateral, ovoid, radiolucent defect near the angle of the mandible below the inferior alveolar canal, and represents a cortical defect caused by an extension of the submandibular salivary gland (Figure 1.21).

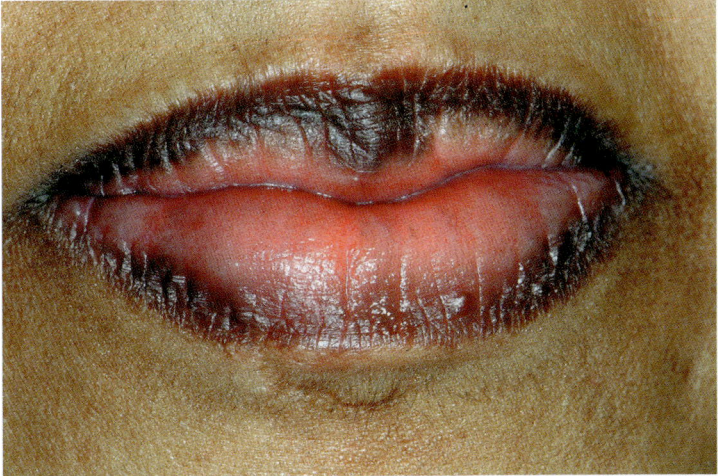

Figure 1.18 Racial pigmentation.

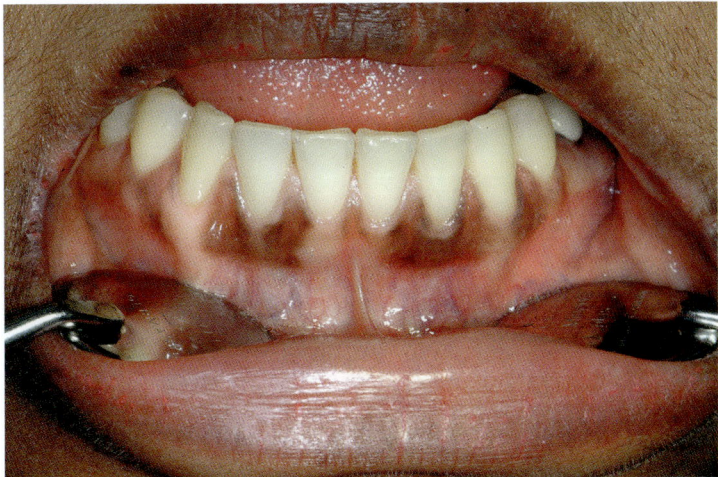

Figure 1.19 Racial pigmentation.

Anatomical features or developmental anomalies (continued)

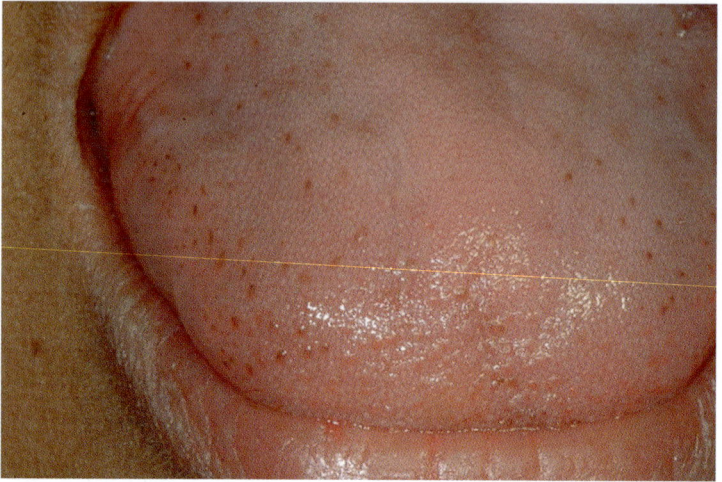

Figure 1.20 Racial pigmentation.

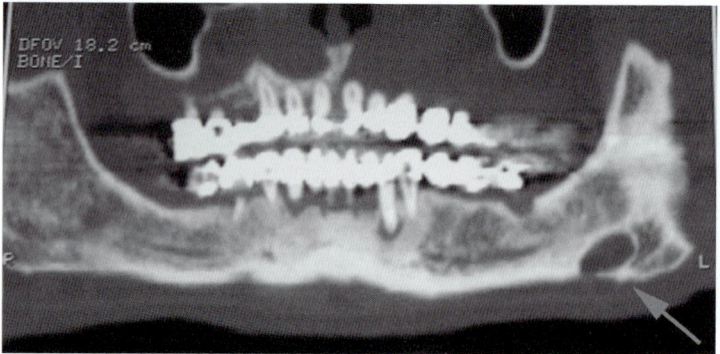

Figure 1.21 Stafne bone cavity in mandible.

Lesion descriptors

Table 1.3 Descriptive terms of oral lesions

Term	Meaning
Bulla	Visible fluid accumulation within or beneath epithelium (blister)
Desquamation	The shedding of the outer layers of the skin/oral mucosa
Ecchymosis	Macular area of haemorrhage >2 cm in diameter (i.e. a bruise)
Erosion	Loss of most of epithelial thickness (often follows a blister)
Erythema	Redness of mucosa
Macule	Flat, circumscribed alteration in colour or texture, not raised
Naevus	A pigmented lesion that is congenital or acquired
Nodule	Solid mass under/within mucosa or skin >0.5 cm in diameter
Papule	Circumscribed palpable elevation <0.5 cm in diameter
Pedunculated	Polyp with a stalk
Petechia	Punctate haemorrhagic spot 1–2 mm in diameter; often multiple
Plaque	Elevated area of mucosa or skin >0.5 cm in diameter
Polyp	Projecting mass of overgrown tissue
Pustule	Visible accumulation of purulent exudate in epithelium
Reticular	Resembles a net
Sessile	Stalkless and attached directly at the base

Continued

Table 1.3 Descriptive terms of oral lesions—cont'd

Term	Meaning
Striae	Thin lines or bands
Telangiectasis	Dilatation of capillaries
Tumour	Enlargement or swelling caused by normal or pathological material or cells
Ulcer	Loss of surface epithelium that extends to the underlying tissues
Vesicle	Small (<0.5 cm) visible fluid accumulation in epithelium

2

Differential diagnosis by signs and symptoms

This chapter discusses the main signs and symptoms of diseases affecting the orofacial region. Specific diseases are discussed in Chapter 3.

Pain is by far the most common symptom affecting the orofacial region (see Pain, page 89). The other most common signs and symptoms of orofacial disease fall into a limited number of categories, namely:

- **C**oloured lesions
- **B**leeding
- **S**oreness
- **W**hite lesions
- **U**lceration
- **L**umps/swelling
- **T**ooth mobility
- **H**alitosis

This can be remembered by the mnemonic **Could Be Someone We Usually Love To Hear.**

Bleeding

Keypoints

- Bleeding may arise from wounds or from the gingival margins, or may be into the tissues – where it appears as petechiae or ecchymoses (purpura).
- Gingival bleeding is usually due to plaque-induced inflammation – gingivitis or periodontitis.
- Gingival bleeding may be aggravated by, and purpura caused by, disorders of haemostasis or drugs interfering with haemostasis.
- Purpura in the mouth is seen mainly at areas of trauma – usually at the occlusal line and junction of the hard and soft palates.
- Bleeding of the lips may be seen where there is a lip fissure, or in erythema multiforme or some types of pemphigus.
- Vascular anomalies such as telangiectasia or angiomas may bleed if traumatized.

Box 2.1 Main causes of gingival bleeding

Gingivitis/periodontitis
Platelet defects
Drugs
Trauma

Causes may include:

- Gingivitis (plaque-induced) – by far the most common cause (Figure 2.1)
- Thrombocytopenia (low blood platelet numbers)
  - aplastic anaemia
  - idiopathic (this means 'of unknown cause' but actually it is autoimmune) thrombocytopenic purpura
  - leukaemia (Figure 2.2)
- Medications that impair haemostasis: anticoagulants, platelet aggregation inhibitors, chemotherapy, some herbal supplements
- Factitial or traumatic injury.

Oral bleeding occasionally arises from a vascular anomaly (Figure 2.3).

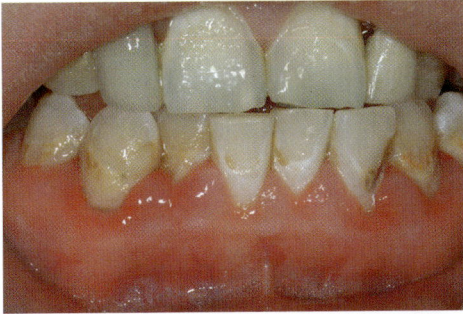

Figure 2.1 Gingivitis – the common cause of gingival bleeding.

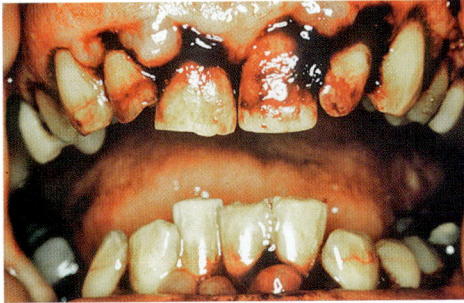

Figure 2.2 Leukaemia may present with gingival bleeding, swelling and/or ulceration.

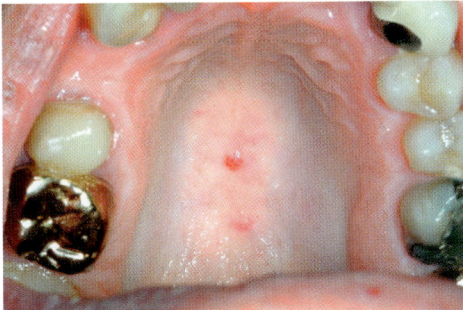

Figure 2.3 Hereditary haemorrhagic telangiectasia may chronically bleed.

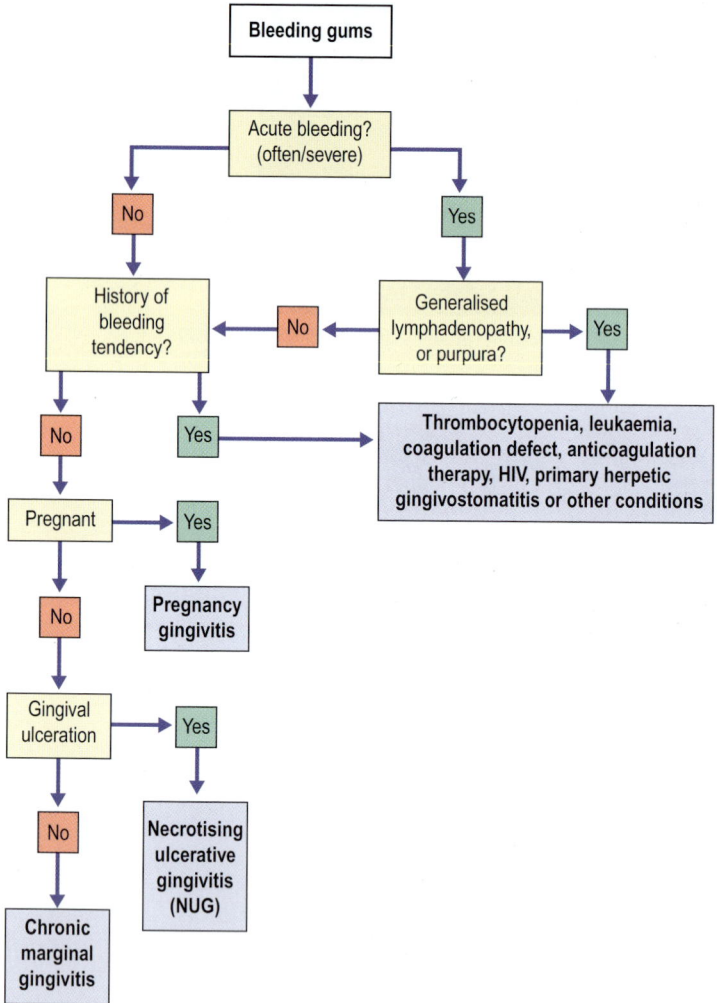

Figure 2.4 Algorithm for bleeding gums diagnosis.

Burning mouth

Keypoints

- Burning mouth (glossodynia) is a common complaint.
- The cause is not usually known but it may be a nerve hypersensitivity.
- Burning mouth is not inherited.
- Burning mouth is not infectious.
- Burning mouth may occasionally be caused by some mouth conditions, dry mouth, deficiencies, diabetes or drugs.
- Burning mouth has no long-term consequences.
- Burning mouth typically affects the anterior tongue bilaterally but may affect other sites such as palate and/or lips.
- Oral examination is important to exclude organic causes of similar discomfort – such as erythema migrans (geographic tongue), candidosis, glossitis and lichen planus (Figure 2.5).

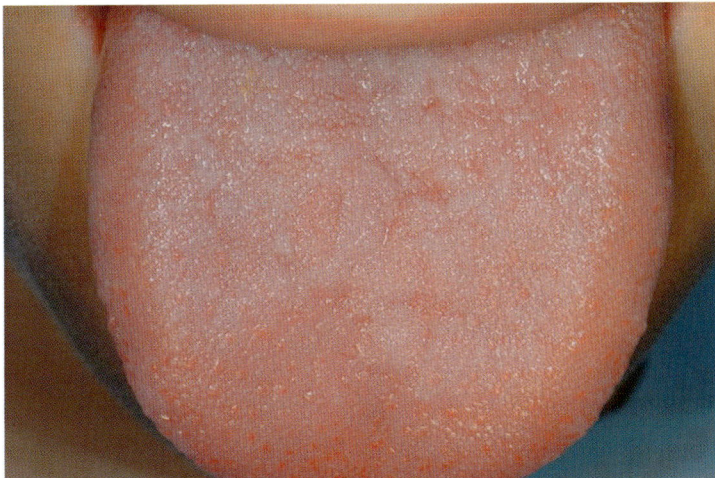

Figure 2.5 Burning mouth caused by lichen planus.

Burning mouth (continued)

- In the absence of a recognizable organic cause (Figure 2.6), the condition is termed 'burning mouth syndrome (BMS)' and the underlying basis may be psychogenic. These patients may also suffer taste disturbances.
- Blood tests, biopsy or other tests may be required.
- Burning mouth syndrome may be controlled by some psychotropic drugs or B vitamin.

Box 2.2 Main causes of burning mouth sensation

Erythema migrans
Lichen planus
Candidosis
Haematinic (iron, folate, vitamin B_{12}) deficiency
Psychogenic

Causes may include (alphabetically):

- Allergies (including oral allergy syndrome)
- Bruxism/tongue thrusting
- Candidosis
- Dermatoses such as lichen planus
- Dry mouth and drugs such as angiotensin-converting enzyme (ACE) inhibitors, proton pump inhibitors (PPIs) and protease inhibitors (PIs)
- Erythema migrans (geographic tongue)
- Fissured tongue
- Gastric reflux, and glossitis such as caused by haematinic deficiency, such as
  - B complex deficiency
  - folate deficiency
  - iron deficiency
  - vitamin B_{12} deficiency
- Hormonal (endocrine) problems such as diabetes and hypothyroidism.

  Once these causes are excluded, the condition is termed 'burning mouth syndrome', when the cause may be psychogenic, and include:

- Anxiety states
- Cancerophobia

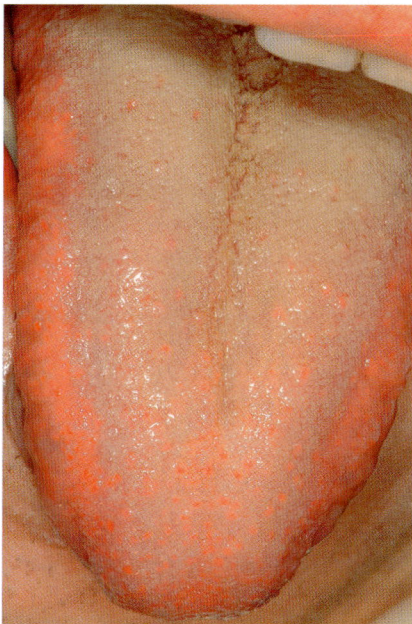

Figure 2.6 Burning mouth syndrome (no lesions discernible apart from mild tongue furring).

- Depression
- Hypochondriasis.

A normal-appearing tongue may be seen in psychogenic causes, and with a burning sensation caused by deficiency states, drugs (e.g. captopril and other ACE inhibitors, proton pump inhibitors) and diabetes mellitus.

This section deals only with a normal-looking but burning tongue.

Burning mouth syndrome

Common, especially in middle-aged females.

Typical orofacial symptoms and signs: invariably persistent burning sensation with no organic disease.

Main oral sites affected: anterior tongue (occasionally palate or lip).

Aetiopathogenesis: see above.

Gender predominance: female.

Age predominance: middle age or older.

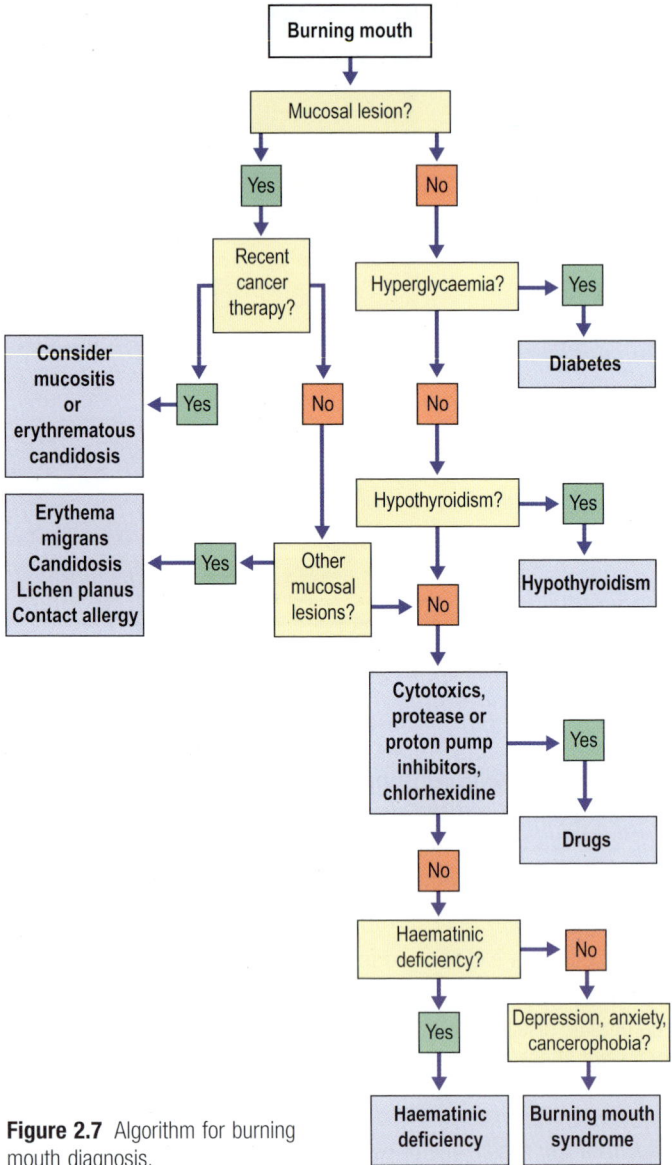

Figure 2.7 Algorithm for burning mouth diagnosis.

Extraoral possible lesions: often psychogenic complaints or anxiety.

Main associated conditions: few profess anxiety about (for example) cancer or sexually shared disease; some admit this on specific questioning.

Differential diagnosis: differentiate from organic causes.

Investigations: blood picture, glucose, thyroid hormone and haematinic assays to exclude organic causes; psychiatric investigation for depression.

Main diagnostic criteria: clinical.

Main treatments: treat any organic cause. Topical anaesthetics and oral distractors such as sucking on ice chips or sugarless candy, and chewing sugarless gum may be temporarily effective. Otherwise, B vitamins, topical capsaicin, psychotherapy (cognitive-behavioural therapy; CBT) or antidepressants are all occasionally helpful.

Desquamative gingivitis

Keypoints

- Desquamative gingivitis is not a disease entity but a clinical term for persistently sore, glazed and red or ulcerated gingivae.
- The usual complaint is of persistently sore gingivae in many areas.
- Lichen planus or pemphigoid are the most common causes.

Box 2.3 Main causes of desquamative gingivitis

Pemphigoid
Lichen planus

Fairly common, it is almost exclusively a disease of middle-aged or older females.

Typical orofacial symptoms and signs: soreness or stinging, especially on eating spices or citrus foods, or taking acidic drinks. Gingivae are red and glazed (patchily or uniformly), especially labially and in several sites. Gingival margins and edentulous ridges tend to be spared. Erythema is exaggerated where oral hygiene is poor.

Main oral sites affected: facial gingivae.

Desquamative gingivitis (continued)

Aetiopathogenesis: lichen planus or mucous membrane pemphigoid, and rarely pemphigus or other dermatoses (skin disorders) (Figures 2.8–2.10).

Gender predominance: female.

Age predominance: adult.

Extraoral possible lesions: cutaneous, mucosal or adnexal lesions of dermatoses may be associated.

Differential diagnosis: differentiate mainly from acute candidosis, chronic marginal gingivitis, and occasionally from plasma cell gingivitis.

Investigations: biopsy with immunostaining.

Main diagnostic criteria: clinical and histology.

Main treatments: improve oral hygiene; topical corticosteroids, or systemic dapsone as appropriate. Corticosteroid creams used overnight in a polythene splint may help. Frequent dental cleanings and periodontal maintenance are important for disease control.

Dry mouth (hyposalivation and xerostomia)

Keypoints

- Xerostomia is a frequent, and the most common, salivary complaint but is not synonymous with hyposalivation.
- Xerostomia is a subjective complaint of oral dryness, and objective evidence of hyposalivation is far less common.
- Hyposalivation (hyposialia) is a reduction in saliva production – usually defined as an unstimulated whole salivary flow rate <0.1 ml/min.
- Causes of hyposalivation are often iatrogenic (doctor-induced), particularly with drugs (medications) or cancer therapy.
- Hyposalivation may also be caused by dehydration, or diseases affecting the salivary glands.
- Xerostomia has similar causes to hyposalivation and, additionally, may be psychogenic.
- Saliva helps swallowing, talking, and taste, and protects the mouth. Where saliva is reduced there is a risk of dental caries and tooth wear, halitosis, altered taste, mouth soreness and infections.

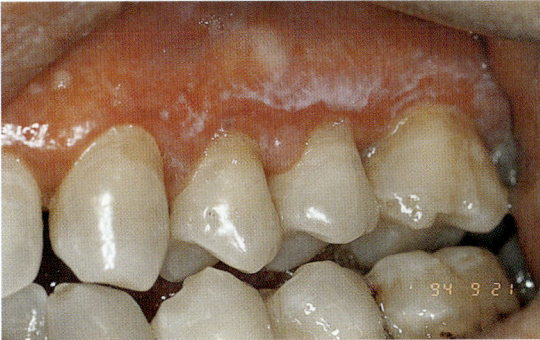

Figure 2.8 Desquamative gingivitis: associated with lichen planus.

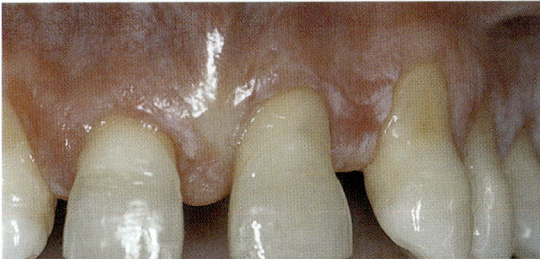

Figure 2.9 Desquamative gingivitis: associated with lichen planus.

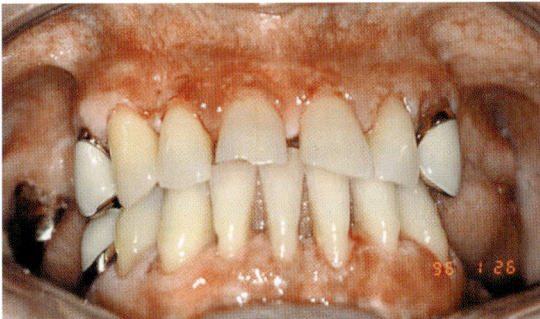

Figure 2.10 Desquamative gingivitis: associated with pemphigoid.

Dry mouth (hyposalivation and xerostomia) (continued)

> **Box 2.4** Main causes of dry mouth sensation
>
> Drugs
> Irradiation of salivary glands
> Sjögren syndrome
> Psychogenic

- Hyposalivation presents with obvious dryness (Figure 2.11) or frothy scant saliva (Figure 2.12), or with complaints of difficulties with speech, swallowing or denture retention; of soreness; or of complications such as candidosis, caries or sialadenitis.

Causes of hyposalivation may include:

- Iatrogenic
  - drugs (medications) with anticholinergic or sympathomimetic effects, such as tricyclic antidepressants, phenothiazines and antihistamines
  - irradiation of major salivary glands
  - cytotoxic agents, bone marrow transplantation and chronic graft-versus-host (GvHD) disease
- Non-iatrogenic
  - dehydration, e.g. uncontrolled diabetes, diabetes insipidus, diarrhoea and vomiting, hypercalcaemia, severe haemorrhage
  - salivary gland disorders
    - a amyloidosis or other deposits
    - b cholinergic dysautonomia
    - c cystic fibrosis
    - d ectodermal dysplasia
    - e HCV infection
    - f HIV infection
    - g IgG4 syndrome
    - h salivary gland aplasia
    - i sarcoidosis
    - j Sjögren syndrome.

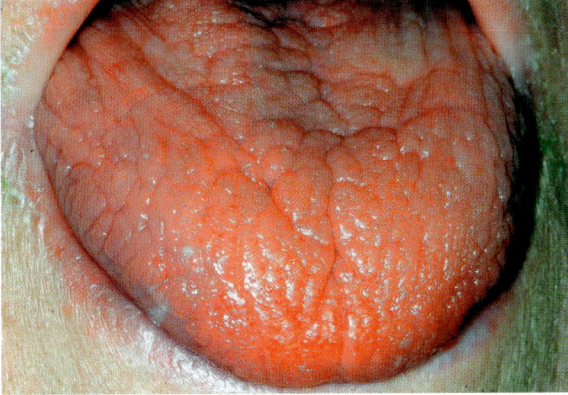

Figure 2.11 Dry mouth, and lobulated tongue which may follow chronic hyposalivation.

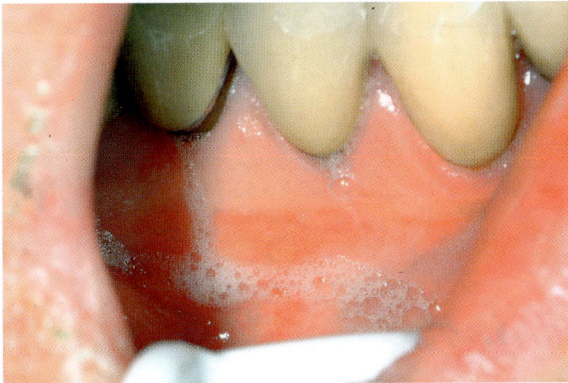

Figure 2.12 Dry mouth manifesting as frothy saliva.

Causes of xerostomia may ALSO include:

- Psychogenic states
    - anxiety states
    - bulimia nervosa
    - depression
    - hypochondriasis.

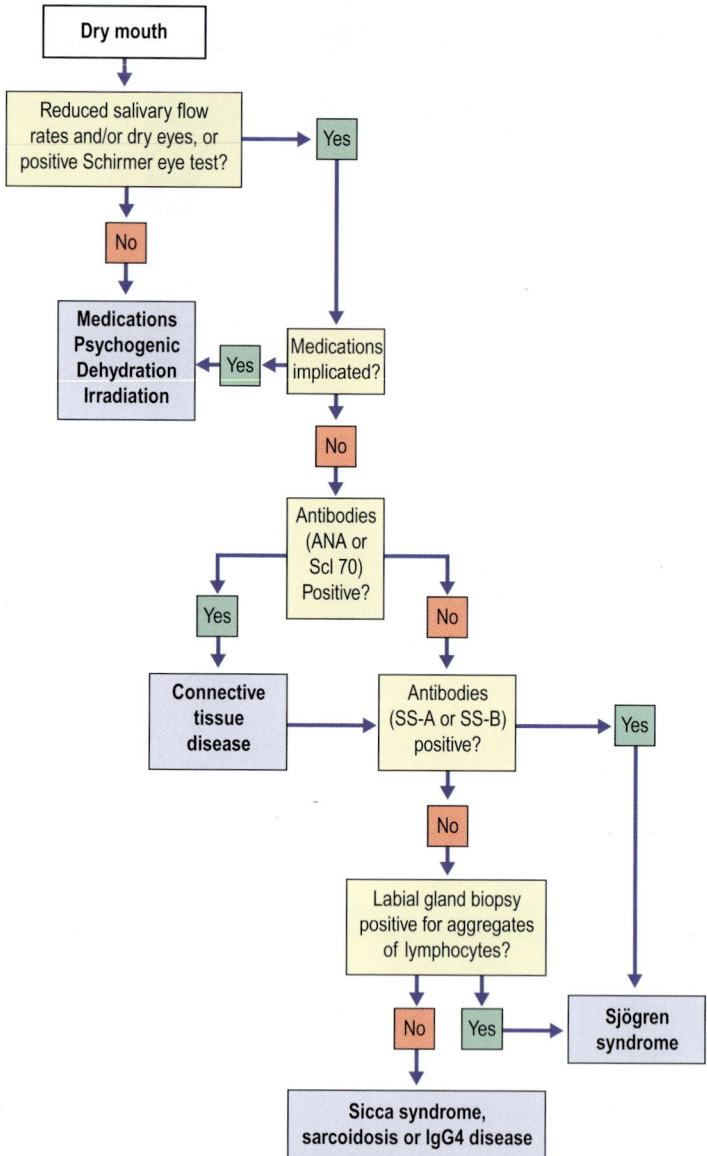

Figure 2.13 Algorithm for dry mouth diagnosis.

Halitosis (oral malodour)

Keypoints

- Oral malodour is a common subjective complaint but often far more obvious to the sufferer than others.
- Malodour 'if real' can be measured with a gas chromatography or a halimeter, but objective evidence for it by measuring volatile sulphur compounds (VSCs) in the breath by halimetry or smelling the breath is far less common.
- Malodour is common on awakening or if there is infrequent eating or starvation, and is then sometimes called 'physiological'.
- It is usually caused by diet, habits, dental plaque or oral disease.
- Oral malodour is to be anticipated in smokers, after eating odiferous foods such as garlic or durian, or drinking excess alcohol or coffee.
- Oral malodour is common where there are oral infections.
- Malodour can sometimes be caused by sinus, nose or throat conditions.
- Oral malodour occasionally arises from metabolic disorders but it is only *rarely* caused by more serious disease.
- In the absence of an identifiable malodour or a defined organic cause, the complaint of malodour may be psychogenic in origin.
- It often significantly improves with oral hygiene and tongue-brushing.
- It may also be helped by:
  - regularly eating yoghurts or ingesting certain probiotics
  - finishing meals with apples, carrots or celery
  - chewing spearmint, tarragon, eucalyptus, rosemary, or cardamom
  - avoiding habits such as smoking and odiferous foods, and avoiding foods such as eggs, legumes, certain meats, fish and foods that contain choline, carnitine, nitrogen and sulphur.

Box 2.5 Main causes of halitosis (oral malodour)

Odiferous foods
Smoking
Poor oral hygiene

Halitosis (oral malodour) (continued)

Causes may include:

- Starvation
- Lifestyle habits
  - ▪ habits
    - a alcohol
    - b amyl nitrites
    - c solvent misuse
    - d tobacco
  - ▪ volatile foodstuffs
    - a durian
    - b garlic
    - c highly spiced foods
    - d onions
- Drugs (see also Chapter 4): amphetamines, aztreonam, cytotoxic drugs, disulfiram, melatonin, mycophenolate sodium, nicotine lozenges, nitrates and phenothiazines
- Oral sepsis
  - ▪ dental or periodontal sepsis (Figure 2.14)
  - ▪ dry socket
  - ▪ food impaction
  - ▪ hyposalivation
  - ▪ necrotizing ulcerative gingivitis
  - ▪ oral malignancy
  - ▪ osteochemonecrosis (bisphosphonates, denosumab, bevacizumab)
  - ▪ osteomyelitis
  - ▪ osteoradionecrosis of the jaw
  - ▪ pericoronitis
  - ▪ ulceration
- Oesophageal disease
  - ▪ pouch
  - ▪ reflux
- Sinusitis
- Nasopharyngeal disease
  - ▪ foreign body
  - ▪ infection
  - ▪ neoplasm

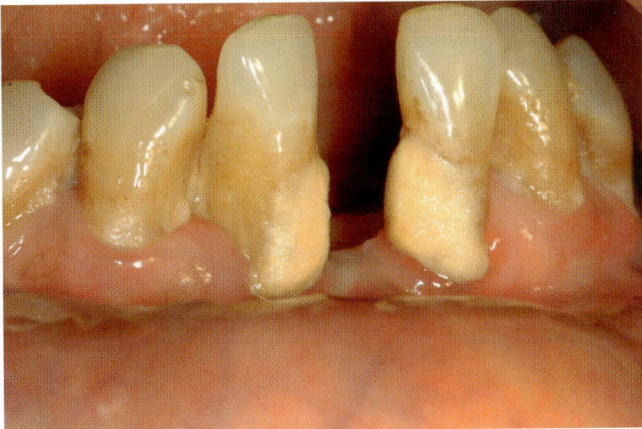

Figure 2.14 Halitosis caused by periodontitis.

- Pharyngeal disease
  - foreign body
  - infection (e.g. tonsillitis, tonsillolith)
  - neoplasm
  - pouch
- Systemic disease
  - acute febrile illness
  - metabolic disorders
    - diabetic ketoacidosis
    - hepatic failure
    - renal failure
    - trimethylaminuria
  - Psychogenic (delusional)
    - neuroses
    - psychoses

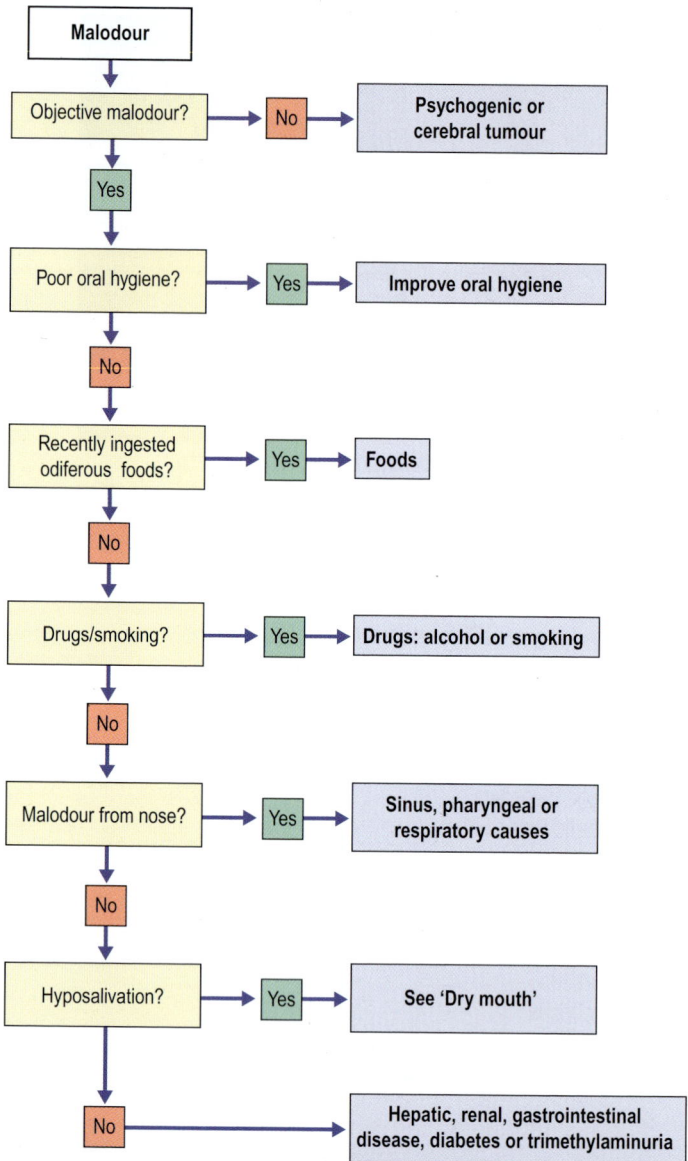

Figure 2.15 Algorithm for halitosis diagnosis.

Mucosal blisters

Keypoints

- A blister, if solitary, may be due to saliva extravasation into the tissues (mucocele).
- Blisters may be due to a subepithelial split, seen mainly in sub-epithelial immune blistering diseases (e.g. pemphigoid) (Figure 2.16).
- Blisters due to intraepithelial vesiculation are less common and caused particularly by pemphigus, and readily break to form erosions.
- Blisters rarely are caused by blood extravasation into the tissues (purpura) (Figure 2.17).

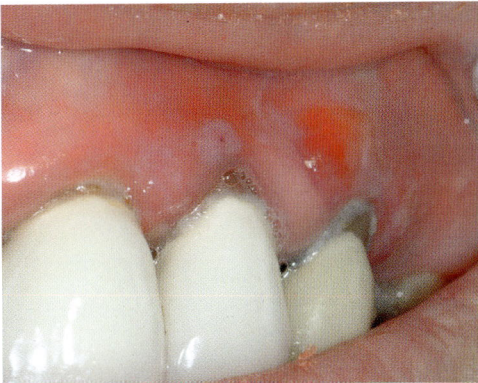

Figure 2.16 Blistering in pemphigoid.

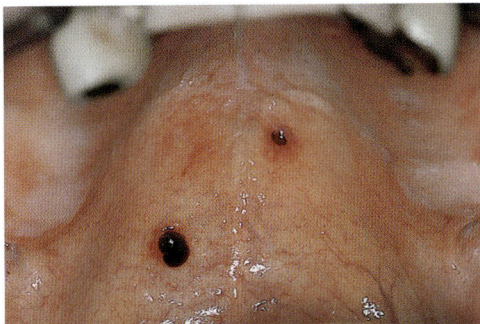

Figure 2.17 Blood blisters in purpura.

Mucosal blisters (continued)

Box 2.6 Main causes of oral blisters

Mucoceles
Angina bullosa haemorrhagica
Pemphigoid
Trauma (mucosal burn)

Causes may include:

- Infections
  - enteroviruses such as Coxsackie viruses and ECHO viruses
  - herpes simplex virus
  - herpes varicella-zoster virus
- Mucoceles
- Purpura, and angina bullosa haemorrhagica (localized oral purpura)
- Burns
- Cysts
- Skin diseases
  - dermatitis herpetiformis
  - epidermolysis bullosa (congenita and acquisita)
  - erythema multiforme and Stevens–Johnson syndrome
  - intraepidermal IgA pustulosis
  - lichen planus (superficial mucoceles)
  - linear IgA disease
  - pemphigoid (usually mucous membrane pemphigoid)
  - pemphigus (usually pemphigus vulgaris)
  - Sweet syndrome
- Drugs
- Paraneoplastic disorders
- Amyloidosis.

Mucosal brown and black lesions

Keypoints

- Mucosal brown and black lesions are common.
- Most mouth pigmentation is inherited. The most common cause of multiple oral brown lesions is racial or ethnic pigmentation, common in people of colour but also seen in some Caucasians and most noticeable on the facial gingivae, or other keratinized areas such as the dorsum of tongue or palate.
- Most pigmented lesions affect only the mouth but they are occasionally seen elsewhere or associated with other conditions.
- Otherwise, the cause is usually embedded amalgam, inflammation, or drugs or social habits.
- The most common cause of single oral brown lesions are naevi (Figure 2.18) or melanotic macules.
- Oral post-inflammatory pigmentation (pigmentary incontinence) is the common cause of multiple oral brown lesions associated with chronic inflammatory disorders (oral lichen planus and lichenoid lesions, pemphigus, or pemphigoid).

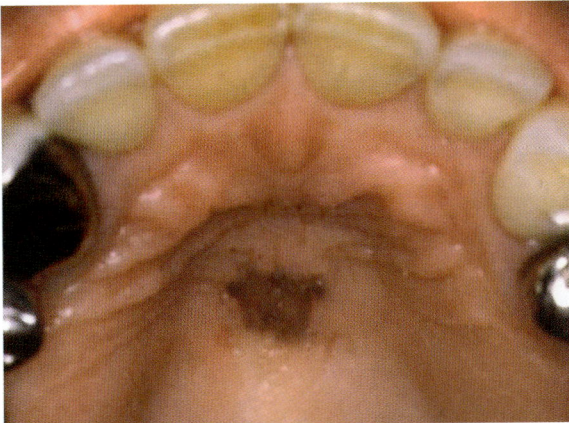

Figure 2.18 Hyperpigmentation: naevus.

Mucosal brown and black lesions (continued)

- The most common cause of single oral grey or black lesions is an amalgam tattoo, where amalgam has become embedded during restorative dental procedures (Figures 2.19, 2.20). A graphite tattoo from a pencil broken in the mouth is uncommon.
- Rare causes of brown or black lesions include drugs (Figure 2.21) or endocrinopathies such as Addisonian hypoadrenalism (Figure 2.22) and neoplasms such as malignant melanoma and Kaposi sarcoma.
- Solitary brown or black lesions may raise concern about the possibility of melanoma.
- Features suggestive of melanoma include (ABCDE):
  Assymetry in shape
  Border irregular
  Colour variations or changes
  Diameter (large size)
  Elevation above mucosa
- Imaging, biopsy or other investigations may be indicated to differentiate the causes.
- Pigmented lesions are often removed by surgery for histopathological examination.
- There are usually no long-term consequences.

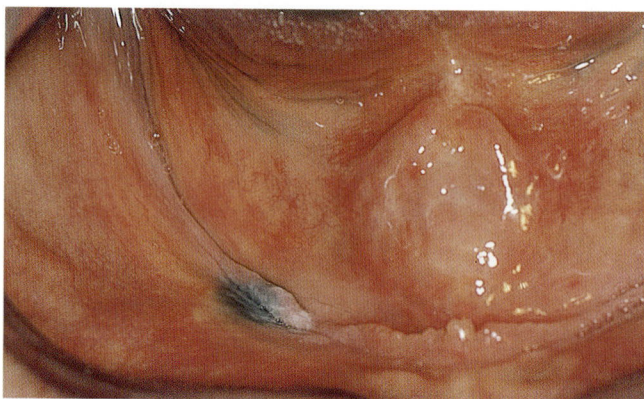

Figure 2.19 Hyperpigmentation: amalgam tattoo.

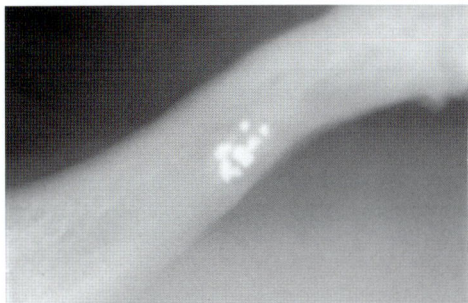

Figure 2.20 Hyperpigmentation: amalgam tattoo (radiographic view).

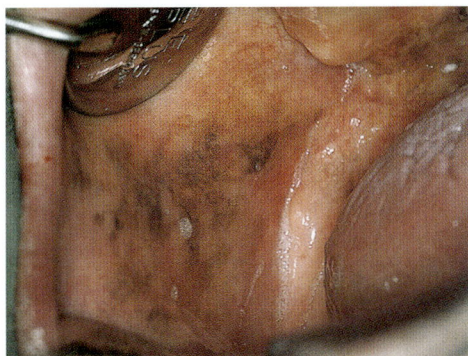

Figure 2.21 Hyperpigmentation: drug-induced (antimalarials, minocycline and others can be responsible).

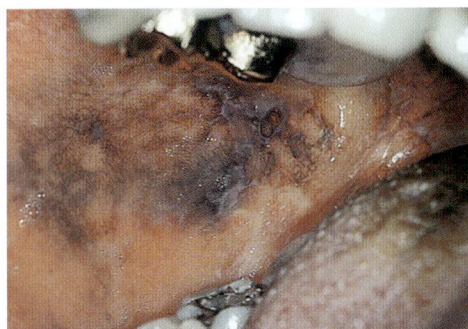

Figure 2.22 Hyperpigmentation: in hypoadrenocorticism (Addison disease).

Mucosal brown and black lesions (continued)

Box 2.7 Main causes of mucosal brown or black lesions

Racial
Naevus
Melanotic macule
Amalgam tattoo
Smoking

Causes may include:

- Racial
- Food/drugs
  - beetroot
  - betel nut
  - chlorhexidine
  - liquorice
  - tobacco
  - systemic drugs, such as minocycline, certain antimalarials and chemotherapeutic agents
- Hormonal
  - pregnancy (chloasma)
  - Addison disease
  - Albright syndrome (fibrous dysplasia)
- Others
  - Kaposi sarcoma
  - leukoplakia with pigmentary incontinence
  - lichen planus with pigmentary incontinence
  - melanoacanthoma
  - melanoma
  - melanotic macule
  - naevus
  - Peutz–Jeghers syndrome.

Table 2.1 Features of most important isolated hyperpigmented oral lesions

Lesion	Usual age of presentation	Morphology	Colour	Main locations	Approximate size	Other comments
Amalgam tattoo	>5 years	Macular	Grey or black	Floor of mouth, mandibular and maxillary gingivae	<1 cm	May be confirmed by radiography
Graphite tattoo	>5 years	Macular	Grey or black	Palate	<0.5 cm	May be revealed by radiography
Kaposi sarcoma	>young adult	Macular becoming nodular	Red, purple or black	Palate, gingivae	Any	Mainly in HIV/ AIDS
Melanoma	Any	Macular becoming nodular	Brown, grey or black	Palate, gingivae	Any	Rare
Melanotic macules	Any	Macular	Brown or black	Lips, gingivae	<1 cm	Usually benign Mostly in Caucasians
Naevi	3rd–4th decade	Raised	Blue or brown	Palate	<1 cm	Usually benign
Purpura	Any	Macular	Red, purple or brown	Palate, buccal or lingual mucosa	Any	Usually traumatic and resolves spontaneously

Mucosal brown and black lesions (continued)

Black or brown hairy tongue

Common, especially in adult men.

Typical orofacial symptoms and signs: persistent brown or black hairy appearance of tongue.

Main oral sites affected: central dorsum of tongue, mainly posteriorly but extending anteriorly.

Aetiopathogenesis: unknown. Smoking, foods such as liquorice, drugs (e.g. iron salts, chlorhexidine, bismuth) and poor oral hygiene (proliferation of chromogenic microorganisms may predispose.

Gender predominance: male.

Age predominance: adult.

Extraoral possible lesions: none.

Main associated conditions: none.

Differential diagnosis: candidosis.

Investigations: history of use of offending agents.

Main diagnostic criteria: clear-cut clinically.

Main treatments: improve oral hygiene; discontinue any drugs responsible; scrape or brush tongue (in evenings with cold water); suck dry peach stone (yes!).

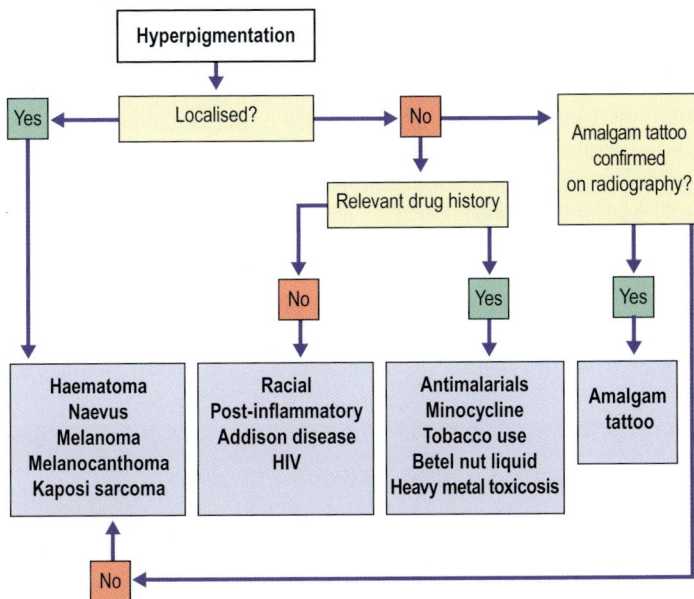

Figure 2.23 Algorithm for hyperpigmentation diagnosis.

Mucosal erosions (see also mucosal ulceration)

Keypoints

- Mucosal damage may lead to inflammation and/or partial-thickness loss of epithelium, both of which appear red, or to loss of most of the epithelium, which then may initially appear red but becomes covered with a yellowish fibrinous slough. Full-thickness loss of epithelium typically causes a grey or yellow lesion (an ulcer).
- Patients often present with a mix of these appearances; mucositis is the term applied to widespread oral erythema, ulceration and soreness.
- Any of the causes of mucosal blisters may result eventually in erosions.

Box 2.8 Main causes of mucosal erosions

Systemic disease (blood, infections, gastrointestinal, skin)
Malignant lesions
Local causes (e.g. burns)
Drugs

Causes may include:

- Any of the causes of mucosal blisters (may result eventually in erosions).
- Erosions are especially seen after burns, caused by drugs (Figure 2.24) and lichen planus (Figure 2.25).
- Mucositis, and sometimes bleeding, is common after chemo- or radio- or chemoradio-therapy, and graft-versus-host disease (GvHD). Sometimes called mucosal barrier injury, mucositis is common during the treatment of cancer but also in the conditioning prior to haematopoietic stem cell transplantation (bone marrow transplants).

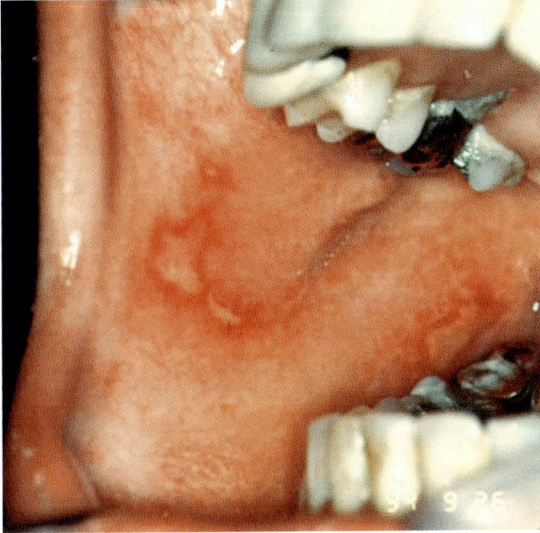

Figure 2.24 Erosion showing fibrinous slough.

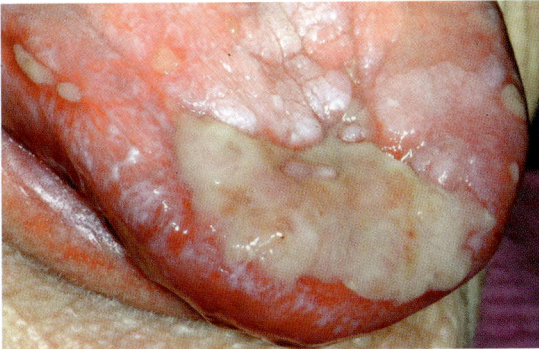

Figure 2.25 Erosions induced by lichenoid adverse drug reaction. Erosions are yellow: the white lesions are lichenoid.

Mucosal fissures or cracks

Keypoints

- Fissures are common on the dorsum of the tongue (Figure 2.26) when they are usually of genetic basis and, as there is no break in the epithelium, they are symptomless unless, as is common, there is an associated geographic tongue (erythema migrans) (Figure 2.27).
- Fissures otherwise are often associated with epithelial breaks and are seen mainly on the lip, usually at the commissures (angular cheilitis or stomatitis), rarely elsewhere (lip fissure).

Box 2.9 Main causes of mucosal fissures

Angular stomatitis
Lip fissure
Any cause of lip swelling (e.g. Crohn disease)

Causes may include:

- Angular stomatitis
- Lip fissure
- Down syndrome
- Crohn disease or orofacial granulomatosis (OFG)
- Actinic cheilitis.

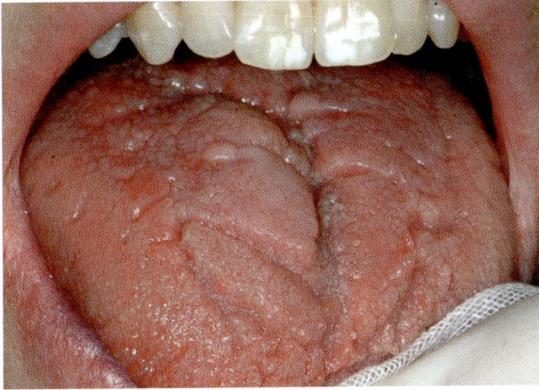

Figure 2.26 Fissured tongue in a patient with Crohn disease.

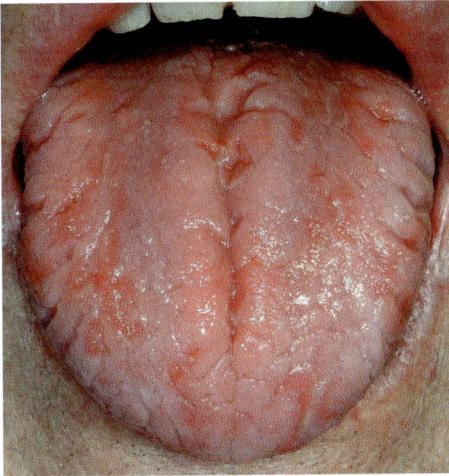

Figure 2.27 Fissured tongue in a patient with erythema migrans (geographic tongue).

Mucosal fissures or cracks (continued)

Angular stomatitis (perleche; angular cheilitis)

Common, especially in older edentulous patients who are denture-wearers.

Typical orofacial symptoms and signs: symmetrical erythematous fissures on skin of commissures (Figures 2.28, 2.29), and (very rarely) commissural leukopakia intraorally.

Main oral sites affected: commissures, bilaterally.

Aetiopathogenesis: usually due to infection with *Candida albicans*. *Staphylococcus aureus* and/or streptococci may also be cultured from lesions. Patients may have denture-related stomatitis or other forms of intraoral candidosis. Other causes include lip incompetence, especially from orthodontic appliances, iron deficiency, hypovitaminoses (especially B), malabsorption states (e.g. Crohn disease), HIV infection and other immune defects.

Gender predominance: none.

Age predominance: older.

Extraoral possible lesions: none usually.

Main associated conditions: see aetiopathogenesis.

Differential diagnosis: see aetiopathogenesis.

Investigations: occasionally, blood picture and haematinic assays; investigations for diabetes and other immune defects; smears for fungal hyphae and bacteriological culture, if refractory.

Main diagnostic criteria: usually clear-cut.

Main treatments: Eliminate any underlying systemic predisposing factors. Treat intraoral candidal infection, in particular denture-related stomatitis. Treat angular stomatitis with topical antifungal such as miconazole or triamcinolone/nystatin combination, or fucidin or mupirocin if staphylococcal.

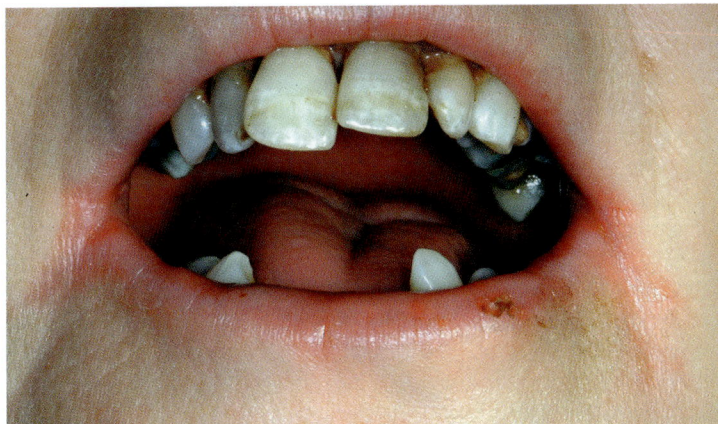

Figure 2.28 Angular stomatitis (cheilitis) causing fissuring at commissures.

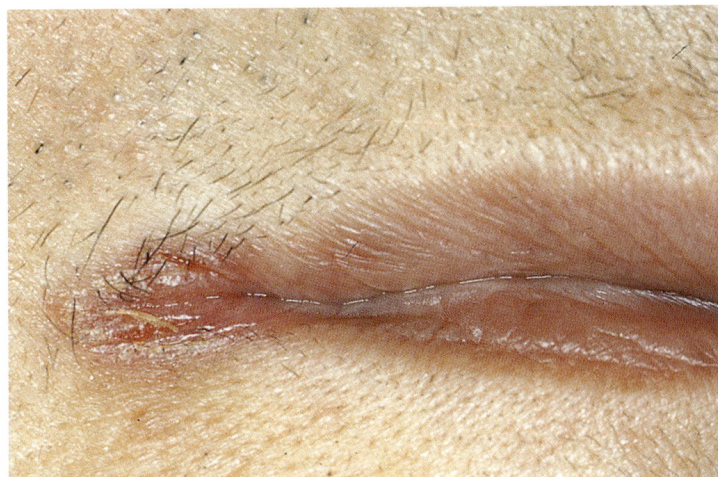

Figure 2.29 Angular stomatitis causing fissuring at commissures.

Mucosal fissures or cracks (continued)

Fissured (cracked) lip

Typical orofacial symptoms and signs: chronic discomfort and, from time to time, some bleeding.

Main oral sites affected: typically in the lower lip (Figure 2.30), usually median.

Aetiopathogenesis: a fissure may develop in the lip where a patient, typically a child, is mouth-breathing. Sun, wind, cold weather and smoking are thought to predispose. A hereditary predisposition for weakness in the first branchial arch fusion may exist. Lip fissures are also common in Down syndrome and when lips swell as, for example, in cheilitis granulomatosa and orofacial granulomatosis/Crohn disease (Figure 2.31).

Gender predominance: males.

Age predominance: young adult.

Extraoral possible lesions: none usually.

Main associated conditions: see aetiopathogenesis.

Differential diagnosis: see aetiopathogenesis.

Investigations: see aetiopathogenesis. If diffuse lip swelling accompanies the fissuring, biopsy is indicated.

Main diagnostic criteria: clinical. Differentiate from angular stomatitis and cheilitis glandularis (occasionally).

Main treatments: predisposing factors should be managed if possible. Bland creams or ointments (e.g. E45) may help the lesion heal spontaneously. Short-term use of low-potency topical corticosteroids with or without anti-fungals or antimicrobials may promote healing. If the fissure fails to heal, excision, preferably with a z-plasty, laser ablation or cryosurgery may be needed.

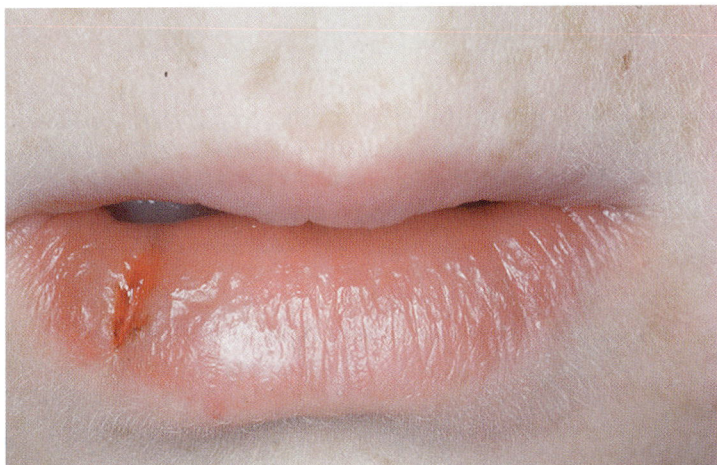

Figure 2.30 Lip fissure.

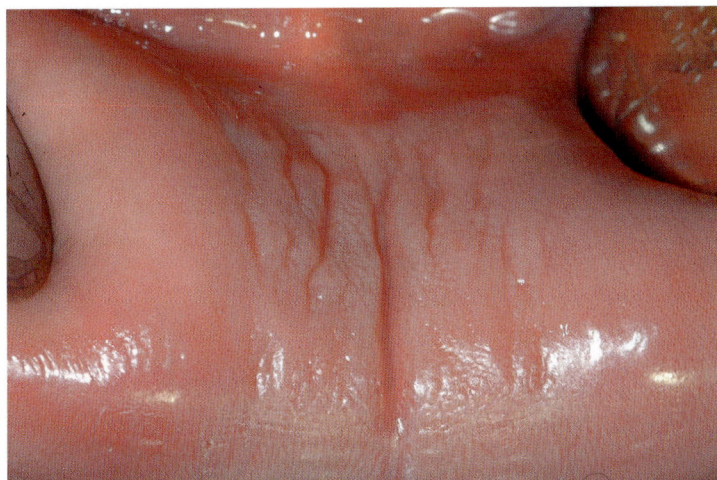

Figure 2.31 Fissured lip in a patient with swelling from Crohn disease.

Mucosal purpura

Keypoints

- Purpura is the accumulation of blood in the mucosa, appearing usually as red or brown macules (Figure 2.32). Purpuric lesions do not blanch on pressure (cf. vascular lesions such as haemangioma, telangiectasia).
- Petechiae are pinpoint-sized haemorrhages from small capillaries in the skin or mucous membranes. Petechia is the term given to the individual small red or red–blue spots which are about 1–5 mm in diameter and make up the rash.
- Purpura is seen mainly in areas prone to trauma, such as at the occlusal line (Figure 2.33) or junction of hard and soft palates.
- Occasional small traumatic petechiae at the occlusal line are common in otherwise healthy patients. Otherwise, oral purpura is uncommon.
- Purpura is usually caused by trauma such as suction, but haemostatic disorders may also present in this manner, so a blood picture (including blood count and platelet count) and haemostatic function may be indicated.

Box 2.10 Main causes of oral purpura

Trauma or suction
Platelet defects

Causes may include:

- Trauma (including suction, forceful coughing or vomiting)
- Thrombocytopenia
  - autoimmune
  - drugs
  - leukaemias
  - viral infections:
    - HIV
    - infectious mononucleosis
    - rubella
- Localized oral purpura (angina bullosa haemorrhagica)
- Amyloidosis
- Mixed connective tissue disease.

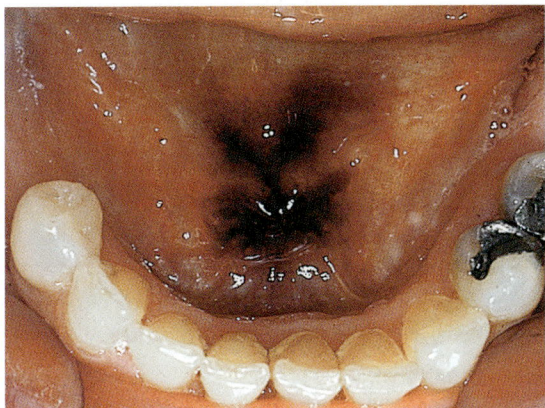

Figure 2.32 Purpura.

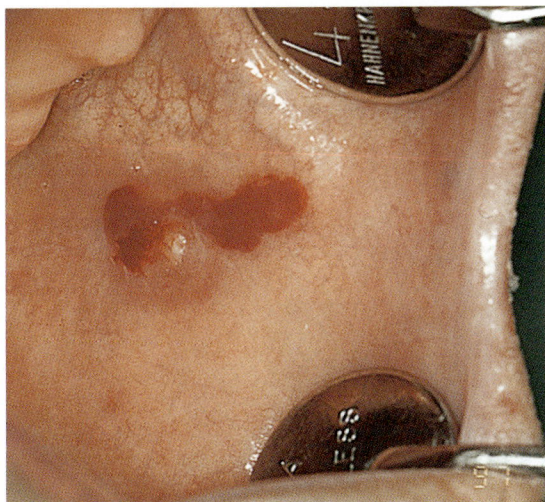

Figure 2.33 Purpura.

Mucosal red lesions

Keypoints

- Mucosal red lesions are usually inflammatory in origin.
- Mucosal red lesions may also be caused by epithelial loss (as in desquamative gingivitis) or atrophy as in erythroplasia (erythroplakia) – which usually represents severe epithelial dysplasia and is potentially malignant, or redness may represent frank carcinoma or other malignant neoplasms.
- Some mucosal red lesions are due to purpura or vascular anomalies such as telangiectasia or haemangiomas (the latter are more commonly purple or blue).

Box 2.11 Main causes of oral red lesions

Any inflammatory condition
Erythroplakia
Angioma

Causes may include:

Generalized redness

- Candidosis (Figure 2.34)
- Mucosal atrophy (e.g. avitaminosis B)
- Mucositis

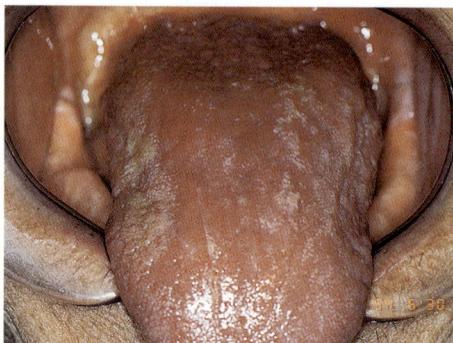

Figure 2.34 Red lesion: candidosis may cause a glossitis.

Localized red patches

- Angiomas (Figures 2.35)
- Avitaminosis B_{12}
- Burns
- Candidosis (erythematous, acute atrophic and denture-related) (Figures 2.36, 2.37)
- Carcinoma (Figure 2.38)
- Contact allergy
- Crohn disease and orofacial granulomatosis (OFG)
- Deep mycoses
- Desquamative gingivitis
- Drug allergies
- Erythroplakia (Figure 2.39)
- Geographic tongue (erythema migrans)
- Kaposi sarcoma
- Lichen planus
- Lichenoid reactions
- Lupus erythematosus
- Median rhomboid glossitis
- Mucositis
- Plasma cell gingivitis
- Purpura
- Sarcoidosis

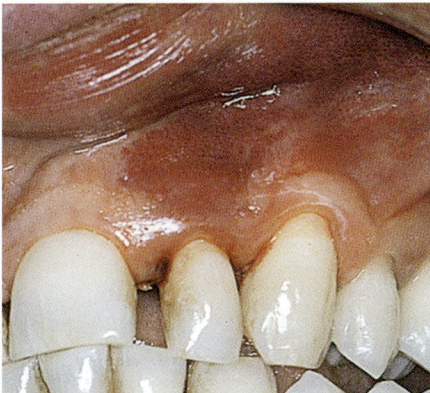

Figure 2.35 Red lesion: angioma extending from lip to gingiva.

Mucosal red lesions (continued)

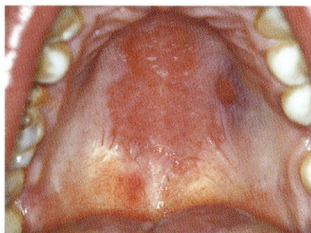

Figure 2.36 Red lesion: candidosis in the palate is common in HIV/AIDS, presenting a 'thumb print' appearance.

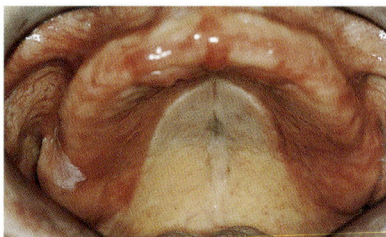

Figure 2.37 Red lesion: candidosis causing denture-related stomatitis.

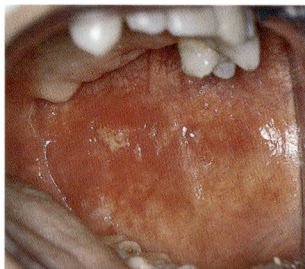

Figure 2.38 Red lesion: carcinoma.

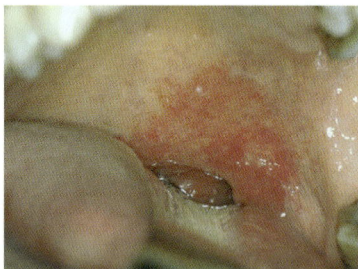

Figure 2.39 Red lesion: erythroplakia.

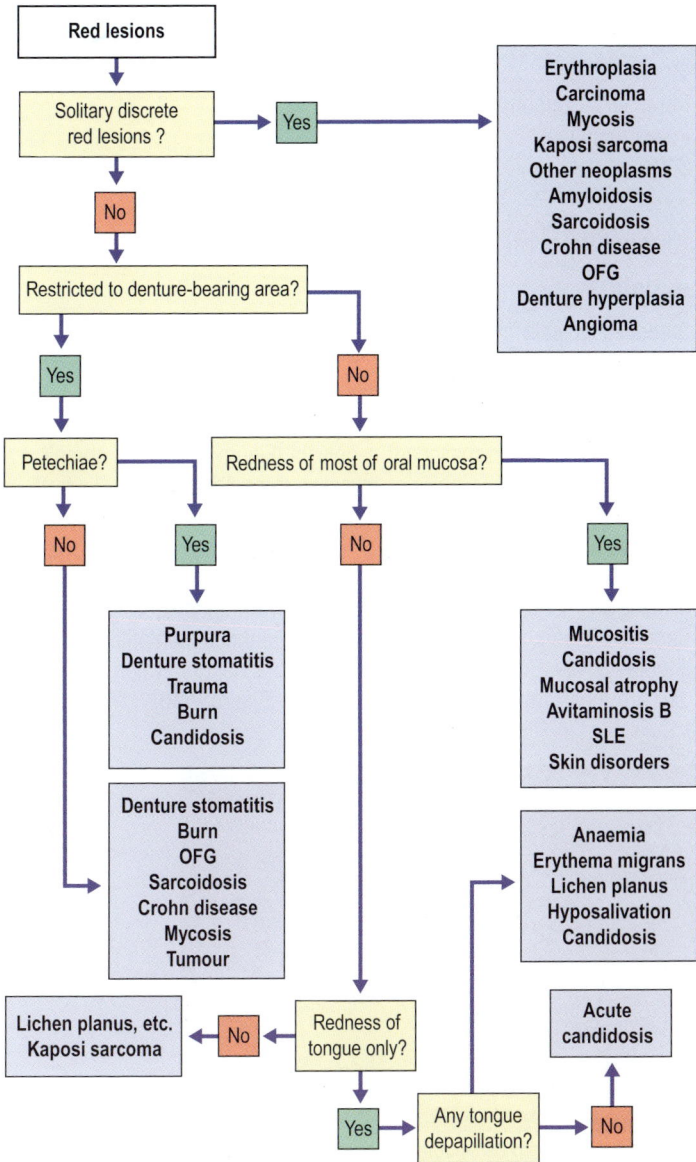

Figure 2.40 Algorithm for red lesions.

Mucosal red lesions (continued)

Telangiectases
- Hereditary haemorrhagic telangiectasia
- Post-irradiation
- Scleroderma

Mucosal ulceration or soreness (see also mucosal erosions)

Keypoints

- Soreness typically indicates a break in epithelial continuity, usually caused by erosions or ulcers.
- Ulcers can have a wide range of causes.
- Single ulcers lasting more than 3 weeks are a special concern since they may represent a malignant neoplasm (Figure 2.41) or a chronic infection such as TB, syphilis or mycoses (fungal infections). Gingival ulcers may be caused by these conditions, or acute necrotizing gingivitis (Figure 2.42).
- Other persistent ulcers may have a systemic cause, such as a skin disease like lichen planus, pemphigoid or even pemphigus.
- Recurrent ulcers may represent recurrent aphthous stomatitis (aphthae) (Figures 2.43–2.45) but occasionally they manifest in systemic disease and are then termed 'aphthous-like' ulcers (Figure 2.46).

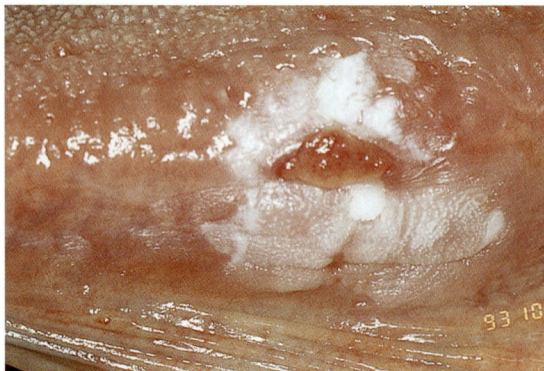

Figure 2.41 Ulceration: carcinoma presenting as an ulcerated white lesion.

Box 2.12 Main causes of oral ulceraton

Systemic disease (blood, infections, gastrointestinal, skin)
Malignant lesions
Local causes (e.g. burns)
Aphthae
Drugs

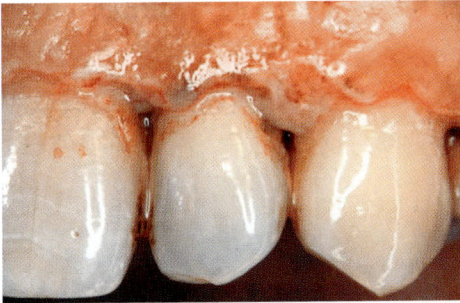

Figure 2.42 Ulceration: necrotizing ulcerative gingivitis (NUG). The papillae are ulcerated.

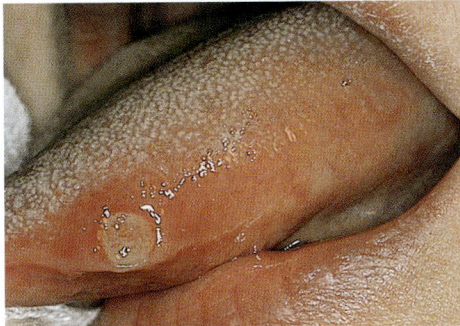

Figure 2.43 Ulceration: recurrent aphthous stomatitis (minor aphthae).

Mucosal ulceration or soreness (continued)

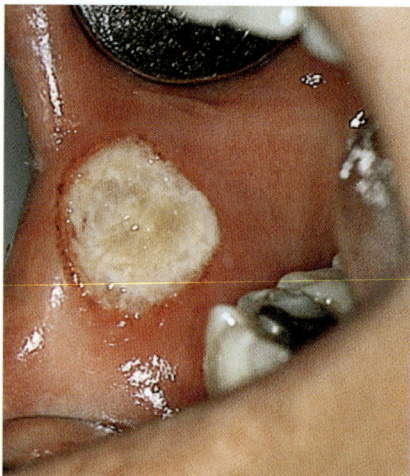

Figure 2.44 Ulceration: recurrent aphthous stomatitis (major aphthae).

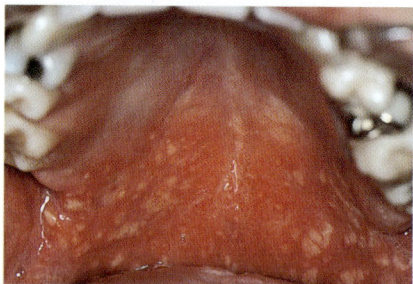

Figure 2.45 Ulceration: recurrent aphthous stomatitis (herpetiform ulcers).

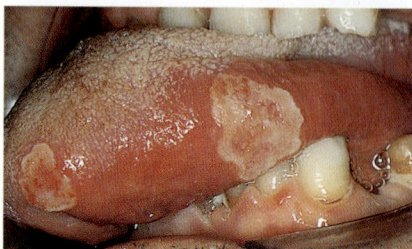

Figure 2.46 Ulceration: Behçet syndrome.

Causes may include:

Causes are diverse and may be remembered by the mnemonic **So Many Laws And Directives**, which includes:

- **S**ystemic
  - blood
  - infections
  - gastrointestinal
  - skin
- **M**alignancy
- **L**ocal
- **A**phthae
- **D**rugs.

Systemic disease

The acronym **BIGS** (**B**lood, **I**nfections, **G**astrointestinal, **S**kin) may be used, to include:

- **B**lood or vascular disorders: anaemia, neutropenias, leukaemias
- **I**nfective: viruses (HIV, herpes simplex, chickenpox, herpes zoster, hand, foot and mouth disease, herpangina, infectious mononucleosis), bacteria (necrotizing ulcerative gingivitis, tuberculosis and atypical mycobacterial infections, syphilis), fungi (e.g. aspergillosis, histoplasmosis), parasites (leishmaniasis)
- **G**astrointestinal: coeliac disease, Crohn disease and OFG, ulcerative colitis
- **S**kin and connective tissue disease: lichen planus, pemphigus, pemphigoid, erythema multiforme, lupus erythematosus.

Malignancy

Carcinoma and other malignant tumours such as lymphoma or salivary neoplasms.

Mucosal ulceration or soreness (continued)

Local causes

- Traumatic (may be artifactual – factitial [self-induced])
- Burns – chemical, electrical, thermal, radiation-induced
- Eosinophilic ulcer (traumatic ulcerative granuloma with stromal eosinophilia – TUGSE)
- Necrotizing sialometaplasia.

Aphthae

Recurrent aphthous stomatitis (RAS), including aphthous-like ulcers as seen in Behçet syndrome, and auto-inflammatory syndromes (e.g. PFAPA – periodic fever, aphthae, pharyngitis, adenitis).

Drugs

- Drugs causing mucositis such as cytotoxic agents, particularly methotrexate.
- Agents producing lichen-planus-like (lichenoid) lesions, such as antihypertensives, antidiabetics, gold salts, non-steroidal anti-inflammatory drugs (NSAIDs), antimalarials and other drugs.
- Agents causing local chemical burns (especially aspirin held in the mouth).
- Drugs causing osteonecrosis. Bisphosphonate-related osteonecrosis of the jaw (BRONJ), and osteochemonecrosis due to other agents (denosumab, bevacizumab) may present as ulceration.

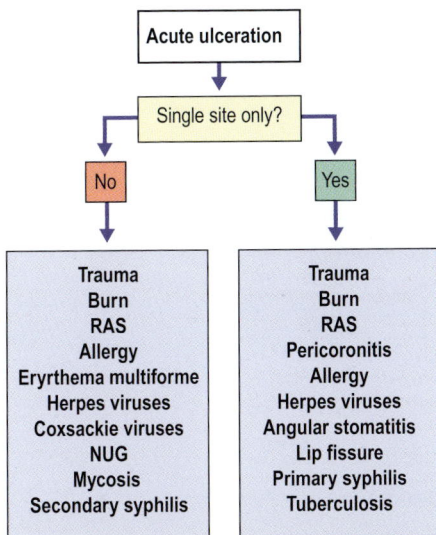

Figure 2.47 Algorithm for acute ulceration diagnosis.

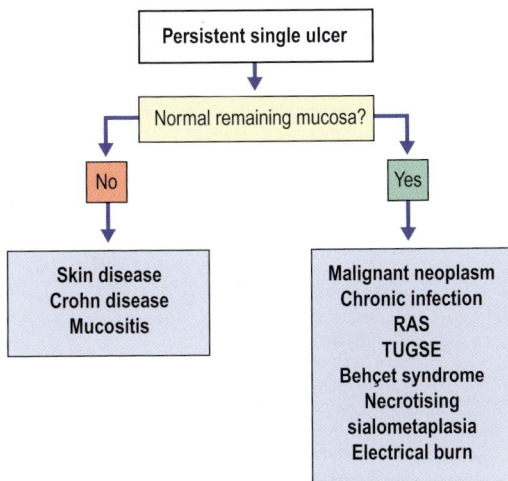

Figure 2.48 Algorithm for persistent single ulcer diagnosis.

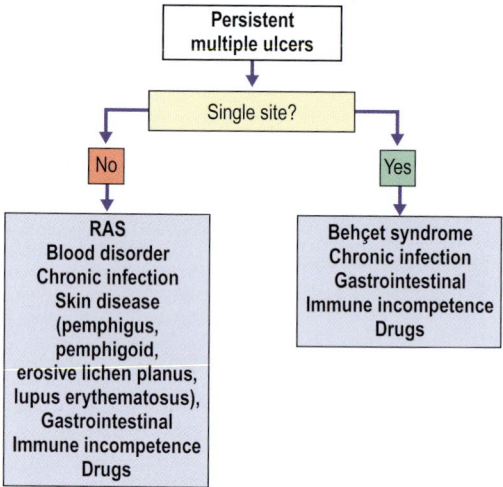

Figure 2.49 Algorithm for persistent multiple ulcers diagnosis.

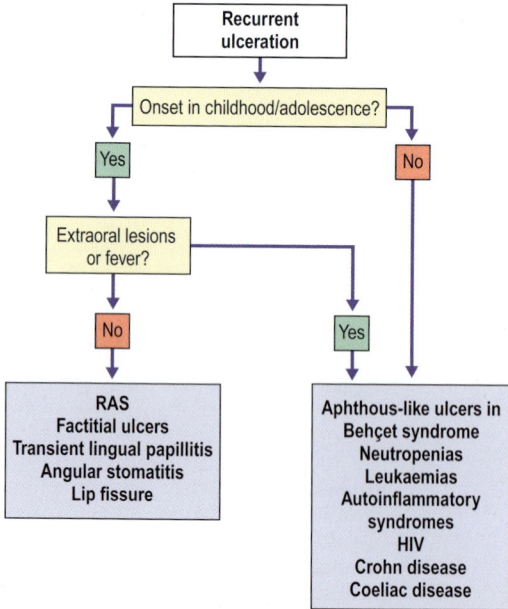

Figure 2.50 Algorithm for recurrent ulcer diagnosis.

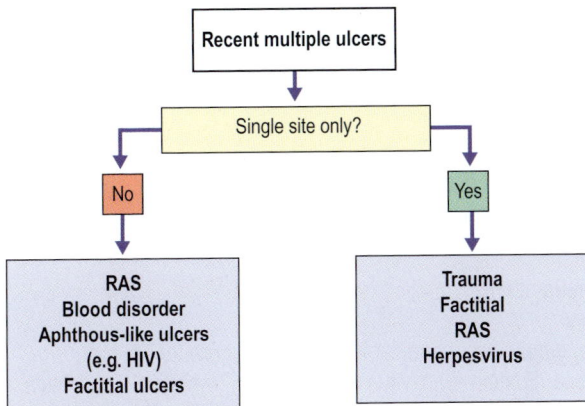

Figure 2.51 Algorithm for recurrent multiple ulcers diagnosis.

Mucosal white lesions

Keypoints

- White lesions are often due to material on the surface of the mucosa, which wipes away with a gauze swab; materia alba (debris) and thrush (candidosis) are the common causes.
- White lesions may be due to increased keratinization, such as in keratosis or lichen planus. These do not wipe off with a gauze swab.

Box 2.13 Main causes of oral white lesions
Materia alba
Candidosis
Lichen planus
Keratosis
Leukoplakia

Mucosal white lesions (continued)

Causes may include:

Hereditary
- Leukoedema
- White sponge naevus (Figure 2.52)
- Others (e.g. dyskeratosis congenita)

Acquired
- Debris (materia alba)
- Inflammatory
  - infective: candidosis, candidal leukoplakia (Figure 2.53), hairy leukoplakia (Epstein–Barr virus [EBV] related), syphilitic leukoplakia, Koplik spots (measles virus), papillomas (human papillomavirus – HPV) (Figure 2.54)

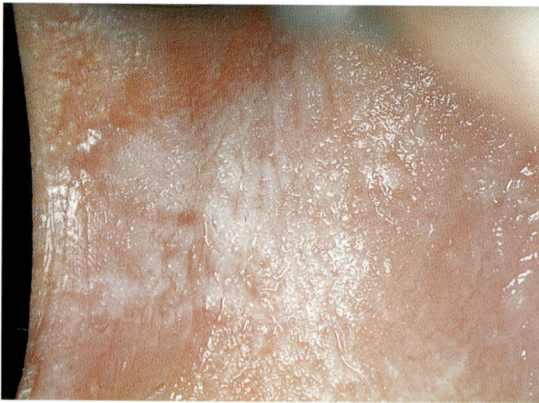

Figure 2.52 White lesion: genetic (white sponge naevus).

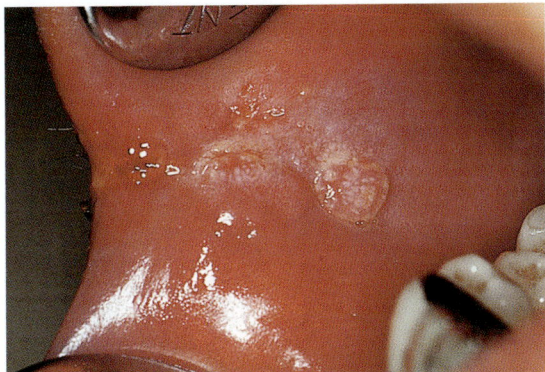

Figure 2.53 White lesion: infective (candidal leukoplakia).

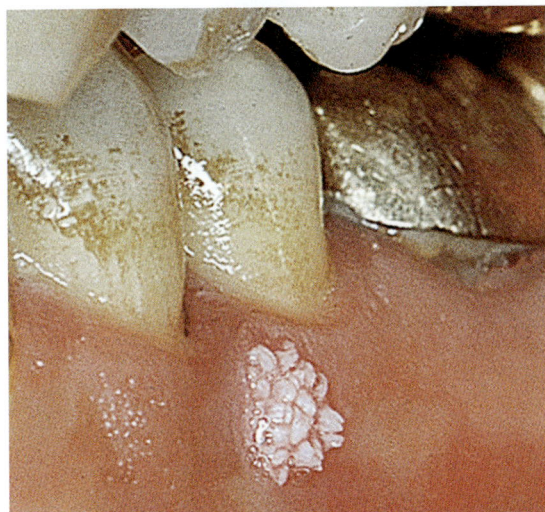

Figure 2.54 White lesion: infective (papilloma).

Mucosal white lesions (continued)

- non-infective: lichen planus and lichenoid lesions (Figure 2.55), lichen sclerosis, lupus erythematosus, contact cinnamon allergy
- Neoplastic and potentially malignant disorders
  - carcinoma (Figures 2.56–2.58)

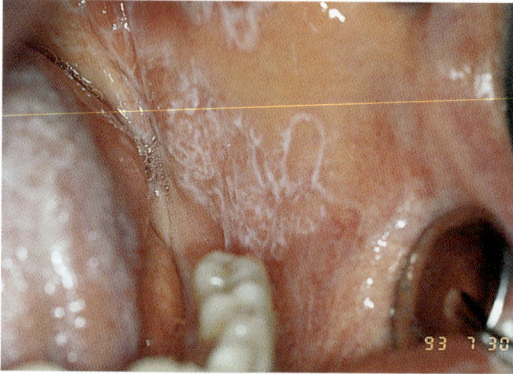

Figure 2.55 White lesion: inflammatory (lichen planus).

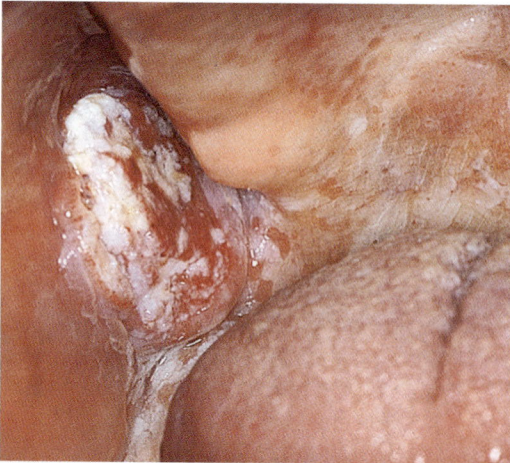

Figure 2.56 White lesion: speckled white and red lump which was a carcinoma.

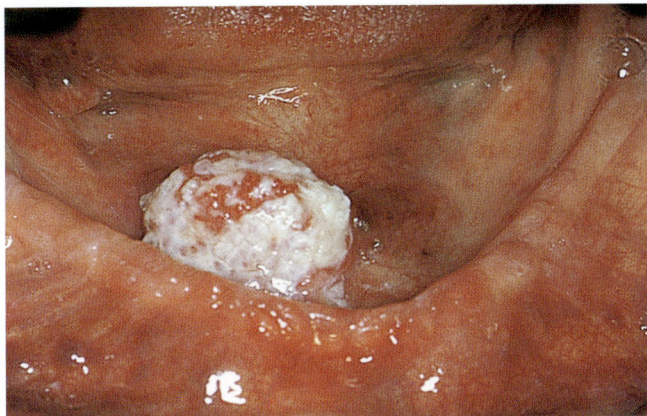

(above) Figure 2.57 White lesion: speckled white and red lump which was a carcinoma.

(right) Figure 2.58 White lesion: verrucous carcinoma.

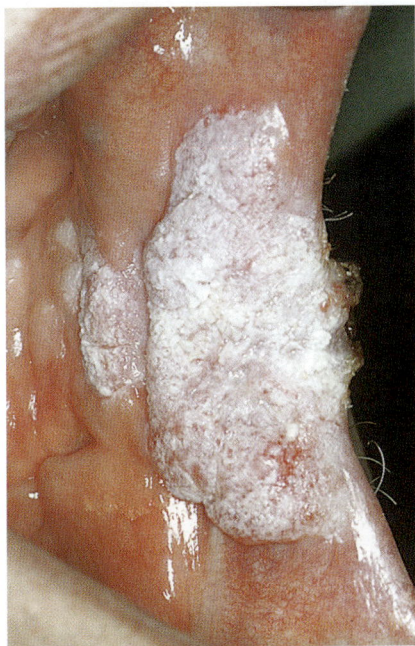

Mucosal white lesions (continued)

- ■ leukoplakias
- ■ verrucous and speckled leukoplakia (Figures 2.59 and 2.60)
- • Drug burns

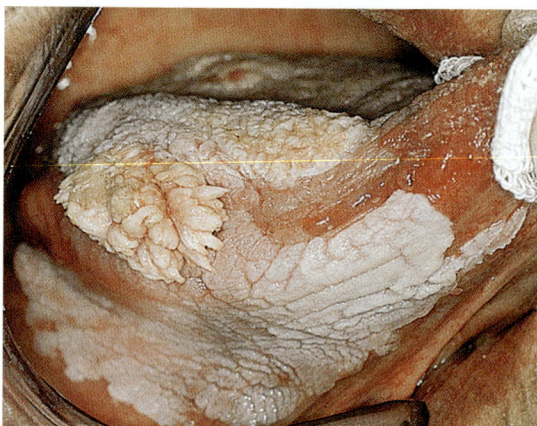

Figure 2.59 White lesion: proliferative verrucous leukoplakia.

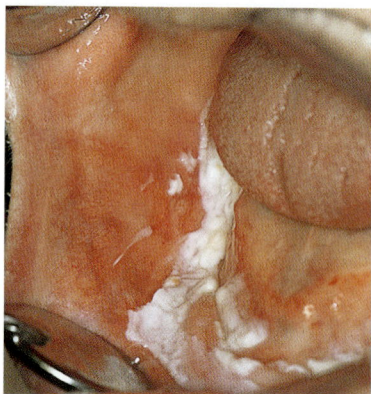

Figure 2.60 White lesion: proliferative verrucous leukoplakia.

- Reactive/traumatic
  - BARK (benign alveolar ridge keratosis)
  - cheek biting (Figure 2.61)
  - frictional hyperkeratosis
  - nicotine stomatitis (stomatitis nicotinia; smokers keratosis) (Figure 2.62).

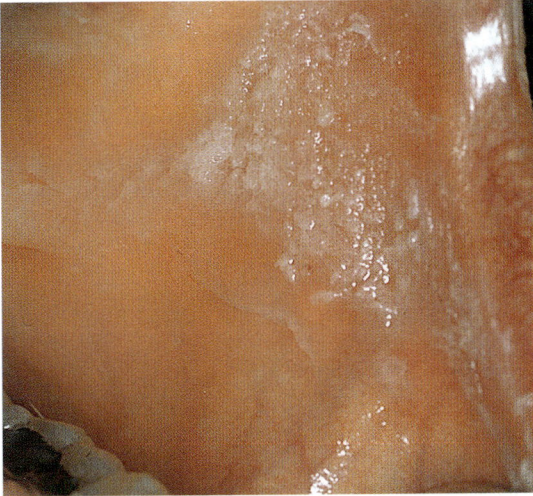

Figure 2.61 White lesion: cheek biting (morsicatio buccarum).

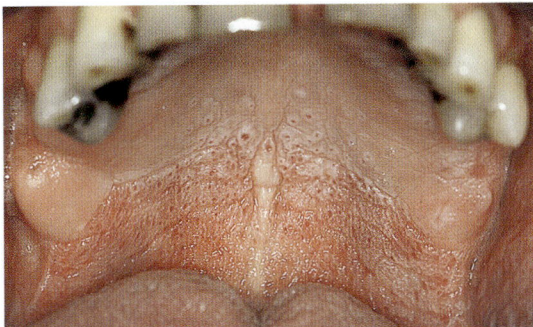

Figure 2.62 White lesion: stomatitis nicotinia (smoker's keratosis).

White patch

Rubs off with gauze? → Yes →
- Candidosis
- Materia alba
- Burn (heat, drug, chemical)

No

Localised to one site? → Yes →
- Keratosis
- Leukoplakia
- Lichenoid lesions
- Hyperplastic candidosis
- Burn
- Carcinoma

No

Plaque? → Yes →
- Leukoplakia
- Keratosis
- Lichen planus
- White sponge naevus
- Hyperplastic candidosis
- Hairy leukoplakia

No

Striated? → Yes →
- Lichen planus
- Linea alba
- Leukoedema
- Lupus erythematosus
- Scar

No

Papular? → Yes →
- Lichen planus
- Syphilis
- Gingival and palatal cysts of newborn
- Fordyce disease
- Koplik spots

No

Abraded? → Yes →
- Cheek chewing

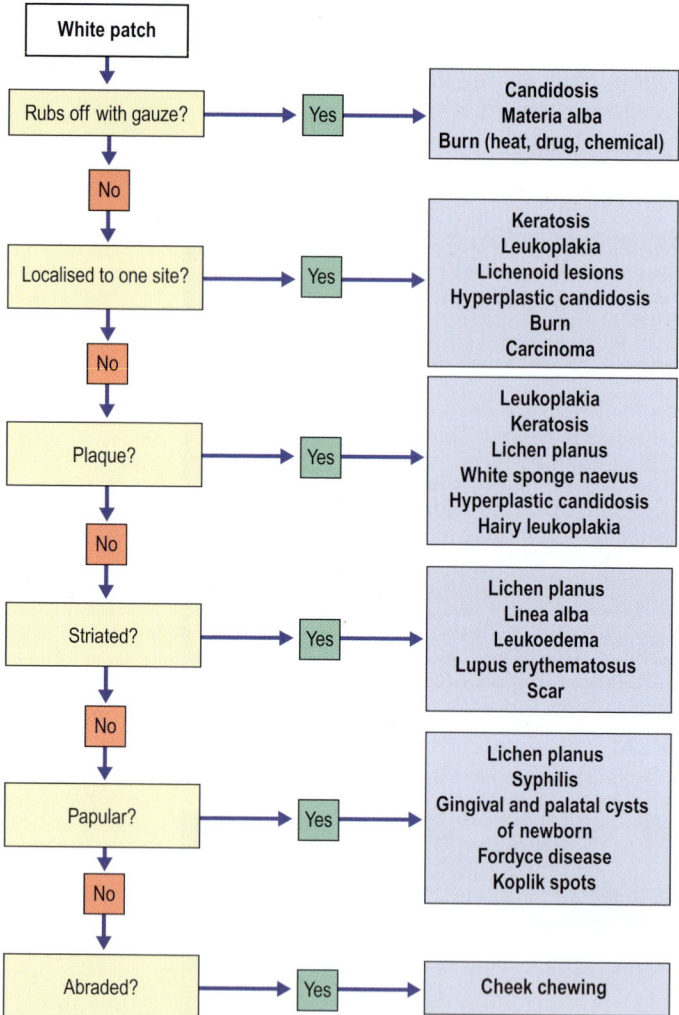

Figure 2.63 Algorithm for white patch diagnosis.

Pain (orofacial)

Keypoints

- Facial or maxillofacial pain is common and most is of local (odontogenic) cause.
- Vascular disorders such as migrainous neuralgia and giant cell arteritis may present with orofacial pain.
- Some facial pain is referred from elsewhere, such as the chest and neck.
- Neurological disorders are an important cause of orofacial pain but, except trigeminal neuralgia, they are uncommon.
- Pain may have a psychogenic basis but this can only be considered when local, neurological, vascular and referred causes of pain have been excluded. Even patients with psychogenic disorders can suffer organic pain: 'hypochondriacs can be ill'!
- History (Box 1.1), examination findings and imaging using radiography, CT, MRI or ultrasonography are important in order not to miss detecting organic disease and thus mislabelling the patient as having psychogenic pain. MRI of the entire trigeminal nerve gives better resolution of brainstem and cranial nerves than does CT, is recommended for all patients, and certainly is mandatory if there are atypical features, sensory or motor disturbances.
- Medical advice may well be indicated, especially if a neurological lesion is at all possible and is **urgently** required if orofacial pain is:
  - accompanied by pain elsewhere (chest, shoulder, neck or arm – may be angina)
  - accompanied by other unexplained symptoms or signs (numbness, weakness, headaches, neck stiffness, nausea or vomiting – may be intracerebral disease)
  - focused in the temple on one side (may be giant cell arteritis – a threat to vision).

Box 2.14 Main causes of orofacial pain

Local
Vascular
Referred
Neurological
Psychogenic

Pain (orofacial) (continued)

Causes may include:

- Local diseases
- Vascular disorders
- Referred pain
- Neurological disorders
- Psychogenic pain.

Remember from the mnemonic **Let Veterans Read Newspapers.**

Local diseases

- Diseases of the teeth
  - dentine sensitivity
  - periapical periodontitis
  - pulpitis
- Diseases of the periodontium
  - lateral (periodontal) abscess
  - necrotizing periodontitis
  - necrotizing ulcerative gingivitis
  - pericoronitis
- Diseases of the jaws
  - dry socket
  - fractures
  - infected cysts
  - malignant neoplasms
  - osteochemonecrosis (bisphosphonate-related, denosumab, bevacizumab)
  - osteomyelitis
  - osteoradionecrosis
- Diseases of the maxillary sinus (antrum)
  - acute sinusitis
  - malignant neoplasms
- Diseases of the temporomandibular joint
  - arthritis
  - temporomandibular pain dysfunction (facial arthromyalgia)
  - others

- Diseases of the salivary glands
  - acute sialadenitis
  - calculi or other obstruction to duct
  - HIV salivary gland disease
  - malignant neoplasms.

Vascular disorders
- Giant cell arteritis
- Migraine
- Migrainous neuralgia.

Referred pain
- Cervical spine
- Chest
- Eyes
- Ears
- Nasopharynx
- Others.

Neurological disorders
- Herpes zoster (including post-herpetic neuralgia)
- HIV neuropathy
- Lyme disease
- Malignant neoplasms involving the trigeminal nerve
- Multiple sclerosis
- Trigeminal neuralgia.

Psychogenic pain (oral dysaesthesia)
- Idiopathic (atypical) facial pain
- Atypical odontalgia, and other oral symptoms associated with anxiety or depression
- Burning mouth syndrome (BMS).

Drugs
For example, vinca alkaloids.

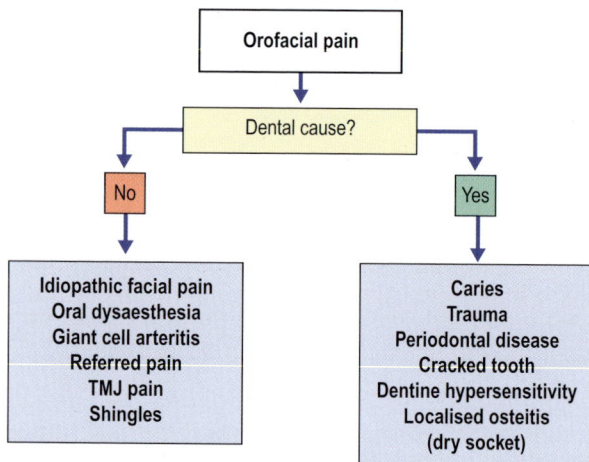

Figure 2.64 Algorithm for pain diagnosis.

Palsy (orofacial)

Keypoints

- Facial palsy (paralysis) is usually due to a facial nerve disorder but myopathies may give the appearance of facial palsy.
- The common causes of facial palsy are a stroke (cerebrovascular event), iatrogenic surgical trauma or Bell palsy.
- Bell palsy is fairly common and affects only the facial nerve; there are no brain or other neurological problems.
- Bell palsy often has an infective cause – often herpes simplex virus (HSV); consider other viruses (VZV, HIV), and bacteria (*Borrelia burgdorferi* causing Lyme disease) mainly. It is not contagious.
- Bell palsy disproportionately attacks pregnant women and people who have diabetes, influenza, a cold, or immune problems.
- There are usually no serious long-term consequences.
- Radiographs, scans and blood tests may be required.
- Treatment takes time and patience; corticosteroids and/or antimicrobials can sometimes help.
- Most patients begin to get significantly better within 2 weeks, and about 80% recover completely within 3 months.
- It rarely recurs, but can do so in ~ 5–10%.

Box 2.15 Main causes of facial paralysis

Stroke (cerebrovascular event)
Bell palsy

Causes may include:

Mostly the cause is neurological – usually a stroke, or Bell palsy.

- Central causes
  - cerebral palsy, tumour or cerebrovascular event (stroke)
  - connective tissue disorders
  - demyelinating disorders (e.g. multiple sclerosis)
  - diabetes mellitus
  - granulomatous diseases
    - a Crohn disease
    - b orofacial granulomatosis
    - c sarcoidosis
- Trauma to facial nerve or its branches, including local anaesthesia
- Infections affecting facial nerve (Bell palsy)
  - viral infections (e.g. herpesviruses, retroviruses, Coxsackie viruses or Guillain–Barré syndrome)
  - bacterial infections (otitis media, Lyme disease)
  - fungal infections (e.g. zygomycosis)
  - parasitic infestations (e.g. toxoplasmosis)
  - possible infections: Kawasaki disease (mucocutaneous lymph node syndrome), Reiter disease (reactive arthritis)
- Middle ear disease
  - cholesteatoma
  - malignancy
  - mastoiditis
  - trauma (including surgery, and barotrauma – as in scuba diving)
- Parotid lesions
  - parotid malignancy
  - parotid trauma.

Clinical features: upper motor neurone lesions (e.g. stroke): unilateral palsy, mainly in lower face may be features of stroke but hearing or taste normal. Lower motor neurone lesions (e.g. Bell palsy): complete unilateral facial

Palsy (orofacial) (continued)

palsy demonstrable when the patient smiles, whistles or tries to show their teeth (Figures 2.65, 2.66); may also be loss of taste and/or hyperacusis.

Investigations: neurological; advanced imaging; blood pressure; blood tests for diabetes and infective agents. Lyme disease, since it is amenable to antibiotics, should be excluded – especially in endemic areas.

Management: Bell palsy: systemic corticosteroids, with or without antivirals; stroke: physiotherapy and rehabilitation.

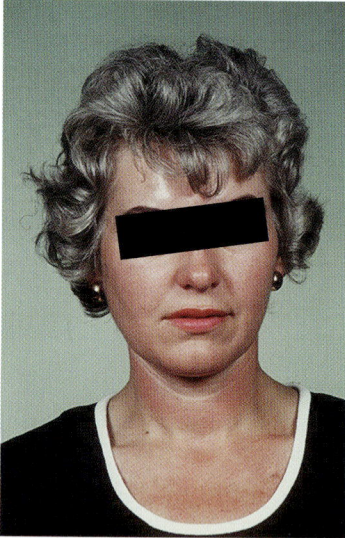

Figure 2.65 Bell palsy (at rest).

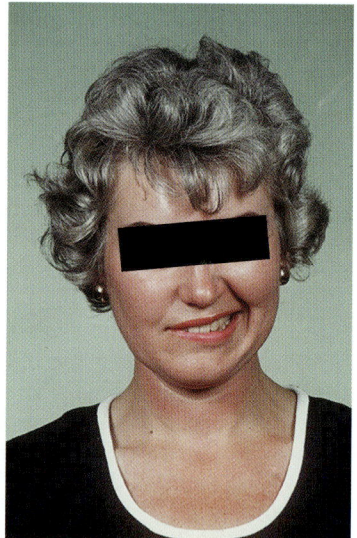

Figure 2.66 Bell palsy (attempting a smile) showing right-sided palsy.

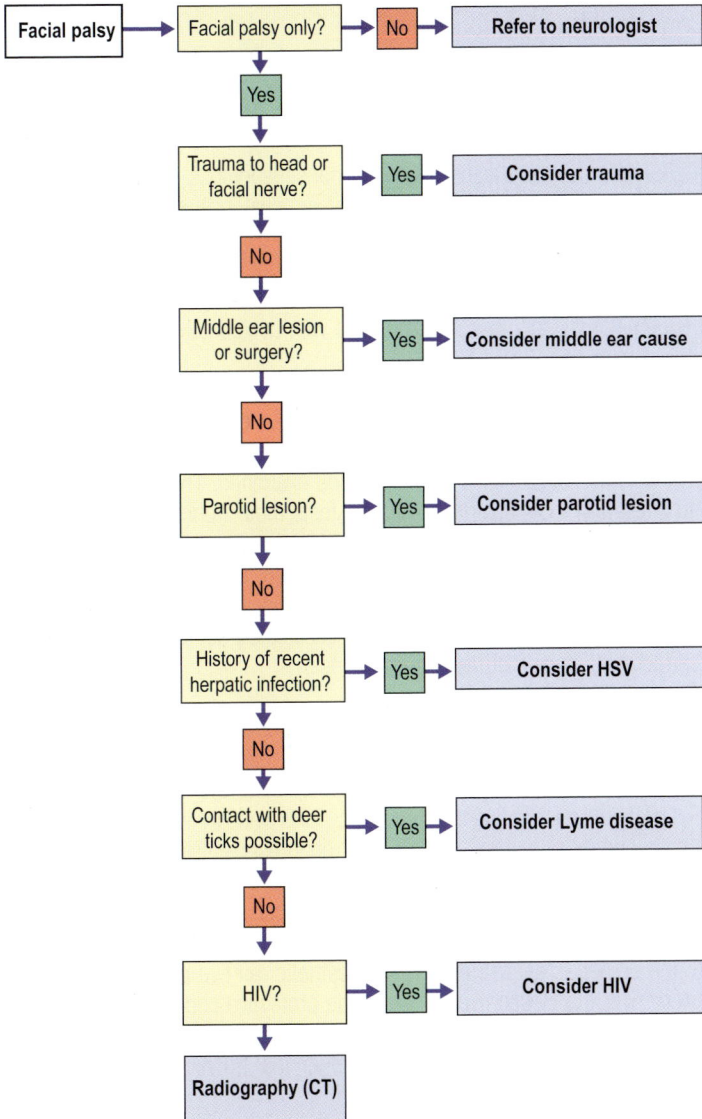

Figure 2.67 Algorithm for facial palsy diagnosis.

Sensory changes (orofacial)

Keypoints

- The trigeminal nerve supplies sensation to most of the maxillofacial region.
- Trauma is the usual cause of trigeminal sensory loss – and is seen especially after mandibular third molar removal, orthognathic or cancer surgery (Figures 2.68, 2.69).
- Other important causes of sensory loss include osteomyelitis and malignant disease, often presenting as 'numb chin syndrome'.
- Trigeminal sensory loss may manifest with accidental self-damage to the skin or lip.
- Clinical tests for trigeminal nerve function include applying gentle touch, pinpricks, or warm or cold objects to areas supplied by the nerve – these are reduced in trigeminal sensory loss. The jaw jerk and eye and corneal reflexes should also be examined. The patient's ability to chew and work against resistance tests motor function.
- In view of the potential seriousness of facial sensory loss, a full neurological assessment must be undertaken, unless the loss is unequivocally related to local trauma and, since other cranial nerves are anatomically close, there may be associated neurological deficits in intracranial causes of facial sensory loss.
- Possible investigations include:
  - imaging (panoral, occipitomental, lateral and postero-anterior skull, and MRI/CT of brain and skull base and mandibular division)
  - a full blood count, erythrocyte sedimentation rate or C-reactive protein, random sugar (glucose), syphilis and HIV serology, autoantibody screen, plasma electrophoresis, calcium, phosphate and alkaline phosphatase levels
  - lumbar puncture – if disseminated sclerosis, carcinomatous meningitis or leptomeningeal metastases are suspected.
- If the cornea is anaesthetic or hypoaesthetic, an eye pad should be worn over the closed eyelids, since the protective corneal reflex is lost and the cornea may easily be damaged. Facial hypoaesthesia results in the loss of protective reflexes and a trigeminal trophic syndrome with facial ulceration can follow.

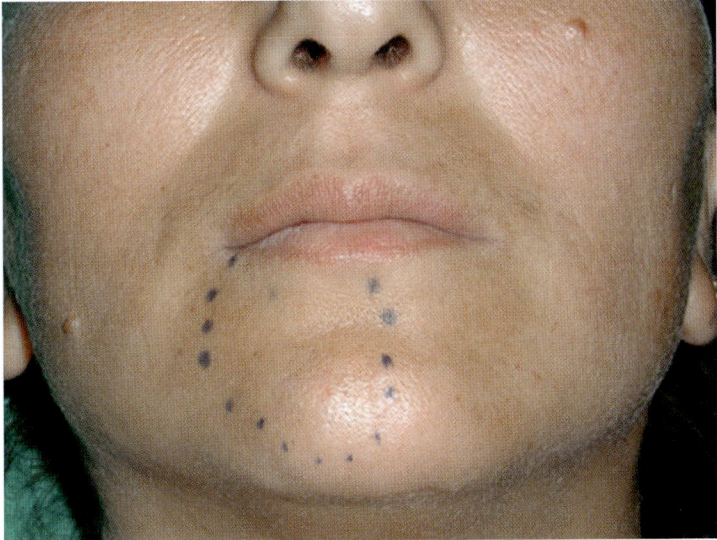

Figure 2.68 Numb chin syndrome, damaged right inferior alveolar nerve during mandibular third molar removal.

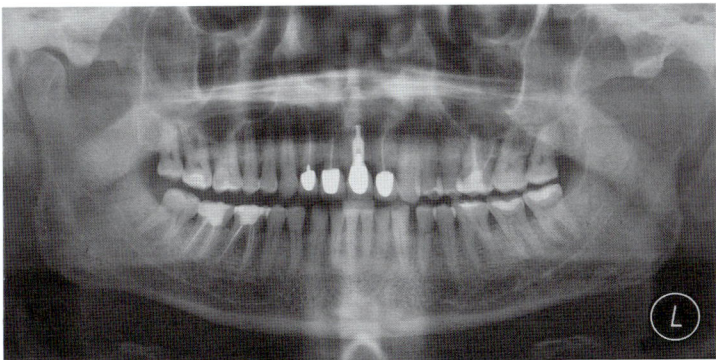

Figure 2.69 Neoplasm in left mandibular ramus (multiple myeloma) presenting with sensory loss.

Sensory changes (orofacial) (continued)

- If there has been neurotmesis (cut nerve), rather than crushing (neuropraxia), surgical correction can achieve good results.
- In benign, reversible causes of sensory loss, the underlying cause should be corrected, and the patient reassured that there should be some, if not full, return of sensation over the subsequent 18 months.

Box 2.16 Main causes of orofacial sensory loss

Trauma
Trigeminal nerve pressure from a lesion
Disseminated sclerosis

Causes may include:

- Trauma
- Numb chin syndrome
- Benign trigeminal neuropathy
- Psychogenic causes
- Congenital causes.

Trauma

Trauma to the mandibular division of the trigeminal nerve and inferior alveolar nerve may be caused by:

- Inferior alveolar local analgesic injections
- Fractures of the mandibular body or angle
- Surgery (particularly cancer and orthognathic surgery or surgical extraction of lower-third molars) or even endodontics or endosseous implants.

Causes of damage to the mental nerve include:

- Surgery in the region
- Trauma from a denture – the mental foramen is close beneath a lower denture and there is ipsilateral anaesthesia of the lower lip.

Causes of damage to the lingual nerve include lower third molar removal, particularly when the lingual split technique is used. Ipsilateral lingual hypo-aesthesia or anaesthesia usually result.

Causes of damage to branches of the maxillary division of the trigeminal nerve include trauma (usually Le Fort II or III middle-third facial fractures).

Numb chin syndrome

Numb chin syndrome (NCS) is unilateral chin numbness which may be caused by:

- Trauma
- Osteomyelitis
- Inferior alveolar nerve malignant infiltration or compression by jaw metastases (mainly lymphomas or breast cancer)
- Nasopharyngeal carcinomas may: invade the pharyngeal wall to infiltrate the mandibular division of the trigeminal nerve, causing pain and sensory loss in the region of the inferior alveolar, lingual and auriculotemporal nerve distributions; invade the levator palati to cause soft palate immobility; occlude the Eustachian tube to cause deafness (Trotter syndrome)
- Metastatic or other deposit in the meninges or at the base of skull
- Sensory stroke.

Bilateral chin numbness, or circumoral numbness may be caused by:

- Hyperventilation
- Hypocalcaemia, including drug-induced (e.g. protease inhibitor, ritonavir)
- Central nervous system toxicity from local anaesthetics
- Syringobulbia.

Benign trigeminal neuropathy

This is a long-standing sensory loss in one or more trigeminal divisions of unknown cause, although it is important to exclude connective tissue diseases and intracranial and extracranial causes before considering this to be the final diagnosis. It seldom occurs until the second decade or affects the corneal reflex. In some cases there is associated pain, which may be responsive to amitryptiline.

Psychogenic causes

Hysteria, and particularly hyperventilation syndrome, may underlie some causes of facial anaesthesia/hypoaesthesia. Typically then, the 'anaesthesia' is bilateral and associated with bizarre neurological complaints.

Congenital causes

Rare cases of facial sensory loss are congenital.

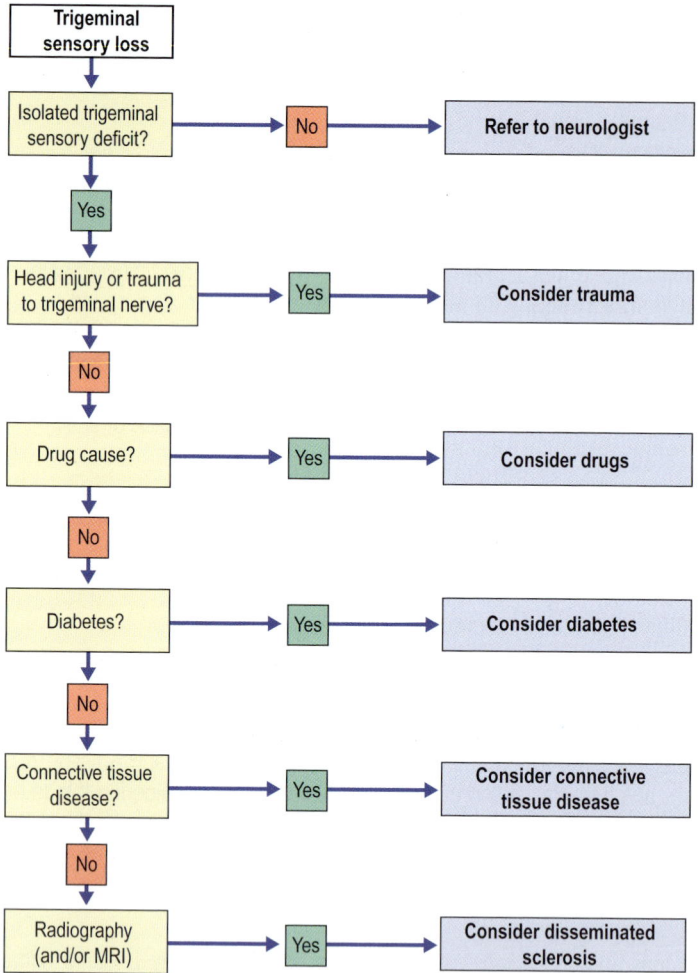

Figure 2.70 Algorithm for trigeminal sensory loss diagnosis.

Sialorrhoea (hypersalivation and drooling)

Keypoints

- Healthy individuals produce and swallow from 0.5 to 1.5 litres of saliva in 24 hours.
- Salivary flow above this is termed sialorrhoea, hypersialia, hypersalivation or ptyalism.
- Most individuals are able to compensate for any increased salivation by swallowing.
- Disturbed control of swallowing because of disorders of the orofacial and/or palatolingual or pharyngeal musculature can lead to the overflow of saliva from the mouth (drooling) (Figure 2.71).
- Drooling is normal in healthy infants, but usually stops by about 18 months of age and is considered abnormal if it persists beyond the age of four years.
- Drooling can soil clothing and cause perioral skin breakdown and infections, disturbed speech and eating, and can occasionally cause aspiration-related and pulmonary complications.

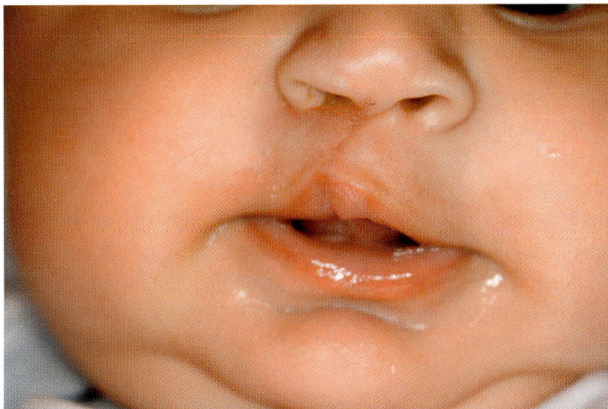

Figure 2.71 Drooling in an infant who has had initial cleft lip repair.

Sialorrhoea (hypersalivation and drooling) (continued)

Box 2.17 Main causes of sensation of sialorrhoea

Poor neuromuscular coordination
Oral painful lesion
Pharygneal or oesophageal obstruction
Psychogenic

Causes may include:

- Psychogenic (usually)
- Painful lesions or foreign bodies in the mouth
- Poor neuromuscular coordination
  - cerebral palsy
  - facial palsy
  - other physical disability
  - Parkinsonism
- Drugs (e.g. bethanecol, clozapine, nitrazepam, pilocarpine, risperidone)
- Poisoning
  - heavy metals
  - insecticides
  - mercury
- Learning impairment
- Obstruction to swallowing
  - pharyngeal
  - oesophageal.

Management options range from conservative therapy (e.g. oral motor training) to medication (e.g. benztropine, glycopyrrolate, scopolamine, botulinum toxoid), radiation, or surgery, and often a combination. A team including at least an otolaryngologist, neurologist, dentist, speech, occupational and physical therapists is needed.

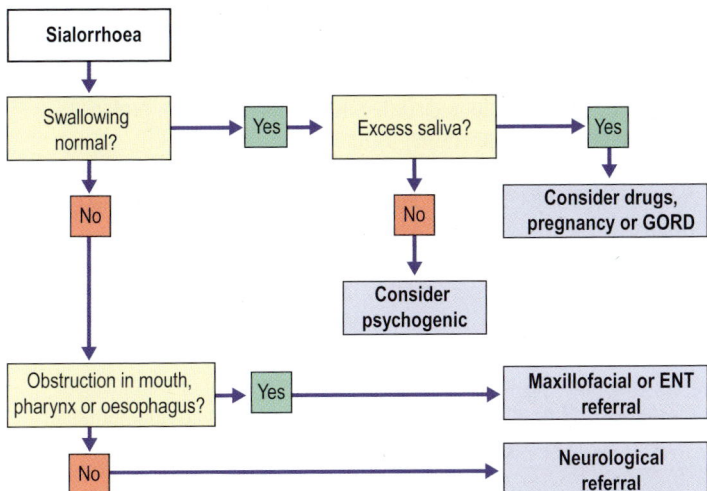

Figure 2.72 Algorithm for sialorrhoea. GORD: gastro-oesophageal reflux disease.

Swellings in the lips or face

Keypoints

- Facial swelling that appears over a few minutes or hours may be caused by angioedema.
- Facial swelling that appears over a few hours or days is most commonly inflammatory in origin, often caused by trauma.
- Facial swelling that appears over a few hours or days may also be caused by cutaneous, dental (odontogenic) or, rarely, systemic infections.
- Facial swelling that appears over days or weeks may be seen in masseteric hypertrophy.

Swellings in the lips or face (continued)

- Facial swelling that appears over days or weeks may occasionally be caused by granulomatous disorders (e.g. Crohn disease, orofacial granulomatosis or sarcoidosis) (Figure 2.73).
- Facial swelling that appears over weeks or months is occasionally due to systemic corticosteroid therapy or endocrine disease (Cushing disease, hypothyroidism, acromegaly, diabetes mellitus).
- Facial swelling is commonly of slow onset in obesity.
- Facial swelling that is persistent is rarely caused by:
  - fluid, as in vascular lesions (Figure 2.74) or lymphangiomas (Figure 2.75)
  - solids, such as primary neoplasms (Figure 2.76) or metastases, deposits (e.g. amyloid) or foreign material (as in lip augmentation with silicone or other fillers).

Box 2.18 Main causes of swelling of lips/face

Allergy
Inflammation
Trauma
Granulomatous condition (e.g. Crohn disease, orofacial granulomatosis or sarcoidosis)
Neoplasm

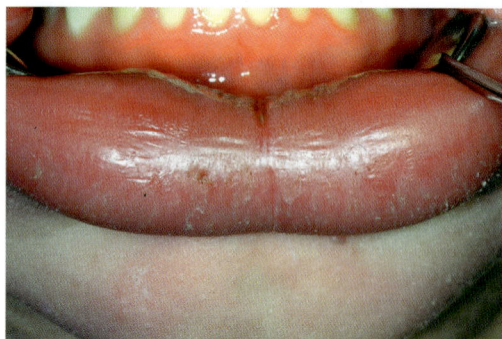

Figure 2.73 Lip swelling: Crohn disease – showing typical lower lip swelling and fissuring, and gingival involvement.

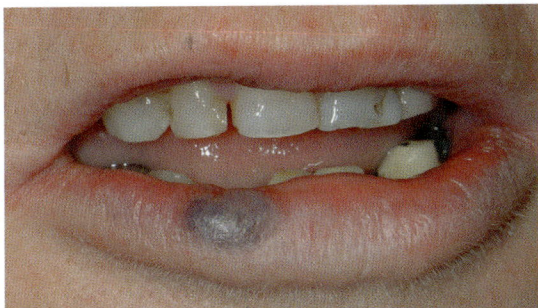

Figure 2.74 Lip swelling: haemangioma.

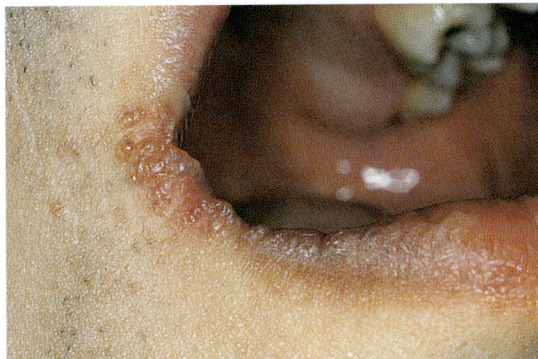

Figure 2.75 Lip swelling: lymphangioma.

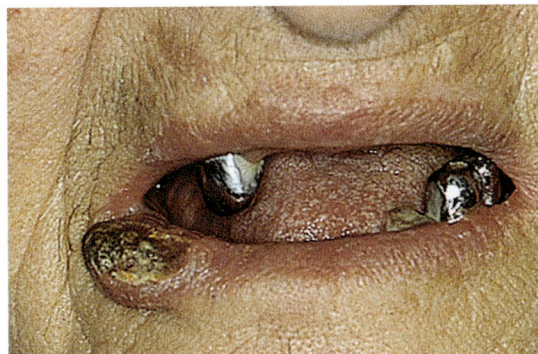

Figure 2.76 Lip swelling: carcinoma.

Swellings in the lips or face (continued)

Causes may include:

Facial swelling is commonly inflammatory in origin – caused by cutaneous or dental (odontogenic) infections or trauma.

- Infective
  - oral or cutaneous infections, cellulitis, fascial space infections
  - insect bites
- Traumatic
  - traumatic or postoperative oedema or haematoma
  - surgical emphysema
- Immunological
  - allergic angioedema
  - C1 esterase inhibitor deficiency (hereditary angioedema)
  - Crohn disease, orofacial granulomatosis (OFG) or sarcoidosis
- Endocrine and metabolic
  - Cushing syndrome and disease
  - myxoedema
  - nephrotic syndrome
  - obesity
  - systemic corticosteroid therapy
- Neoplasms
  - congenital (e.g. lymphangioma)
  - lymphoma
  - oral and antral tumours
- Foreign bodies (including cosmetic fillers)
- Deposits
  - amyloidosis
  - others
- Cysts in soft tissues or bone
- Masseteric hypertrophy
- Bone disease
  - fibrous dysplasia
  - Paget disease.

Swellings in the mouth

Keypoints

- Swellings in the mouth are often caused by infection or trauma (e.g. oedema, haematoma, odontogenic infections, pyogenic granulomas) (Figures 2.77, 2.78).

Box 2.19 Main causes of oral lumps or swelling

Allergy
Inflammation
Trauma
Granulomatous disorders (e.g. Crohn disease, orofacial granulomatosis or sarcoidosis)
Neoplasm
Drugs

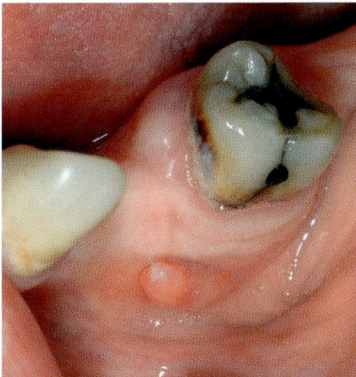

Figure 2.77 Intraoral swelling: periapical abscess.

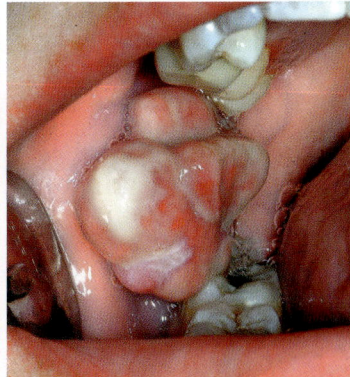

Figure 2.78 Intraoral swelling: pregnancy tumour (pyogenic granuloma).

Swellings in the mouth (continued)

- Swellings in the mouth may occasionally be caused by:
  - neoplastic lesions (e.g. fibrous lumps [fibro-epithelial polyps], carcinoma or lymphoma) (Figures 2.79–2.88).

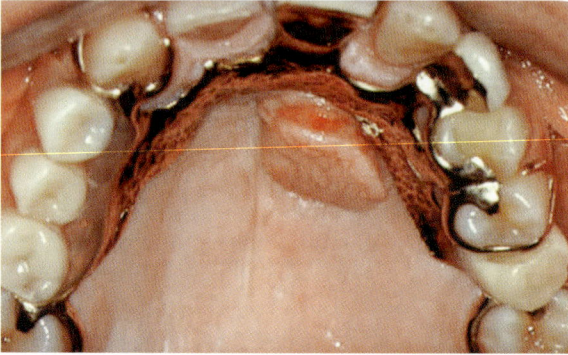

Figure 2.79 Intraoral swelling: fibrous lump.

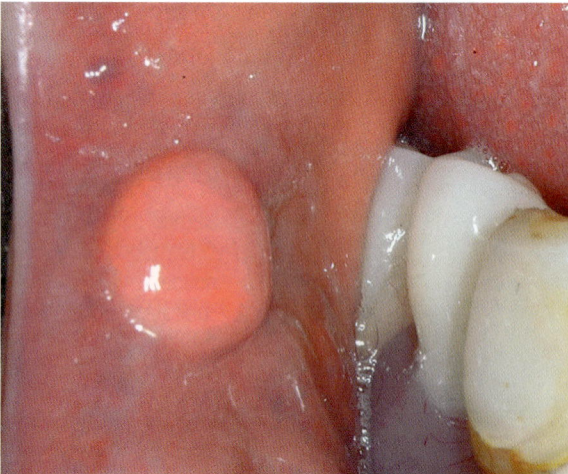

Figure 2.80 Intraoral swelling: fibrous lump.

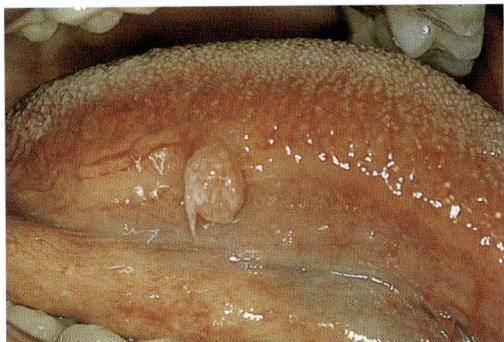

Figure 2.81 Intraoral swelling: papilloma.

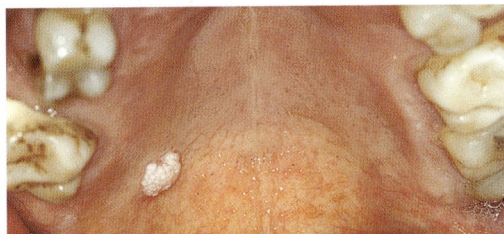

Figure 2.82 Intraoral swelling: papilloma.

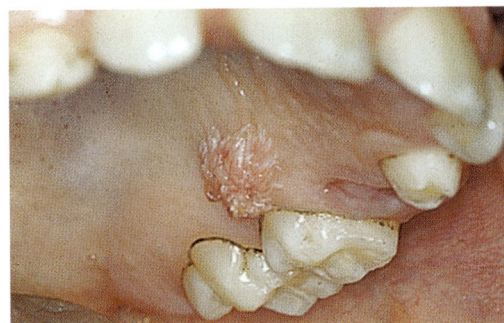

Figure 2.83 Intraoral swelling: papilloma (note also unrelated black stain on teeth).

Swellings in the mouth (continued)

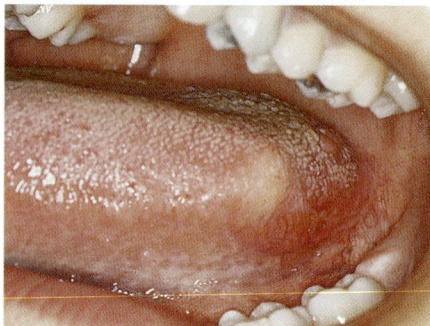

Figure 2.84 Intraoral swelling: granular cell myoblastoma (can be confused histologically with carcinoma).

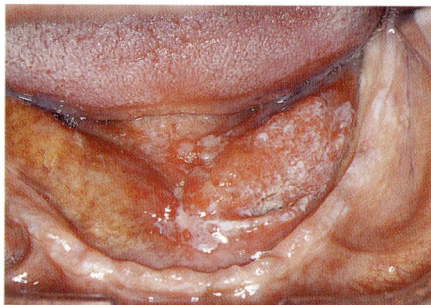

Figure 2.85 Intraoral swelling: carcinoma.

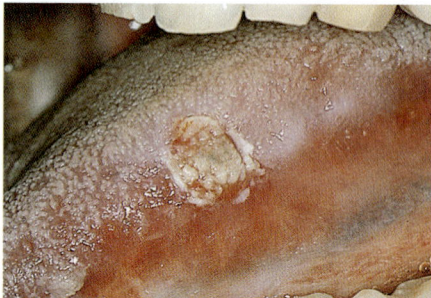

Figure 2.86 Intraoral swelling: carcinoma arising from a white lesion.

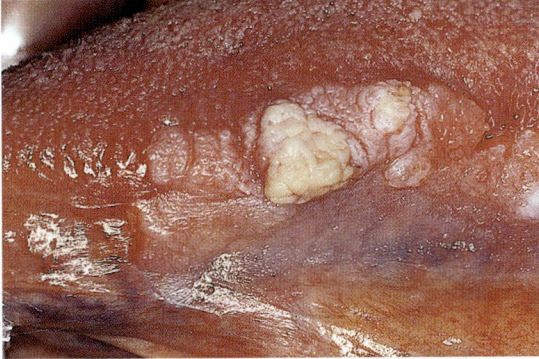

Figure 2.87 Intraoral swelling: carcinoma arising from a white lesion.

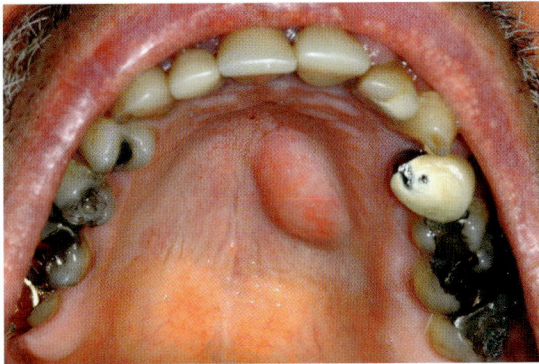

Figure 2.88 Intraoral swelling: salivary neoplasm originally thought to be a dental abscess.

Swellings in the mouth (continued)

- granulomatous disorders (e.g. Crohn disease, orofacial granulomatous disease (OFG), sarcoidosis) (Figures 2.89–2.91).

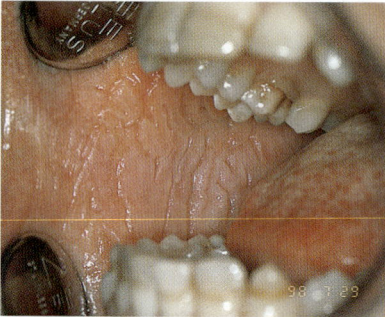

Figure 2.89 Intraoral swelling: Crohn disease 'cobblestoning' of mucosa (same patient as 2.90).

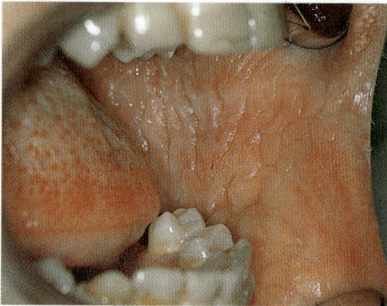

Figure 2.90 Intraoral swelling: Crohn disease.

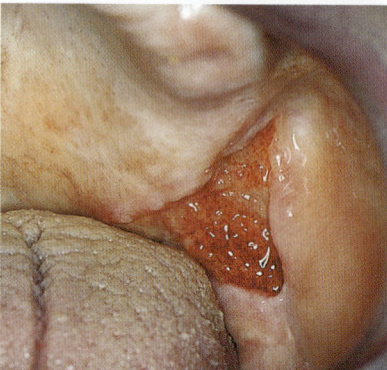

Figure 2.91 Intraoral swelling: Crohn disease swelling and chronic ulceration.

- Swellings in the mouth are rarely caused by:
  - fluid, as in angiomas (Figures 2.92–2.94) or angioedema

Figure 2.92
Intraoral swelling:
haemangioma and
lymphangioma.

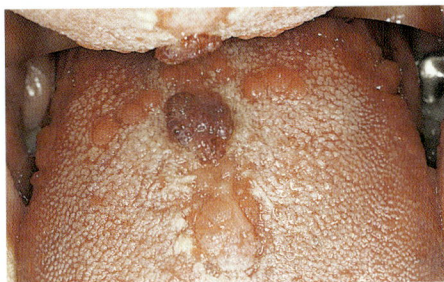

Figure 2.93 Intraoral
swelling: lymphangioma.

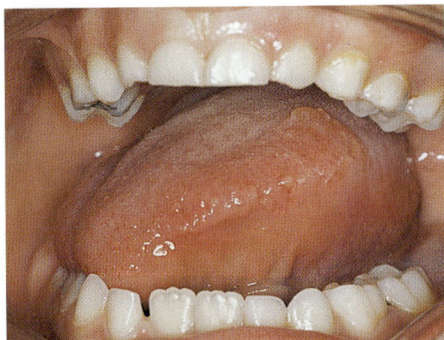

Figure 2.94 Intraoral
swelling: lymphangioma.

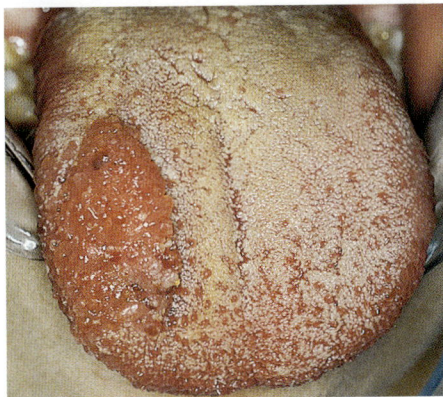

Swellings in the mouth (continued)

- solids, such as some congenital neoplasms (Figure 2.95), foreign material, metastases (Figure 2.96) or deposits (e.g. amyloid).
- Wegener granulomatosis – this can present an almost pathognomonic 'strawberry' appearance of the gingival, or lumps or ulcers elsewhere. There may be lung and kidney lesions, and serum antineutrophil cytoplasmic antibodies (ANCA). Chemotherapy or co-trimoxazole are indicated.
- tongue swelling (macroglossia) is discussed below. In macroglossia, the tongue is indented by teeth, or too large to be contained in the mouth. Ultrasound or MRI may be indicated; biopsy if there is discrete swelling, but not if it is a vascular lesion.
- Gingival swelling is fairly common, often localized to the maxillary anterior gingivae in hyperplastic gingivitis arising as a consequence of mouth-breathing:
  - epulides are localized gingival swellings – rarely are they true neoplasms (Figure 2.97).
  - generalized gingival swelling is commonly drug-induced, usually aggravated by poor oral hygiene and starting interdentally, especially labially. Papillae are firm, pale and enlarge to form false vertical clefts
  - generalized gingival swelling may occasionally be congenital (hereditary gingival fibromatosis), deposits or due to leukaemia.

Epulides

Epulis is a term applied to any discrete swelling arising from the gingiva.

Typical orofacial symptoms and signs: fibrous epulides (irritation fibromas) are most common; they typically form narrow, firm, pale swellings of an anterior interdental papilla and may ulcerate. Pyogenic granulomas, giant cell or neoplastic epulides are often softer, and a deeper red colour but they cannot be distinguished clinically with certainty from fibrous epulides.
Main oral sites affected: facial gingivae.

Aetiopathogenesis: fibrous epulides may result from local gingival irritation, leading to fibrous hyperplasia. Pyogenic granulomas are common lesions, especially in children and teens where there are local factors, including inadequate oral hygiene, malocclusion and orthodontic appliances, and in pregnancy (pregnancy epulides) (the lesions themselves are not

Figure 2.95 Intraoral swelling: neurofibroma (in generalized neurofibromatosis).

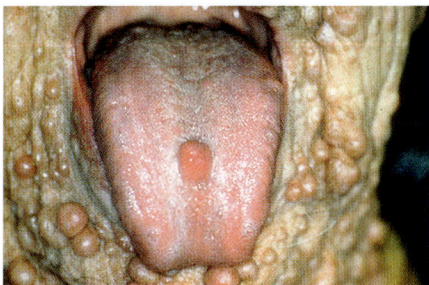

Figure 2.96 Intraoral swelling: metastatic carcinoma (from breast cancer.)

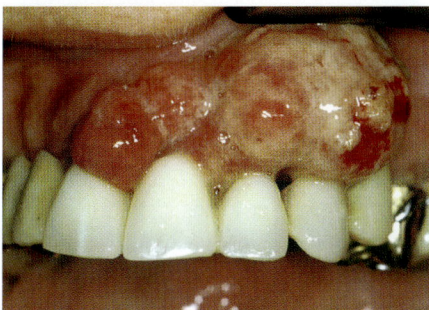

Figure 2.97 Intraoral swelling: fibrous epulis arising adjacent to imbricated teeth.

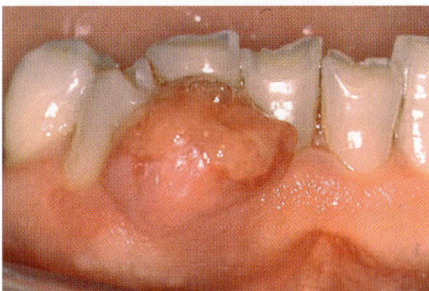

histologically distinguishable). Giant cell epulides (giant cell granulomas) are reactive lesions seen mainly in children caused by local irritation or may result from proliferation of giant cells persisting after resorption of deciduous teeth. Rarely, epulides represent metastatic disease or other tumors.

Investigations: excision biopsy; radiography.

Main treatments: excision; remove local irritants (e.g. calculus).

Swellings in the neck
Keypoints

- Swellings in the neck can arise from any tissue but most commonly from the lymph nodes, salivary or thyroid glands.
- Cervical lymph node swellings may be mainly:
  - inflammatory
  - malignant (Figure 2.98).
- Salivary gland swellings may be caused mainly by:
  - calculi or other obstruction to salivary flow
  - IgG4 syndrome
  - sarcoidosis
  - sialadenitis (usually bacterial or viral)
  - sialosis
  - Sjögren syndrome
  - tumours.
- Thyroid gland swellings are mostly caused by an inadequate intake of iodine; other causes include:
  - benign and malignant thyroid tumours
  - Graves disease (non-painful generalized swelling of the thyroid gland plus hyperthyroidism)
  - thyroiditis: some types of thyroiditis are extremely painful, may disturb thyroid function and may culminate in hypothyroidism
    - a pregnancy (postpartum thyroiditis)
    - b Hashimoto disease (chronic autoimmune thyroiditis)
    - c acute and subacute thyroiditis
    - d silent thyroiditis.
- Skin swellings are mainly:
  - epidermoid/dermoid cyst
  - intraoral abscess with cutaneous sinus tract
  - Ludwig angina (submandibular and sublingual fascial spaces infection).

Box 2.20 Main causes of neck swelling
Allergy
Inflammation
Neoplasm

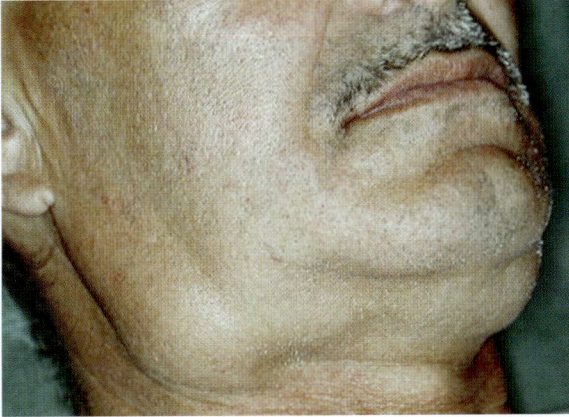

Figure 2.98 Cervical lymph node metastases from ipsilateral oral carcinoma.

Swellings in the side of the neck

Apart from lymph node or salivary gland swellings, these may include:

- Actinomycosis
- Branchial cyst
- Parapharyngeal cellulitis
- Pharyngeal pouch
- Cystic hygroma
- Carotid body tumours or aneurysms
- Muscle or other soft tissue neoplasm
- Focal myositis
- Myositis ossificans
- Proliferative myositis
- Nodular pseudosarcomatous fasciitis.

Swellings in the midline of the neck

These may be due to submental lymphadenopathy, or

- Ectopic thyroid
- Epidermoid/dermoid cyst
- Thyroglossal cyst
- Thyroid tumours or goitre
- 'Plunging' ranula.

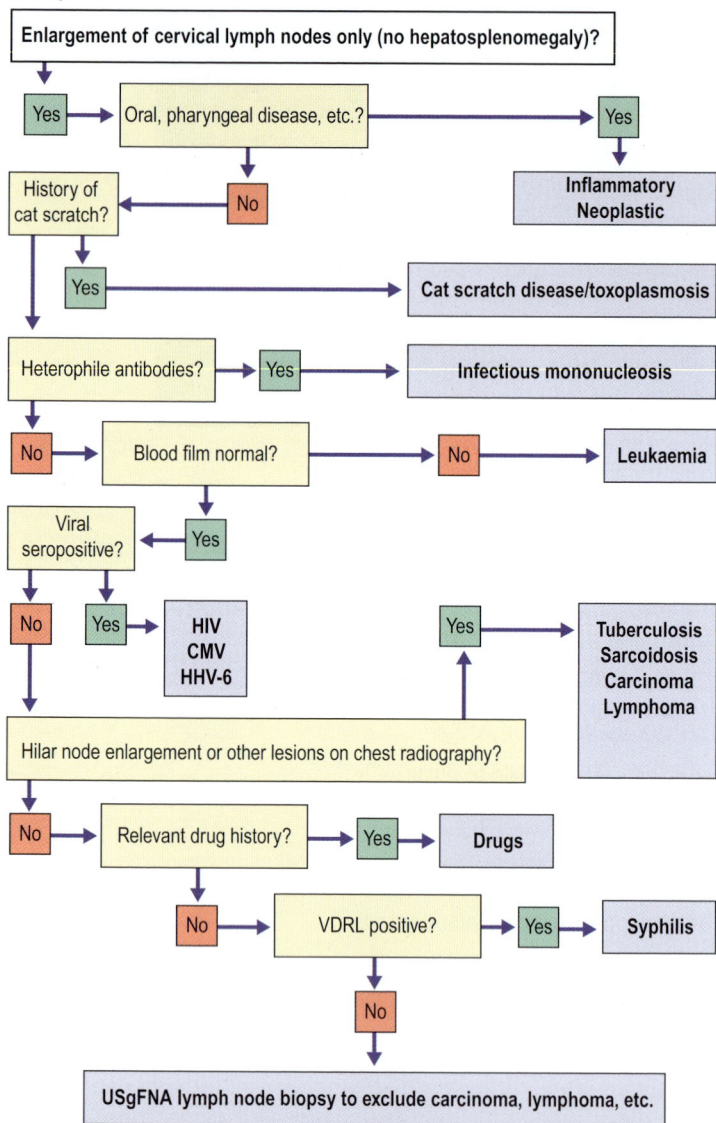

Figure 2.99 Algorithm for cervical lymph node enlargement. USgFNA: ultrasound-guided fine needle aspiration; VDRL: veneral disease research laboratory test.

Swellings of the jaws

Keypoints

- Jaw swelling is most often caused by developmental enlargements (e.g. tori or buccal exostoses), which are benign, painless, broad-based and self-limiting, usually with normal overlying mucosa.
- Jaw swelling is less commonly due to odontogenic causes (unerupted teeth, infections, cysts or neoplasms).
- Metastasis to the mouth is rare but is typically to the jaws, especially the posterior mandible. Most metastases originate from cancers of the breast, lung, kidney, thyroid, stomach, liver, colon, bone or prostate via lymphatic or haematogenous spread, and present as lumps, ulceration, tooth loosening, sensory change or pathological fracture.
- Jaw swelling may occasionally be caused by other inflammatory or neoplastic disorders, or metabolic or fibro-osseous diseases.
- Imaging is almost invariably required to assist the diagnosis.

Box 2.21 Main causes of jaw swelling
Congenital
Odontogenic infections, cysts or neoplasms

Causes may include:

- Congenital (e.g. torus)
- Odontogenic
  - unerupted teeth
  - infections
  - cysts

Swellings of the jaws (continued)

- neoplasms (Figure 2.100)
- postoperative or post-traumatic oedema or haematoma
- Foreign bodies
- Bone disease
  - fibrous dysplasia
  - Paget disease
  - cherubism.

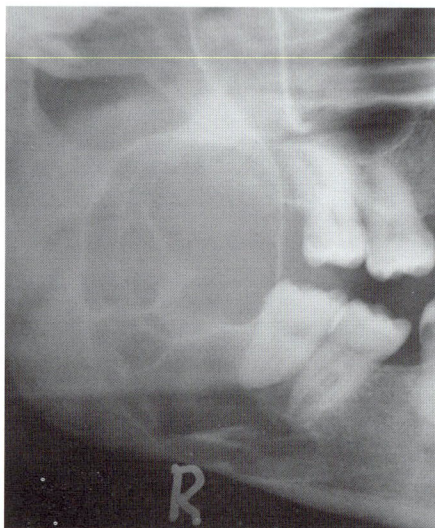

Figure 2.100 Jaw swelling: ameloblastoma showing multilocularity on radiography, seen in the typical location (posterior mandible).

Swelling of the salivary glands
Keypoints

- The most common salivary lesion is the mucocele, usually caused by extravasation of saliva from a damaged minor salivary gland duct and seen in the lower labial mucosa, sometimes caused by retention within a gland.
- In children and young people, the most common cause of swelling of one or more of the major glands is viral sialadenitis (mumps). Recurrent

sialadenitis may be termed juvenile recurrent parotitis, but this is probably a group of conditions variously caused by genetic factors, ductal obstruction, ductal ectasia (dilatations), or diseases such as Sjögren syndrome or sarcoidosis.

- In adults, salivary swelling is most commonly obstructive (e.g. by a salivary stone or calculus [sialolith]) (Figures 2.101, 2.102) or

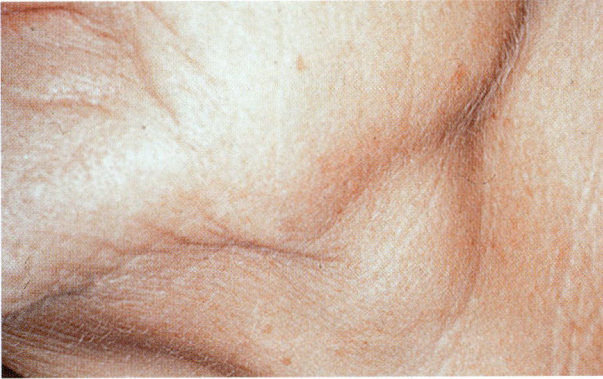

Figure 2.101 Salivary gland swelling: obstruction from submandibular salivary calculus.

Figure 2.102 Salivary gland swelling: obstruction in parotid duct is often due to mucous plugs.

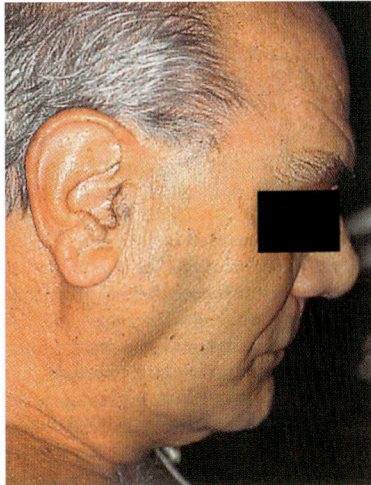

Swelling of the salivary glands (continued)

inflammatory in origin (e.g. infective sialadenitis, sclerosing sialadenitis [IgG4 syndrome], Sjögren syndrome, sarcoidosis) (Figures 2.103–2.105).
- Salivary swelling may be caused by salivary, or rarely systemic, infections.
- Salivary swelling may occasionally be caused by neoplastic (Figures 2.106, 2.107) or other disorders (e.g. sialosis).

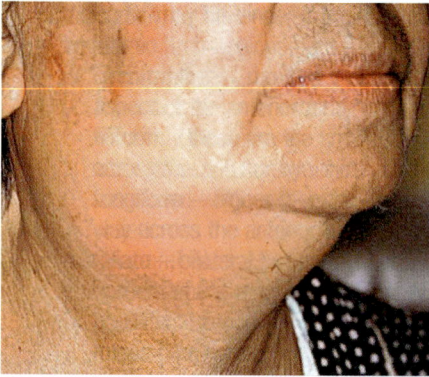

Fig 2.103 Salivary gland swelling: infection of acute sialadenitis produces pain, swelling and erythema.

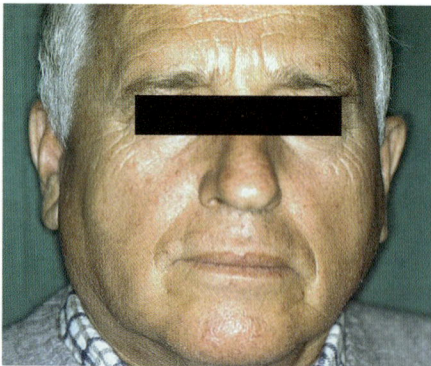

Figure 2.104 Salivary gland swelling; bilateral parotid inflammation in Mikulicz disease (IgG4 syndrome).

Figure 2.105 Salivary gland swelling: parotitis. The gland is painful and swollen, the skin erythematous, and mouth opening is restricted.

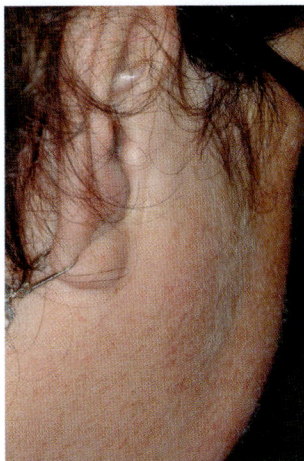

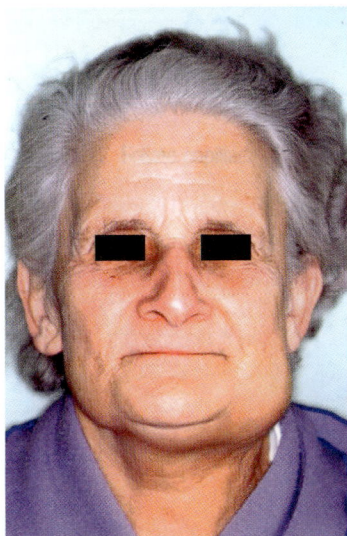

Figure 2.106 Salivary gland swelling: neoplasm (adenoid cystic carcinoma).

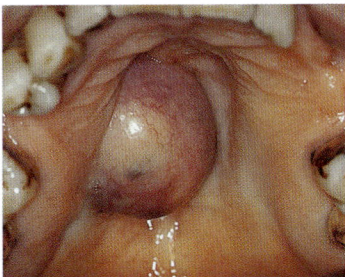

Figure 2.107 Salivary gland swelling: neoplasm (pleomorphic adenoma).

Swelling of the salivary glands (continued)

- Salivary swelling is also caused by:
  - fluid, as in trauma (oedema or haematoma), mucocele (Figures 2.108, 2.109) or vascular lesions
  - solids such as deposits (e.g. amyloid) or foreign material
  - swelling of intra-salivary lymph nodes.

Box 2.22 Main causes of salivary gland swelling
Obstruction
Sialadenitis
Sjögren syndrome
Sialosis
Neoplasm

Causes may include:

- IgG4 syndrome
- Mucocele/ranula
- Neoplasms
- Sarcoidosis
- Sialadenitis
- Sialosis
- Sjögren syndrome.

Obstruction

Fairly common in submandibular duct or gland; rare in parotid.

Typical orofacial symptoms and signs: may be asymptomatic but typically there is pain and swelling of gland at meals (Figures 2.106, 2.107, 2.116) and there can be a consequent bacterial sialadenitis. Obstruction of a minor salivary gland duct or a ductal tear may produce a mucocele.

Main oral sites affected: submandibular mainly, in the duct or gland, or both sites.

Aetiopathogenesis: calculus – the usual cause in the submandibular; more likely to be a mucous plug, fibrous stricture or neoplasm in the parotid.

Gender predominance: male.

Figure 2.108
Salivary gland
swellings: mucoceles
are usually solitary
but occasionally
multiple as here.

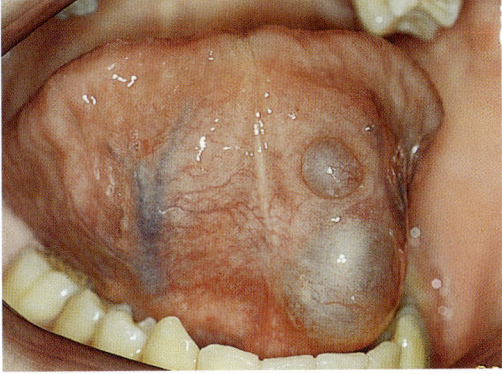

Fig 2.109 Salivary
gland swelling:
submandibular
obstruction (as here)
can mimic a
mucocele.

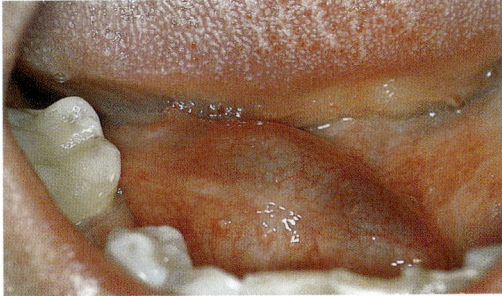

Age predominance: adult.

Extraoral possible lesions: none.

Main associated conditions: none.

Differential diagnosis: differentiate from other causes of salivary swelling: inflammatory – mumps, bacterial sialadenitis, IgG4 syndrome, Sjögren syndrome, sarcoidosis; duct obstruction; neoplasms; others including sialosis, drugs and Mikulicz disease (IgG4 disease: sclerosing sialadenitis).

Investigations: ultrasound, radiography (but 40% of stones are radiolucent); sialography if necessary.

Main diagnostic criteria: clinical and imaging.

Main treatments: surgical removal of obstruction (lithotripsy, endoscopic removal, or incisional removal).

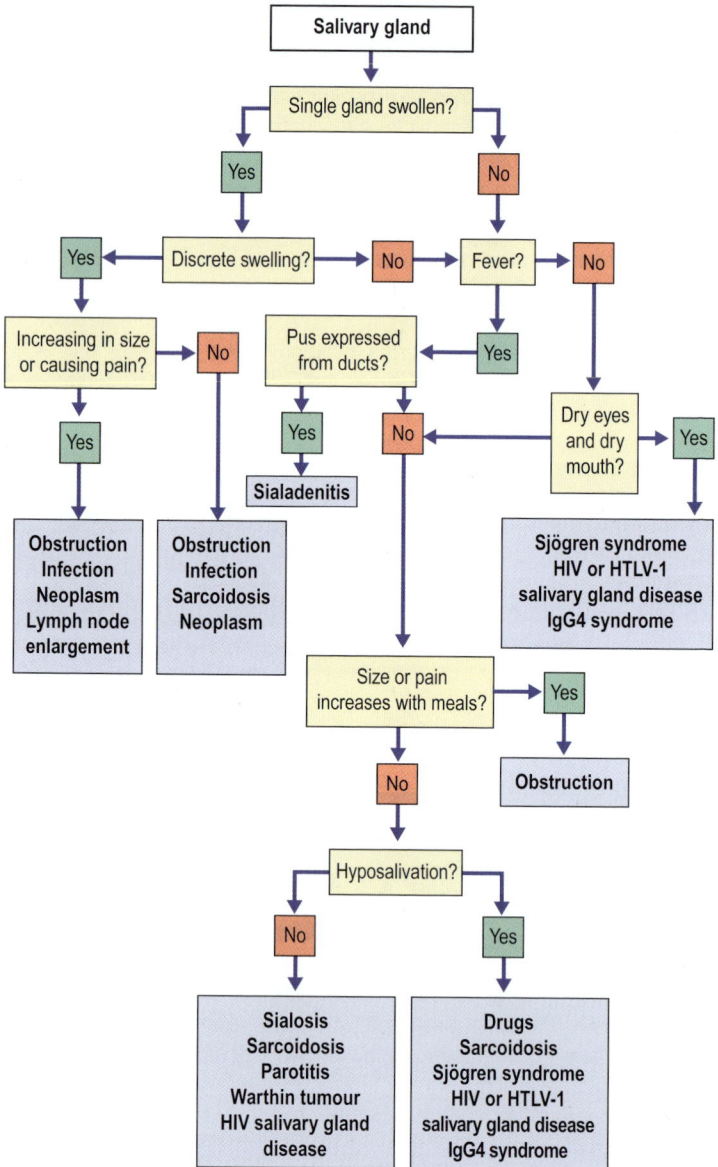

Figure 2.110 Algorithm for salivary gland swelling.

Taste disturbance

Keypoints

- Taste cells scattered across the tongue are sensitive to the five tastes – sweet, sour, bitter, salty and umami.
- Saliva is also essential to taste.
- Three tastes (sweet, bitter and umami) are mediated by receptors from the G protein-coupled receptor family, while salt and sour are tasted using ion channels.
- Taste is transmitted by three different cranial nerves:
  - facial nerve from the anterior two-thirds of the tongue
  - glossopharyngeal nerve from the posterior one-third of the tongue
  - vagus nerve from the epiglottis.
- Taste disturbances are a common complaint, especially with advancing age.
- Taste disturbance is termed dysgeusia, while loss is termed ageusia if complete, hypogeusia if partial; bad taste is termed cacogeusia.
- Taste loss as proven objectively is uncommon.
- Many people who think they have a taste disorder actually have a problem with smell, sometimes caused by nose, sinus or throat conditions.
- Ageusia results mainly from tongue mucosal disorders, neurological damage, B vitamin or zinc deficiency, or drugs.
- Dysgeusia may be caused by oral infections, hyposalivation, chemotherapy, drugs, zinc deficiency or psychogenic causes.
- Patients who suffer from burning mouth syndrome often also suffer from dysgeusia.
- History and clinical examination includes inspection of the oral cavity and ear canal, as lesions of the chorda tympani have a predilection for this site.
- Possible treatments include artificial saliva, pilocarpine (or cevimeline), increased oral hygiene, zinc supplementation, alterations in drug therapy, and alpha lipoic acid.

Taste disturbance (continued)

Box 2.23 Main causes of taste disturbances

Anosmia
Endocrine (e.g. diabetes, hypothyroidism)
Glossitis
Hyposalivation
Iatrogenic (see Table 4.6)
Neurological disease (e.g. trauma, disseminated sclerosis, Bell palsy)
Old age
Zinc or vitamin deficiency

Causes may include:

Loss of taste

- Anosmia causing apparent loss of taste
  - maxillofacial or head injuries (tearing of olfactory nerves)
  - upper respiratory tract infections and sinus disease
- Neurological disease
  - Bell palsy
  - cerebral metastases
  - cerebrovascular disease
  - fractured base of skull
  - frontal lobe tumour
  - lesions of chorda tympani
  - middle ear surgery
  - multiple sclerosis
  - posterior cranial fossa tumours
  - trigeminal sensory neuropathy
- Psychogenic
  - anxiety states
  - depression
  - psychoses
- Drugs
- Others

Cacogeusia

- Oral disease
  - acute necrotizing ulcerative gingivitis

- bisphosphonate-related osteonecrosis of the jaw (BRONJ)
- chronic dental abscesses
- chronic periodontitis
- dry socket
- food impaction
- neoplasms
- osteochemonecrosis (denosumab, bevacizumab)
- osteomyelitis
- osteoradionecrosis
- pericoronitis
- sialadenitis
- Hyposalivation
  - drugs
  - irradiation damage
  - sarcoidosis
  - Sjögren syndrome
- Psychogenic causes
  - anxiety states
  - depression
  - hypochondriasis
  - psychoses
- Drugs
  - Chinese pine nuts
  - smoking
- Nasal or pharyngeal disease
  - chronic sinusitis
  - nasal foreign body
  - neoplasm
  - oroantral fistula
  - pharyngeal disease
  - pharyngeal pouch
  - tonsillitis
- Diabetes
- Respiratory disease
  - bronchiectasis
  - neoplasm
- Gastrointestinal disease
  - gastric regurgitation

Taste disturbance (continued)

- Liver disease
  - liver failure
- Central nervous system disease
  - temporal lobe epilepsy
  - temporal lobe tumours
- Renal disease
  - uraemia

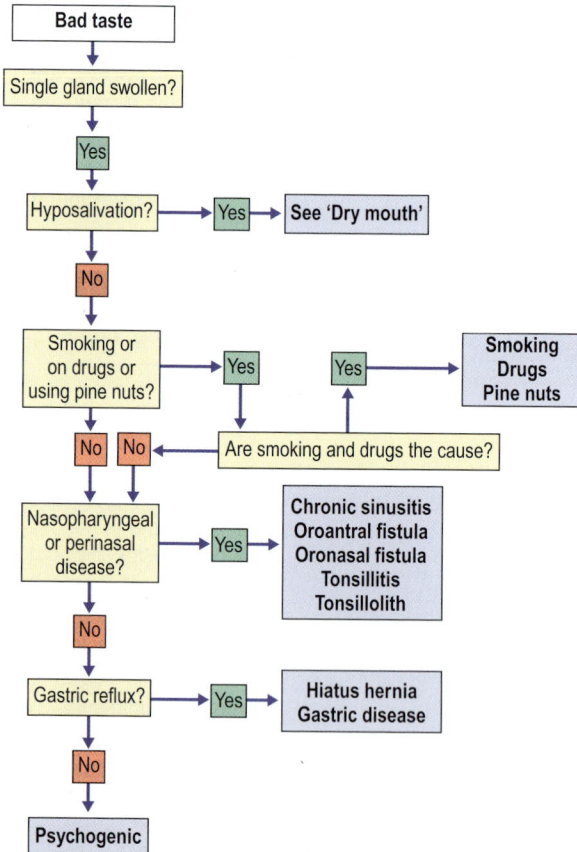

Figure 2.111 Algorithm for bad taste.

Tongue: furred

Keypoints

- A furred tongue in a healthy child is very uncommon.
- A furred tongue in a healthy adult is not uncommon and usually due to the accumulation of debris, including microorganisms on the dorsum (Figure 2.112).
- Dehydration or soft diet allows debris and bacteria to accumulate. An upper denture also does not clean the tongue as effectively as palatal rugae.
- The tongue when furred has a whitish or yellowish 'fur' which may be further discoloured by feverish illnesses (e.g. herpetic stomatitis) (Figure 2.113), hyposalivation, or by foods, drugs or lifestyle habits (e.g.

Figure 2.112 Tongue coated for no apparent reason. Much of this is due to debris which can be removed by brushing or scraping.

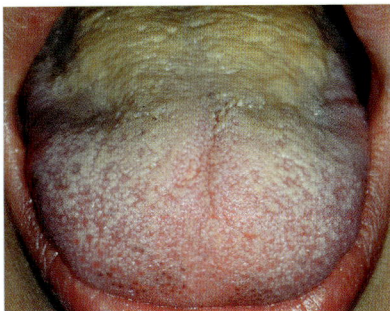

Figure 2.113 Tongue coated and ulcerated in acute herpetic stomatitis.

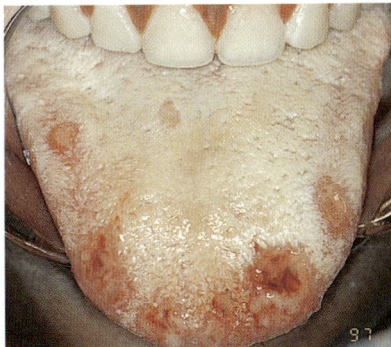

Tongue: furred (continued)

tobacco or betel) and may even be brown or black (Figures 2.114–2.116).

- Thrush, chronic candidosis, hairy leukoplakia (lateral borders of tongue) or other leukoplakias should be excluded.
- The underlying condition should be treated and the tongue brushed or scraped at night before retiring to bed.

Box 2.24 Main causes of furred tongue

Poor oral hygiene
Hyposalivation
Smoking

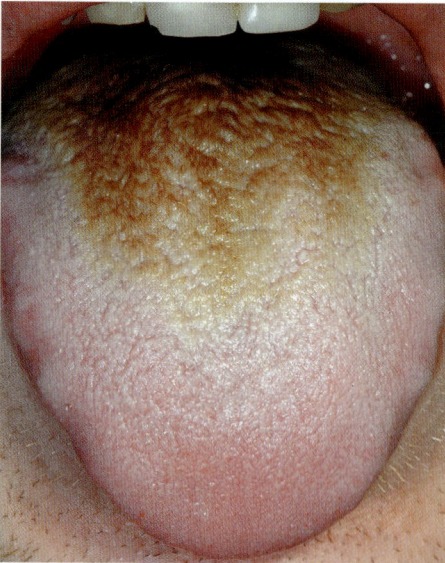

Figure 2.114 Tongue coated – brown hairy tongue. This typically affects the posterior tongue.

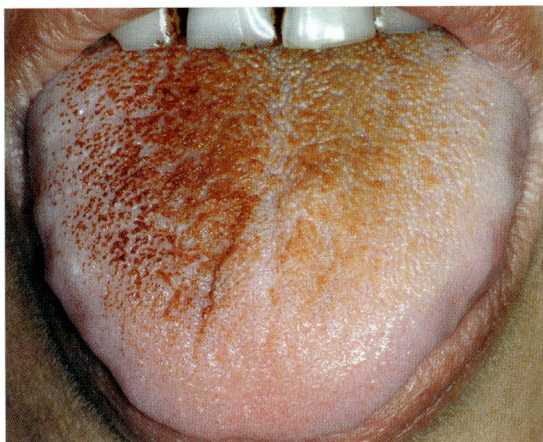

Figure 2.115 Tongue coated – stained by betel use.

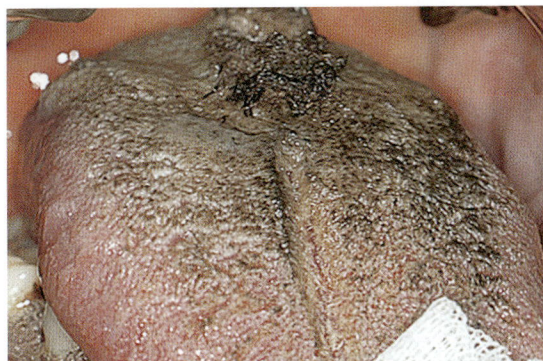

Figure 2.116 Tongue coated and stained by chlorhexidine mouthwash use.

Tongue: smooth (glossitis)

Keypoints

- Glossitis is the term given to a smooth depapillated tongue and is not a specific disorder.
- Glossitis can be caused by deficiencies of iron, folic acid, vitamin B_{12} (rarely other B vitamins), which can cause a sore tongue that may appear normal, or may be red and depapillated (Figure 2.117); by erythema migrans (geographic tongue); by lichen planus; by candidosis (Figures 2.118, 2.119); and by Sjögren syndrome (Figure 2.120).

Box 2.25 Main causes of glossitis

Erythema migrans
Lichen planus
Hyposalivation
Candidosis
Haematinic deficiency

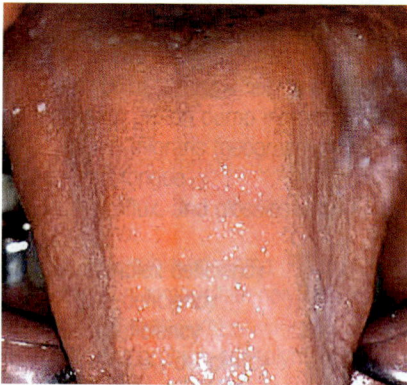

Figure 2.117 Tongue: glossitis; vitamin deficiency.

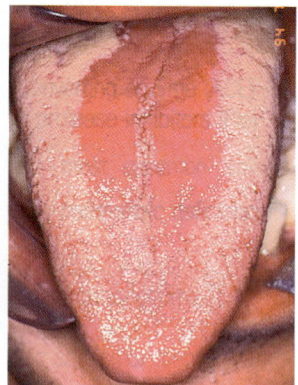

Figure 2.118 Tongue: glossitis; candidosis.

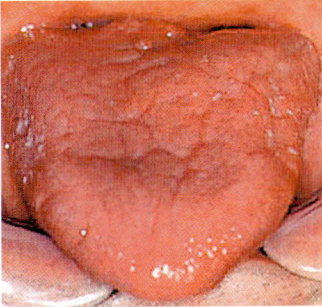

Figure 2.119 Tongue: glossitis; candidosis.

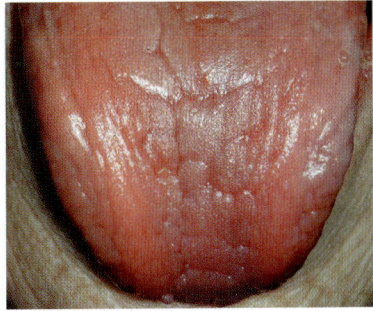

Figure 2.120 Tongue: glossitis; Sjögren syndrome in scleroderma.

Glossitis may be seen in:

- Erythema migrans
- Candidosis
- Sjögren syndrome
- Lichen planus
- Deficiency states.

Deficiency states

The tongue may appear completely normal or there may be linear or patchy red lesions (especially in vitamin B_{12} deficiency), depapillation with erythema (in deficiencies of iron, folic acid or B vitamins) or pallor (iron deficiency). Lingual depapillation begins at the tip and margins of the dorsum but later involves the whole dorsum. Various patterns are described. There may also be oral ulceration and angular stomatitis.

- Rare types of deficiency include:
  - riboflavin: papillae enlarge initially but are later lost
  - niacin: red, swollen, enlarged 'beefy' tongue
  - pyridoxine: swollen, purplish tongue.
- Diagnosis is from the blood picture (full blood picture, whole blood folate, serum vitamin B_{12}, ferritin). Vitamin assays or biopsy are rarely indicated.
- Replacement therapy is indicated after the underlying cause of deficiency is established and rectified.

Tongue swelling

- Tongue swelling (macroglossia) is usually acquired and caused by trauma, infection or allergy (angioedema).
- Uncommon congenital causes of macroglossia include: lymphangioma; haemangioma; neurofibromatosis; Down syndrome; cretinism; and Hurler syndrome (a mucopolysaccharidosis) (Figure 2.121).
- Rare acquired causes include amyloidosis and other deposits.
- In macroglossia, the tongue is indented by teeth, or too large to be contained in the mouth.

Box 2.26 Main causes of enlarged tongue
Allergy
Trauma
Infection
Angioma
Neoplasm

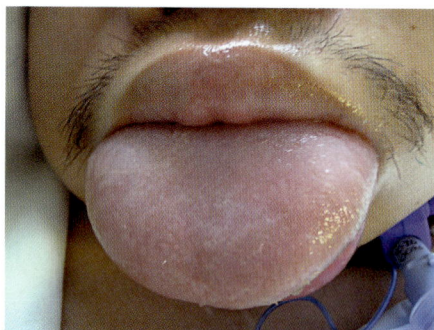

Figure 2.121 Tongue enlarged (macroglossia): in Hurler syndrome – an inborn metabolic error.

Tooth abrasion

Keypoints

- Abrasion is a common form of tooth surface loss at the cervical margin, caused mechanically by exogenous factors, typically toothbrushing.
- Abrasion also causes gingival attachment loss.
- Initially there is gingival recession labially and the neck of the tooth is exposed, sometimes with hypersensitivity. A groove forms as cementum and dentine is abraded, especially on the maxillary canines. Abrasion, if extreme, causes teeth to snap off (Figure 2.122) but otherwise the pulp is rarely exposed since reactionary dentine is deposited.
- Desensitizing agents may help relieve symptoms. If aesthetically displeasing or causing hypersensitivity, the abrasion may be restored with composites or glass ionomer cements.

Box 2.27 Main causes of tooth abrasion
Overenthusiastic horizontal toothbrushing

Causes may include:

Usually, vigorous toothbrushing, especially horizontally with abrasive dentifrices and hard brushes.

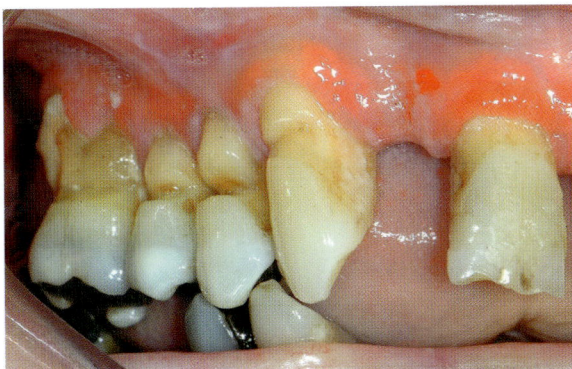

Figure 2.122 Teeth abrasion (also the patient has an unrelated desquamative gingivitis).

Tooth attrition

Keypoints

- Attrition is the most common form of tooth surface loss.
- Attrition is the mechanical wearing down of tooth surfaces by tooth–tooth or tooth–prosthesis contact.
- Attrition is most common in people who suffer bruxism, or eat an abrasive diet.
- The incisal edges, cusps and occlusal surfaces wear (Figure 2.123) and, characteristically, opposing tooth facets will match perfectly in occlusion.
- If the enamel is breached there is more loss of the softer dentine than enamel, leading to a flat or hollowed surface – a facet.
- Unless attrition is rapid, the pulp is generally protected by obliteration with secondary dentine formation and thus attrition rarely causes dentine hypersensitivity.
- Restorative dentistry and occlusal splint therapy may be indicated.

Box 2.28 Main causes of attrition
Bruxism
Coarse diet

Causes may include:

The wearing away of tooth biting (occlusal) surfaces by mastication is most obvious where there are excessive occlusal forces/movements such as in:

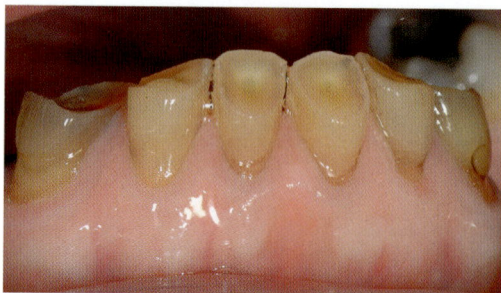

Figure 2.123 Teeth; attrition: secondary dentine deposition tends to avoid hypersensitivity and pulp exposure.

- a parafunctional habit such as bruxism (seen especially in profound vegetative states, Rett syndrome or Fragile X syndrome)
- where the diet is particularly coarse (as in some unrefined diets) or
- where the teeth are of weaker composition (such as amelogenesis imperfecta or dentinogenesis imperfecta). Interproximal attrition is far less common.

Tooth discolouration

Keypoints

- Teeth may be discoloured, most commonly from superficial (extrinsic) staining by bad oral hygiene, lifestyle habits such as use of tobacco or betel, or drugs such as chlorhexidine (Figures 2.124, 2.125).

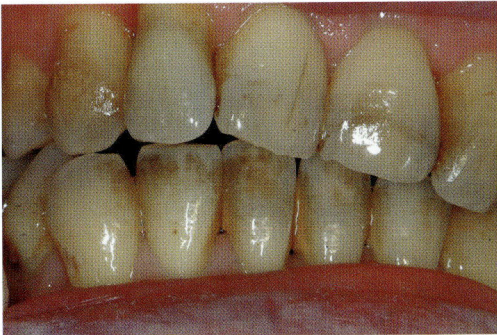

Figure 2.124 Tooth discoloration: from smoking and poor oral hygiene.

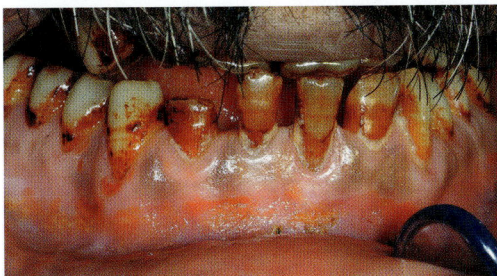

Figure 2.125 Tooth discoloration: from betel chewing. There is also tooth surface loss.

Tooth discolouration (continued)

- Extrinsic staining typically affects many teeth, predominantly in the cervical third of the teeth.
- Less commonly, staining is internal (intrinsic) – usually from caries, trauma or tooth restorations (Figure 2.126), or because the tooth has become non-vital (Figures 2.127, 2.128).
- Intrinsic discolouration usually but not invariably affects the whole of one or a few teeth or only parts of the teeth.

Box 2.29 Main causes of tooth discoloration

Superficial (extrinsic) staining is mainly from smoking, poor oral hygiene, drugs, or betel use

Intrinsic staining is seen in non-vital teeth, from caries or restorations, or tetracycline

---

Causes may include:

Extrinsic causes
- Brown/black stain
  - betel
  - chlorhexidine
  - doxycycline
  - iron medications
  - stannous fluoride
  - tea, coffee, wine and other beverages
  - tobacco products
- Green stain
  - chromogenic bacteria
  - metals
- Orange stain
  - chromogenic bacteria
  - metals

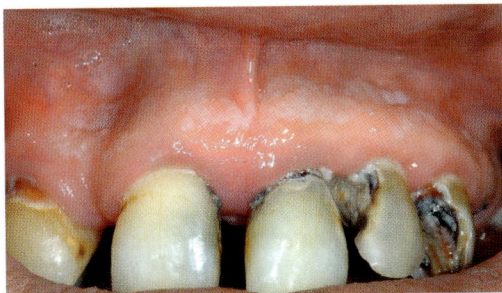

Figure 2.126 Tooth discolouration: from caries.

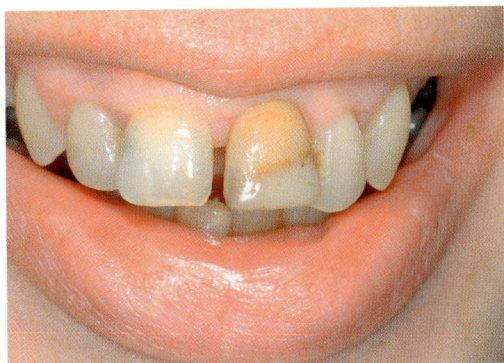

Figure 2.127 Tooth discolouration: a traumatized non-vital tooth in a person who suffers seizures.

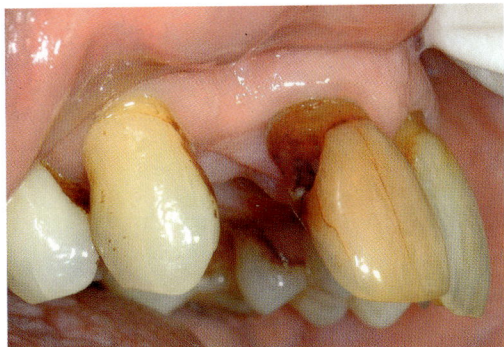

Figure 2.128 Tooth discolouration: a non-vital tooth from caries.

Tooth discolouration (continued)

Intrinsic causes

- White (opaque) stain
  - incipient caries (primary or secondary teeth)
  - mild trauma to teeth during enamel formation/amelogenesis (secondary teeth), e.g., Turner tooth
  - periapical infection of primary tooth predecessor
- Yellow stain
  - amelogenesis imperfecta
  - dentinogenesis imperfecta
  - composites or glass ionomer or acrylic restorations
  - tetracycline
  - moderate trauma to teeth during amelogenesis (secondary teeth), e.g., Turner tooth
  - periapical infection of primary tooth predecessor
  - trauma without haemorrhage
  - traumatic injury to primary tooth or teeth
- Brown stain
  - amelogenesis imperfecta
  - dentinogenesis imperfecta
  - severe trauma to teeth during amelogenesis (secondary teeth), e.g., Turner tooth
  - tetracyclines
  - periapical infection of primary predecessor
  - traumatic injury to primary tooth
  - composite, glass ionomer, or acrylic restorations
  - caries
  - pulpal trauma with haemorrhage (necrotic tooth)
- Blue, grey, or black stain
  - amalgam restoration
  - dentinogenesis imperfecta
  - metal crown margin associated with porcelain fused to metal crown
  - tetracyclines
  - trauma
- Green stain
  - hyperbilirubinaemia (e.g., haemolytic disease of the newborn, biliary atresia)

- Pink stain
  - internal resorption
  - recent tooth trauma
  - porphyria.

Tooth erosion

Keypoints

- Erosion is tooth surface loss as a consequence of chemical activity.
- Erosion typically affects several teeth and leaves smooth tooth surfaces.
- Ingestion of acidic materials such as carbonated beverages (carbonic acid, e.g. cola) or fruit juices (citric acid) or vinegar (acetic acid) produces smooth depressions on labial surfaces of anterior teeth (Figure 2.129).
- In gastric regurgitation, palatal and lingual surfaces are eroded by the gastric hydrochloric acid.
- A careful history is usually adequate to differentiate erosion from abrasion, dentinogenesis imperfecta and amelogenesis imperfecta.
- Prevent the habit or treat regurgitation. Use a straw to drink acidic fluids. Use desensitizers. If erosion is aesthetically unacceptable, restore.

Box 2.30 Main causes of tooth erosion
Consumption of acidic beverages and foods
Gastric acid reflux

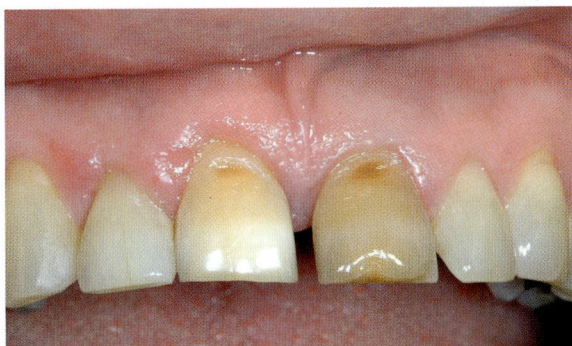

Figure 2.129 Tooth surface loss: erosion (the left central incisor is nonvital because of trauma).

Tooth erosion (continued)

Causes may include:

Repeated and prolonged exposure to:

- acids (beverages such as carbonated [carbonic acid] and citrus [citric acid] juices); foods rich in citrus fruits or containing vinegar (acetic acid); or acidic atmospheres (e.g. carbonic or sulphuric acid); sodas, sports drinks, energy drinks and alcoholic drinks, including wine, may also be culpable
- gastric contents (gastro-oesophageal reflux disease [GORD]), pyloric stenosis or bulimia [hydrochloric acid])
- alcoholic patients in particular are predisposed to erosion.

Tooth hypoplasia

Keypoints

- Hypoplasia of single teeth (Turner tooth): usually disturbed odontogenesis caused by periapical infection of a deciduous predecessor. It affects premolars mainly, especially mandibular. The crown is opaque, yellow-brown and hypoplastic (Figure 2.130).
- Hypoplasia of multiple teeth; generally acquired as a result of fluorosis (Figure 2.131), systemic illness or intervention (such as cancer treatments) during the period of tooth development (chronological hypoplasia). Pitting hypoplasia affects parts of developing crowns and, since systemic disturbances are especially common during the first year of life, defects usually affect tips of permanent incisors and first molars (Figure 2.132).

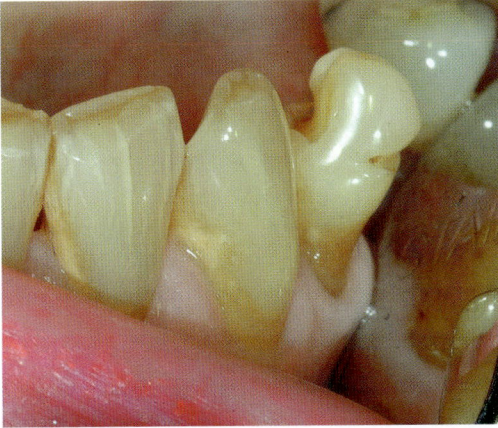

Figure 2.130 Tooth hypoplasia: a Turner premolar tooth.

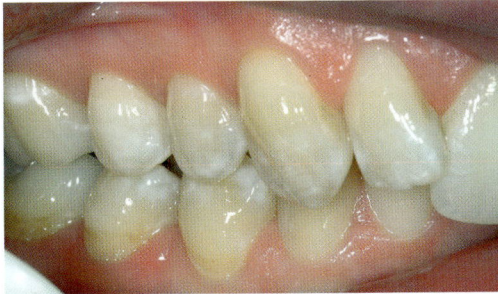

Figure 2.131 Tooth hypoplasia: in fluorosis.

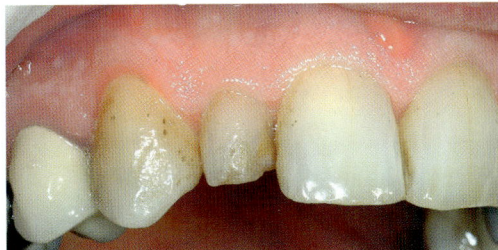

Figure 2.132 Tooth hypoplasia and microdontia of lateral incisor.

Tooth hypoplasia (continued)

- Congenital syphilis is a rare cause of hypoplasia, producing notched screwdriver-shaped incisors (Hutchinson incisors (Figure 2.133; and abnormal molars (Moon or mulberry molars).
- Genetically determined causes of tooth hypoplasia may be seen rarely.

Box 2.31 Main causes of hypoplastic teeth

Trauma
Infection
Cancer therapy

Causes may include:

Congenital
- Amelogenesis imperfecta
- Cleidocranial dysplasia
- Epidermolysis bullosa
- Vitamin D resistant rickets (hypophosphataemia)
- Congenital hypoparathyroidism, Down and other syndromes
- Intrauterine infections (rubella; syphilis).

Acquired
Exposure of developing teeth to

- Trauma
- Infection
- Prematurity
- Hyperbilirubinaemia (kernicterus)
- Hypocalcaemia
- Severe infections
- Radiotherapy
- Cytotoxic chemotherapy
- Endocrinopathies (especially hypoparathyroidism)
- Severe nutritional deficiencies (as in coeliac disease)
- Nephrotic syndrome
- Severe fluorosis
- Molar – incisor hypomineralization (? caused by dioxin).

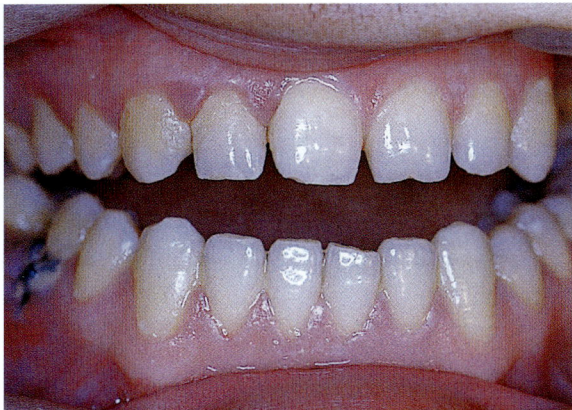

Figure 2.133 Tooth hypoplasia: screwdriver-shaped incisors (Hutchinson incisors) in congenital syphilis.

Tooth mobility or premature loss

Keypoints

- Most tooth mobility arises from plaque-related periodontitis or trauma, and these can cause premature tooth loss.
- Tooth mobility in the absence of periodontitis may be caused by trauma (including abuse) or a neoplasm.
- Early tooth loss usually has an obvious cause, such as trauma (in sports, assaults or other injuries, extraction as a result of dental caries) or for orthodontic reasons or, in adults, periodontal disease.
- Unexplained early tooth loss in children or adults may be a feature in:
  - non-accidental injury
  - immune defects (e.g. Down syndrome, diabetes mellitus, HIV/AIDS), or cathepsin C deficiency (this includes Papillon–Lefèvre syndrome [palmo-plantar hyperkeratosis] or leucocyte adhesion defects [LAD])
  - hypophosphatasia
  - neoplasms, or eosinophilic granuloma.
- Periodontitis that is disproportionate to the degree of plaque accumulation may signify an underlying immune defect.

Tooth mobility or premature loss (continued)

Box 2.32 Main causes of premature tooth mobility/loss

Trauma
Immune defects

Tooth number anomalies

Keypoints

- Definitions are:
  - hypodontia: less than six missing teeth (excluding the third molars)
  - oligodontia: six or more missing teeth (excluding the third molars)
  - anodontia: no teeth present (typically seen in ectodermal dysplasia)
  - hyperdontia: extra teeth (supernumerary teeth) present.
- Hypodontia is not uncommon.
  - Most cases where teeth are missing from the arch (hypodontia) are because the tooth has impacted, or been extracted or lost for other reasons.
  - Hypodontia is seen mainly in the second dentition.
  - Hypodontia most often affects permanent third molars; up to 10–30% of the population may miss these teeth. After that, incisor-premolar hypodontia (IPH) is most common, affecting mainly mandibular second premolars and then maxillary lateral incisors. Maxillary second premolars and maxillary and mandibular first molars and canines are then affected.
  - Teeth may sometimes be missing as part of systemic disease such as ectodermal dysplasia, or as a consequence of cancer treatments.
  - Hypodontia is often associated with retention of the deciduous predecessor, and may be associated with delayed eruption, a reduction in size of teeth, ectopic teeth, short roots, taurodontism, tooth rotation, or hypocalcification.
- Hyperdontia, or additional (supernumerary) teeth, is not common.
  - When normal permanent teeth erupt before the deciduous incisors have exfoliated (i.e. the mixed dentition), it is not uncommon to see what appear to be two rows of teeth in the lower incisor region, particularly when there is inadequate space to accommodate the

larger permanent teeth, but this is not true hyperdontia. The situation here normally resolves as primary incisors are lost and the mandible grows.

- Hyperdontia may occur in isolation but sometimes in cleft lip–palate or as part of a syndrome such as craniofacial dysplasia. Extra teeth may be found especially in the anterior maxilla and most typically occur alone in otherwise healthy individuals.

- Most extra teeth are small and/or conical or tuberculate (supernumerary teeth) and are seen in the maxillary midline where they may remain unerupted and may cause a permanent incisor to impact (mesiodens). Although a mesiodens may erupt, sometimes it is inverted. Tuberculate supernumeraries are uncommon, often paired, usually located palatal to the central incisors and they rarely erupt.

- Some additional teeth are of normal form (supplemental teeth) but these are uncommon, of unknown cause, and most frequently seen in the maxillary lateral incisor region.

- Extra maxillary molars are sometimes termed distodens (they may also be called paramolars or fourth molars if distal to the third, some also call them distomolars).

- Additional teeth often erupt in an abnormal position and may cause malocclusion, occasionally impede tooth eruption, or, rarely, are the site of dentigerous cyst formation.

Table 2.2 Dental findings at various ages

Age	Should be visible on radiography
Birth	All primary teeth Crypts of first molars
Age 2 years	Crowns of premolars and second molars begin
Age 6 years	Crowns of all permanent teeth except third molars
Age 18 years	All permanent teeth

Tooth number anomalies (continued)

Causes of hypodontia may include:

- Failure to erupt
- Premature loss
- Failure to develop – agenesis.

Hypodontia is usually seen in otherwise apparently healthy people, but can also be a feature of local growth disorders such as:

- Cleft palate
- After radiotherapy to the area
- After chemotherapy
- Thalidomide exposure.

Hypodontia may also be seen in several syndromes, such as:

- Ectodermal dysplasia
- Incontinentia pigmenti
- Down syndrome
- Ehlers–Danlos syndrome.

Causes of hyperdontia may include:

- Supernumerary teeth may be seen in syndromic conditions typically in association with:
  - cleft lip/palate
  - craniofacial (cleidocranial) dysplasia
  - Gardner syndrome
  - Sturge–Weber syndrome.

Box 2.33 Main causes of abnormal tooth numbers

Hypodontia – impacted tooth, cancer therapies, or genetic
Hyperdontia – genetic

Tooth shape anomalies

Keypoints

- Most anomalies of tooth shape are acquired but some are genetically determined.

- Acquired anomalies are usually termed hypoplasia.
- Genetic anomalies may include:
  - conical teeth (Figure 2.134)
  - connation (double tooth); affects deciduous teeth
  - dens in dente
  - enamel clefts
  - macrodontia – all teeth enlarged
  - microdontia – all teeth small
  - taurodontism.
- Developmental dental anomalies may:
  - exist in isolation or
  - be associated with extraoral clinical manifestations in syndromes; and they can be
  - due to the action of teratogens, or
  - of genetic origin.
- Dilaceration: bent root/tooth is typically acquired and affects mainly the permanent incisors.
- In some cultures, tooth shape is deliberately altered for cosmetic or other reasons.

Box 2.34 Main causes of anomalies of tooth shape
Infections
Trauma
Cancer therapies
Genetic

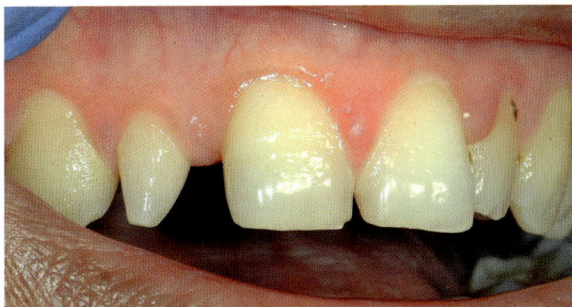

Figure 2.134 Tooth shape anomaly: peg-shaped lateral incisor.

Tooth shape anomalies (continued)

Causes of genetic dental anomalies may include:

- Any interference with developmental processes can lead to clinical anomalies and defects and some occasionally even result in tumours arising from dental epithelial cells (odontogenic tumours).
- Genetic anomalies of enamel or dentine formation include defects of:
  - structural proteins of enamel or dentine matrices, or
  - the mineralization process.
- Amelogenesis imperfecta (AI) – the genetic disorder of enamel formation has several forms. Defective enamel may also be seen in several syndromes, and in metabolic disorders with known gene mutations.
- Dentinogenesis imperfecta (DI) is a group of inherited alterations in dentine formation. Abnormal dentine may also be a variable feature of syndromes such as osteogenesis imperfecta.

Causes of acquired dental anomalies may include:

- Trauma
- Childhood infections
- Anticancer treatments
- Chronic fluoride intoxication
- Molar–incisor hypomineralization (MIH), which is defined as a hypomineralization of systemic origin of one to four permanent first molars frequently associated with affected incisors. MIH molars are fragile and caries can develop very easily in them.

Trismus

Keypoints

- Trismus is an inability to open the mouth due to muscle spasm, but the term is commonly used for any cause of restriction in mouth opening/mandibular movement.
- Limited opening of the jaw is usually due to extra-articular disease with masticatory muscle spasm secondary to stress, trauma or local infection (e.g. pericoronitis around a partially erupted mandibular third molar).

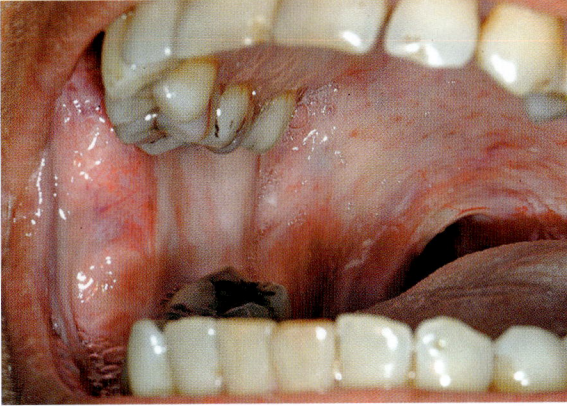

Figure 2.135 Trismus in oral submucous fibrosis in a betel chewer. The palate is also affected.

- Occasionally, trismus is caused by joint (intra-articular) disease, or conditions affecting the soft tissues such as scarring, infiltrating neoplasms or oral submucous fibrosis (OSMF) (Figure 2.135).

Box 2.35 Main causes of trismus
Infections
Trauma
Submucous fibrosis
Neoplasms

Causes of acute trismus may include:

- Infection
  - pericoronitis
  - odontogenic abscess with soft tissue spread involving masticatory muscles
  - infratemporal fossa
  - submasseteric space
  - lateral pharyngeal space
  - submandibular space
  - sublingual space

Trismus (continued)

- extension to neck
- Ludwig angina
- tonsillar or pharyngeal infection
- otitis
- tetanus
- Trauma
  - mandible
  - mid-face
  - zygomatic arch impingement
  - facial soft tissues
  - postoperative
    - wisdom teeth removal
    - other jaw and oral surgery
    - associated with haematoma
- Drug related
  - extra-pyramidal reaction to anti-emetics
  - malignant hyperthermia
- TMD – myofacial pain, bruxism.

Causes of subacute trismus may include:

- Tumour infiltration of muscles
  - buccal
  - retromolar
  - tonsillar
  - floor of mouth
  - infratemporal fossa.

Causes of chronic trismus may include:

- Scar formation
  - post-trauma or burn
  - post-surgery
  - post-radiotherapy
- Submucous fibrosis
- Scleroderma
- Post-traumatic (TMJ)
- TMJ ankylosis.

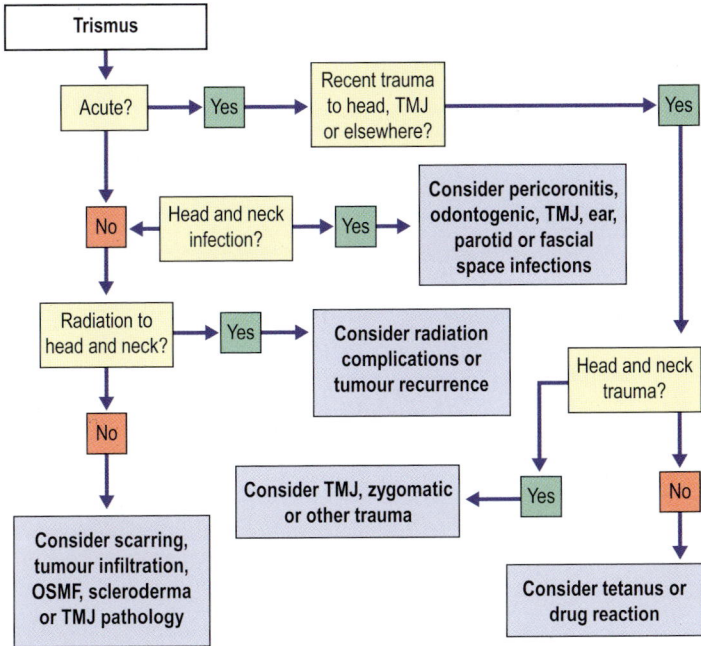

Figure 2.136 Algorithm for trismus.

3

Differential diagnosis by site

Keypoints

- Few lesions affect only a single oral site: for example, cleft palate affects only the palate.
- Some lesions affect mainly one site; erythema migrans (geographic tongue), for example, almost exclusively affects the dorsum of tongue.
- Other conditions have a predilection for a limited number of sites; pemphigoid, for example, affects mainly the gingivae while burning mouth syndrome affects mainly the anterior tongue.
- Many disorders can affect almost any oral site; lichen planus, for example, can affect most oral sites, and oral pain can appear in any area.

Cervical lymph node disease

Cervical lymph nodes must be examined in every patient. Though most causes of enlargement (lymphadenopathy) are inflammatory (lymphadenitis), especially arising from local infection; others may be caused by malignant disease (Figure 3.1) – either local, distant or systemic – or other serious causes.

Infection (the usual cause) may be:

- local viral or bacterial (dental, face, scalp, ear, nose or throat): including staphylococcal and non-tuberculous mycobacterial lymphadenitis
- systemic
  - viral glandular fever syndromes (EBV, CMV, HIV, HHV-6 [human herpesvirus 6]), and rubella
  - tuberculosis or other mycobacterial infections, other bacterial infections (brucella, cat-scratch fever, syphilis)
  - parasitic, e.g. toxoplasmosis
  - others, e.g. Kawasaki disease (mucocutaneous lymph node syndrome; MLNS).

Other inflammatory causes may be:

- granulomatous disorders (e.g. sarcoidosis, Crohn disease, orofacial granulomatosis)
- connective tissue diseases.

Malignant disease may be:

- local (oral, scalp, parotid, ear, nose or throat usually; rarely thyroid)
- systemic: carcinomas, lymphomas, leukaemias, Langerhans cell histiocytosis – especially Letterer–Siwe disease, Wegener granulomatosis.

Drugs – particularly phenytoin – may also be a cause.

Keypoints

- Lymphadenopathy is the term used when one or more lymph nodes enlarge or swell.
- Lymph nodes swell mainly in inflammatory or neoplastic disorders.
- Lymph nodes that swell because of an inflammatory cause are often tender but remain mobile (lymphadenitis).
- Lymph nodes that swell because of malignant involvement may become hard and fixed.

- It is crucial to establish whether only the regional (cervical) lymph nodes alone are involved, or if there is generalized lymphadenopathy.
- Cervical lymph nodes may enlarge in some systemic disorders – when there is typically generalized lymphadenopathy, and there may also be hepato- and/or splenomegaly.

Causes may include:

- Inflammatory causes:
  - infection (the usual cause)
  - local viral (e.g. herpes simplex infections) or bacterial (dental, scalp, ear, nose or throat) – including cat-scratch fever, staphylococcal lymphadenitis and cervicofacial actinomycosis (Figure 3.2)

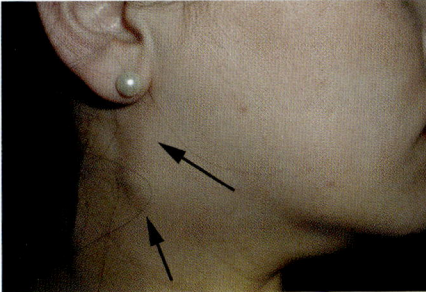

Figure 3.1 Neck lesion: lymphoma presenting as upper cervical lymph node enlargement.

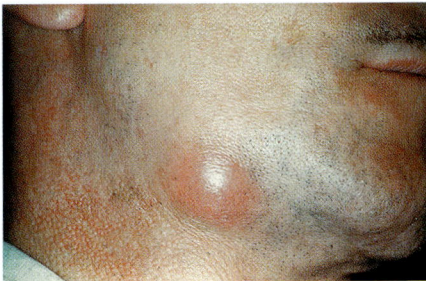

Figure 3.2 Neck lesion: actinomycosis showing purplish swelling in the typical location.

Cervical lymph node disease (continued)

- systemic: viral, e.g. infectious mononucleosis, cytomegalovirus, or HIV infection; bacterial, including syphilis, tuberculosis, brucellosis; fungal, rarely; parasitic, toxoplasmosis; Kawasaki disease (mucocutaneous lymph node syndrome)
- others: sarcoidosis, Crohn disease, orofacial granulomatosis, connective tissue diseases
- Malignant disease:
  - local (oral, scalp, ear, nose or throat usually; rarely thyroid)
  - systemic: leukaemias and lymphomas, carcinomas, Letterer–Siwe disease
- Drugs:
  - particularly phenytoin.

Clinical features:

- lymphadenitis: discrete tender, mobile, enlarged firm nodes; rarely suppurate
- metastases: discrete or matted, fixed, enlarged, hard nodes (rubbery in lymphomas); may ulcerate.

Investigations:

- culture and sensitivity testing, if infection is suspected
- search for lesion in drainage area (imaging if necessary)
- blood picture; monospot test or toxoplasma serological profile (TSP)
- fine needle aspiration biopsy (FNAB) or biopsy if neoplasm suspected.

Diagnosis: see above.

Management:

- treat cause
- if oral disease is ruled out, then referral to appropriate health provider is needed

Salivary gland disease
Keypoints

- Salivary gland disease may present with swelling, pain or mouth dryness (hyposalivation).
- Swelling may be obstructive, inflammatory, neoplastic or idiopathic (e.g. sialosis).
- Pain may be due to obstructive, inflammatory, or neoplastic conditions.
- Dryness may be iatrogenic – for example after salivary gland irradiation, chemotherapy or graft-versus-host disease, or due to inflammatory disease such as Sjögren syndrome, or sarcoidosis.

Causes may include:

- Swellings:
  - ductal obstruction (e.g. by calculus or tumour)
  - inflammatory
    - a actinomycosis
    - b ascending (acute suppurative) sialadenitis
    - c HIV salivary gland disease
    - d IgG4 syndrome
    - e lymphadenitis
    - f mumps
    - g recurrent sialadenitis
    - h sarcoidosis
    - i Sjögren syndrome
    - j tuberculosis
  - neoplasms
  - other causes
    - a deposits: amyloidosis; haemochromatosis
    - b Mikulicz disease (lymphoepithelial lesion and syndrome, now known to be IgG_4 syndrome)
    - c sialosis (sialadenosis)
    - d drug-associated (see also)
- Salivary gland pain:
  - duct obstruction (stones or other causes)
  - inflammatory
    - a acute bacterial sialadenitis

Salivary gland disease (continued)

    b viral sialadenitis: HIV sialadenitis; EBV sialadenitis; HCV sialadenitis; mumps
    c recurrent sialadenitis
    d Sjögren syndrome
- ▪ neoplastic (salivary gland malignant tumours)
- ▪ drug-associated (e.g. chlorhexidine, see also)
- Dryness:
  - ▪ dehydration
  - ▪ iatrogenic
    - drugs
    - irradiation
    - graft-versus-host disease
  - ▪ diseases affecting salivary glands
    - sarcoidosis
    - Sjögren syndrome and IgG4 syndrome
    - viral infections (e.g. EBV; HCV; HIV).

Acute bacterial (ascending) sialadenitis

Rare, except when following hyposalivation.

Typical orofacial symptoms and signs: painful swelling of one gland only, with red, shiny overlying skin, trismus, and purulent discharge from duct (Figures 3.3, 3.4).

Main oral sites affected: parotid gland.

Aetiopathogenesis: usually a bacterial infection ascends the duct of a reduced- or non-functioning salivary gland. Infectious agents include pneumococci, *Staphylococcus aureus* or viridans streptococci.

Gender predominance: male.

Age predominance: older adults.

Extraoral possible lesions: none.

Main associated conditions: dehydration; poor oral hygiene.

Differential diagnosis: other causes of sialadenitis: mainly mumps.

Investigations: purulent exudate for culture and sensitivities.

Main diagnostic criteria: clinical features.

Main treatments: antimicrobials (flucloxacillin if staphylococcal and not allergic to penicillin); sialogogues (saliva stimulants such as chewing gum or pilocarpine).

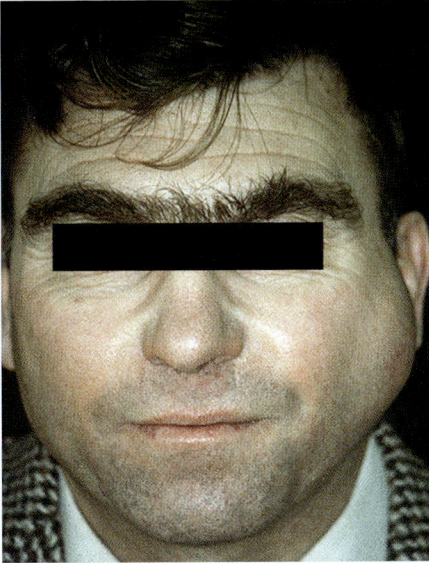

Figure 3.3 Salivary disease: parotitis showing enlarged left parotid gland.

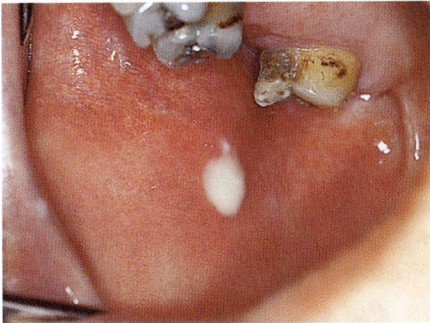

Figure 3.4 Salivary disease: parotitis, intraorally showing purulent discharge from Stensen duct.

Salivary gland disease (continued)

Mucocele

Common.

Typical orofacial symptoms and signs: dome-shaped, bluish, translucent, fluctuant, painless swelling, usually <10 mm diameter (Figure 3.5) which may rupture. Recur frequently. Deeper mucoceles are less common, more persistent and are often retention cysts (Figure 3.6).

Main oral sites affected: lower lip mainly. Superficial mucoceles are small intra-epithelial lesions (<5 mm diameter) sometimes simulating a vesiculobullous disorder but usually producing a small vesicle only; seen often in the soft palate. Ranula is the term used for the 'frog belly' appearance of a large retention mucocele in the floor of the mouth often arising from the sublingual gland and, rarely, burrowing through the mylohyoid muscle (plunging ranula).

Aetiopathogenesis: usually extravasation of mucus from a damaged minor salivary gland duct; rarely retention of mucus within a salivary gland or its duct.

Gender predominance: none.

Age predominance: young people.

Extraoral possible lesions: none except neck swelling and airway obstruction if plunging ranula.

Main associated conditions: superficial mucoceles may be seen in lichen planus or Graft versus host disease.

Differential diagnosis: diagnosis is clear-cut but neoplasm must be excluded, particularly in the upper lip.

Investigations: microscopic features.

Main diagnostic criteria: clinical history and features.

Main treatments: if asymptomatic and small, observe; otherwise, use cryo-surgery, laser ablation, micro-marsupialization or excision. Some lesions spontaneously resolve. Systemic gamma linolenic acid (evening primrose oil) has also been used.

Mumps (acute viral sialadenitis)

This is more common in childhood if vaccination with MMR (mumps, measles and rubella vaccine) is not taken.

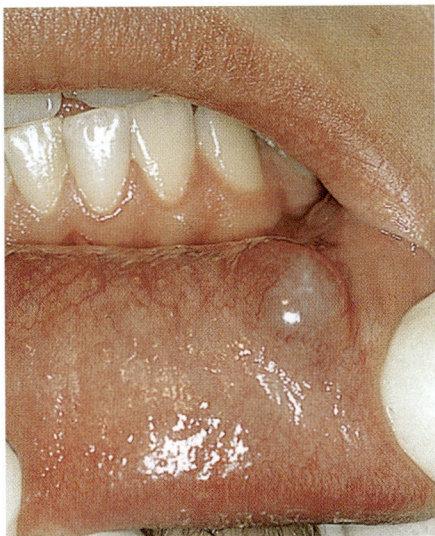

Figure 3.5 Salivary disease: mucocele in a typical location – the lower labial mucosa.

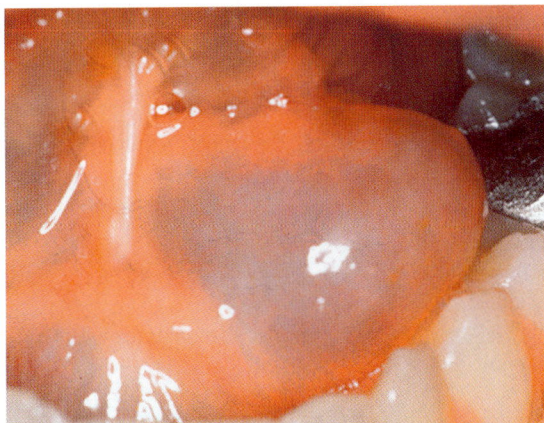

Figure 3.6 Salivary disease: mucocele in the floor of mouth (ranula).

Salivary gland disease (continued)

Typical orofacial symptoms and signs: incubation period 14–21 days. Infections are often subclinical. Malaise, fever, anorexia and sialadenitis – painful, diffuse swelling of one/both parotids and sometimes submandibulars may be seen (Figure 3.7). Saliva is non-purulent but the duct is inflamed. Trismus and occasionally dry mouth may be present.

Main oral sites affected: parotids bilaterally usually.

Aetiopathogenesis: mumps virus; rarely Coxsackie, ECHO, EBV or HIV infection.

Gender predominance: none.

Age predominance: typically in children.

Extraoral possible lesions: complications are uncommon but may include pancreatitis, encephalitis, orchitis, oophoritis and deafness.

Main associated conditions: as above.

Differential diagnosis: differentiate from obstructive and/or bacterial sialadenitis and recurrent juvenile parotitis mainly.

Investigations: mumps antibody titres (rarely needed); serum amylases or lipases (occasionally); ultrasound.

Main diagnostic criteria: clinical history and features.

Main treatments: symptomatic (reduce fever, pain and malaise with paracetamol, and maintain hydration).

Necrotizing sialometaplasia (see page 289)

Salivary gland neoplasms

These are uncommon. Classification of the most common salivary neoplasms is:

- Adenomas:
  - pleomorphic adenoma (PA: mixed tumour)
  - Warthin tumour (adenolymphoma or papillary cystadenoma lymphomatosum)
  - 'monomorphic': adenolymphoma/oncocytic adenoma/ (canalicular, basal cell, others)
- Others:
  - polymorphous low-grade adenocarcinoma
  - mucoepidermoid carcinoma
  - acinic cell carcinoma
  - adenoid cystic and other carcinomas.

Typical orofacial symptoms and signs: asymptomatic, firm and sometimes nodular swelling in one gland (usually parotid) and possible eversion of ear lobe (Figures 3.8). Warthin tumour may be bilateral. No hyposalivation. Malignant neoplasms classically may grow rapidly, may cause pain, may ulcerate and may involve nerves (e.g. facial palsy).

Figure 3.7 Salivary disease: mumps – bilateral sialadenitis.

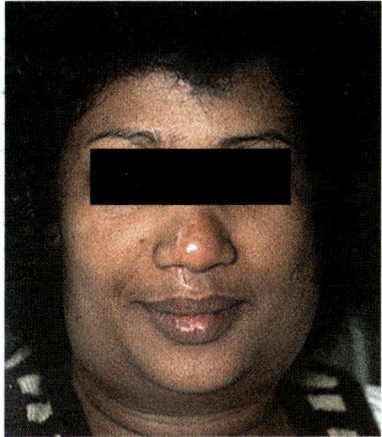

Figure 3.8 Salivary disease: neoplasm; pleomorphic adenoma in tail of parotid.

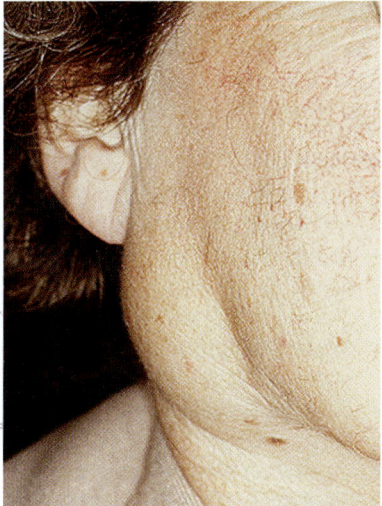

Salivary gland disease (continued)

Main oral sites affected: most tumours involve the parotid (75%), where most are benign pleomorphic adenomas (60%). Most other salivary tumours are in the minor glands, where many are malignant (60%), often arising from palatal glands (Figures 3.9–3.11). Few tumours are in the submandibular or sublingual glands. Submandibular tumours can be benign or malignant. Most sublingual gland tumours are malignant.

Neoplasms in major salivary glands

Aetiopathogenesis: unknown, but age smoking, irradiation and viruses have been implicated; more controversial is the possible effect of mobile telephones.

Gender predominance: none.

Age predominance: middle and old age.

Extraoral possible lesions: none except for enlarged lymph nodes due to metastasis.

Main associated conditions: usually none but a weak association with breast cancer.

Differential diagnosis: differentiate from other neoplasms such as lymphomas or metastases, and from non-neoplastic salivary gland swellings.

Investigations: ultrasound and fine needle aspiration biopsy (FNAB). Microscopy after parotidectomy (open biopsy may allow seeding and recurrence).

Main diagnostic criteria: clinical, advanced imaging and microscopy.

Main treatments: surgical excision; radiotherapy also for some.

Intraoral (minor) salivary gland neoplasms

- Intraoral salivary gland neoplasms are less common than neoplasms in major glands, but a higher proportion are malignant.
- Mucoepidermoid carcinoma is the most common intraoral salivary neoplasm, but adenoid cystic carcinoma and pleomorphic adenoma (PA) are relatively common in the mouth.
- Salivary gland tumours in the tongue are usually malignant – and are especially adenoid cystic carcinoma.
- Salivary gland tumours in the sublingual gland are usually malignant but are rare.
- Salivary gland tumours in the lips are usually seen in the upper lip but are typically benign (pleomorphic or other adenoma).

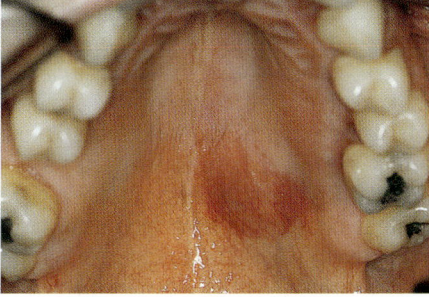

Figure 3.9 Salivary disease: neoplasm in palatal minor glands.

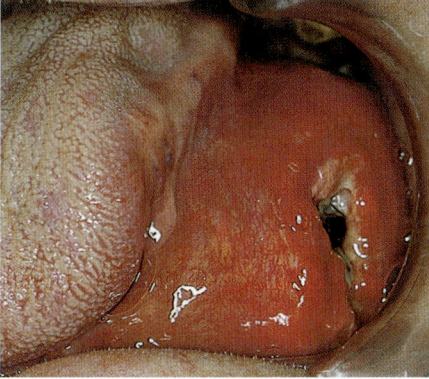

Figure 3.10 Salivary disease: neoplasm – malignant tumour in sublingual gland. Most tumours arising there are malignant.

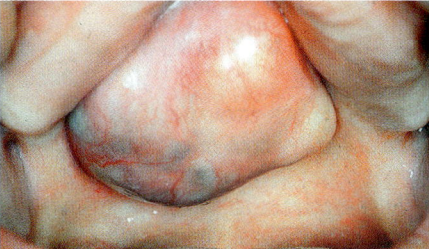

Figure 3.11 Salivary disease: neoplasm.

Salivary gland disease (continued)

Typical orofacial symptoms and signs: Pleomorphic adenomas are typically rubbery and often lobulated (Figures 3.12, 3.13); benign neoplasms form painless swellings. Malignant tumours are not initially distinguishable clinically from benign tumours but, in their later stages, are often painful and ulcerate, invade perineurally and they metastasize to upper cervical lymph nodes.

Main oral sites affected: the palate is the intraoral site of predilection.

Aetiopathogenesis: unknown.

Gender predominance: females.

Age predominance: older persons.

Extraoral possible lesions: none.

Main associated conditions: none.

Differential diagnosis: from other causes of lumps or ulcers, particularly:

- lower lip salivary tumours – from mucocele, benign connective tissue tumours
- tongue salivary tumours – from carcinoma, benign connective tissue tumours
- palatal salivary tumours – from oral carcinoma, benign connective tissue tumours, lymphomas, antral carcinoma or necrotizing sialometaplasia.

Main diagnostic criteria: ultrasound, advanced imaging and microscopy.

Main treatments: wide excision; radiation treatment if perineural invasion, and microscopic examination.

Sarcoidosis

Uncommon granulomatous condition.

Typical orofacial symptoms and signs: salivary gland swelling usually painless, bilateral (Figure 3.14). Often hyposalivation is present. May be cervical lymphoadenopathy; mucosal nodules; gingival hyperplasia; or labial swelling.

Main oral sites affected: lips, palate, major salivary glands.

Aetiopathogenesis: unknown.

Gender predominance: female.

Age predominance: adult.

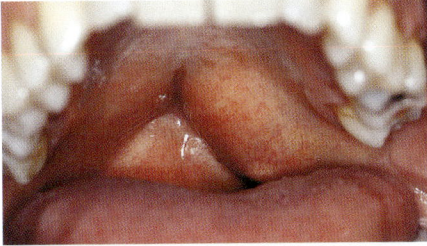

Figure 3.12 Salivary disease: neoplasm presenting as palatal swelling.

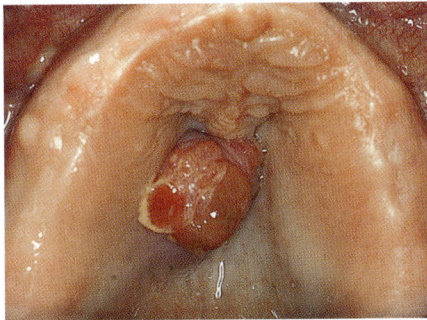

Figure 3.13 Salivary disease: neoplasm.

Figure 3.14 Salivary disease: sarcoidosis presenting with parotid swelling.

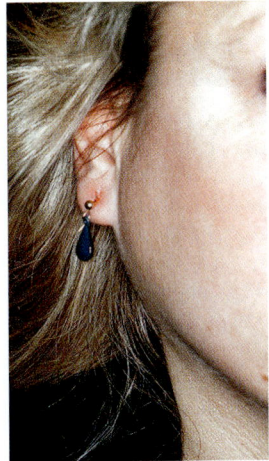

Salivary gland disease (continued)

Extraoral possible lesions: can affect any organ, typically lungs and lymph nodes (e.g. hilar nodes); also ocular (e.g. uveitis) and skin (e.g. erythema nodosum) lesions. The rare combination of parotitis, anterior uveitis, VIIth cranial nerve paralysis and fever is termed uveoparotid fever (Heerfordt–Waldenstrom) syndrome.

Main associated conditions: sometimes autoimmune disorders.

Differential diagnosis: from other causes of salivary gland swelling (particularly sialosis, Sjögren syndrome and IgG$_4$ disease, hyposalivation, metastatic disease, lymphomas, Wegener granulomatosis, rheumatoid nodules, varicella–zoster infection and atypical infections such as *Mycobacterium avium* complex, cytomegalovirus, and cryptococcosis.

Investigations: lesional biopsy; chest radiograph; gallium scan, raised serum angiotensin-converting enzyme (SACE) and adenosine deaminase. Vitamin D and prolactin levels are often increased.

Main diagnostic criteria: microscopy and SACE.

Main treatments: corticosteroids, methotrexate or other immunosuppressive drugs if lungs or eyes are involved, or if there is hypercalcaemia.

Sialosis

Typical orofacial symptoms and signs: painless, usually bilateral salivary gland swelling (Figure 3.15).

Main oral sites affected: parotids.

Aetiopathogenesis: the common feature is autonomic dysfunction. Frequently idiopathic; known causes include:

- neurogenic: various drugs, such as isoprenaline
- dystrophic-metabolic: anorexia–bulimia, alcoholic cirrhosis, diabetes, malnutrition, thyroid disease, acromegaly and pregnancy.

Gender predominance: male but depends on cause.

Age predominance: older patients.

Extraoral possible lesions: dependent upon aetiopathogenesis.

Main associated conditions: see aetiopathogenesis.

Differential diagnosis: sarcoidosis, Sjögren syndrome, IgG$_4$ disease and Warthin tumour mainly.

Investigations: ultrasound, MRI; blood glucose, liver function tests, immunoglobulins; possibly growth hormone levels.

Main diagnostic criteria: clinical, ultrasound, MRI and exclusion of other diagnoses.

Main treatments: identify and treat predisposing cause.

Sjögren syndrome

Uncommon, the cause is unknown but it is immunological and possibly viral. The common features are dry mouth and dry eyes: joint and other problems *may* be associated.

Typical orofacial symptoms and signs: saliva is frothy and not pooling; the mucosa may be parchment-like with food debris (Figure 3.16), the lips

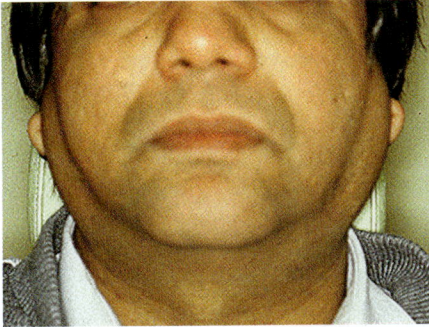

Figure 3.15 Salivary disease: sialosis (sialadenosis) – bilateral painless swellings.

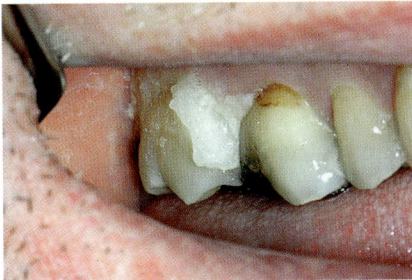

Figure 3.16 Salivary disease: Sjögren syndrome; dry mouth and food residues.

Salivary gland disease (continued)

often dry (Figure 3.17) and the tongue lobulated and depapillated (Figure 3.18). There may be complaints of dry mouth (hyposalivation): difficulty in eating dry foods, disturbed taste, and disturbed speech and swallowing.

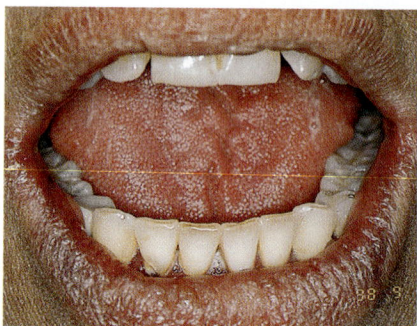

Figure 3.17 Salivary disease: Sjögren syndrome; dry lips.

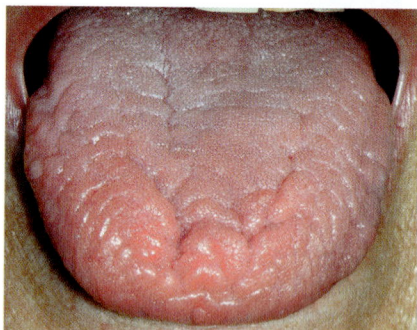

Figure 3.18 Salivary disease: Sjögren syndrome; dry and lobulated tongue.

Rampant caries, candidosis and recurrent sialadenitis may be seen (Figures 3.19 and 3.20). Salivary and lachrymal glands may sometimes swell

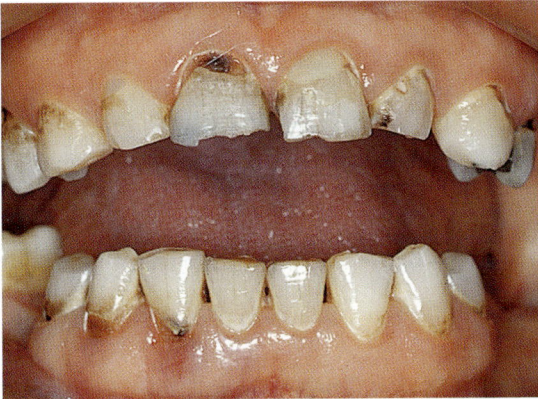

Figure 3.19 Salivary disease: Sjögren syndrome; caries.

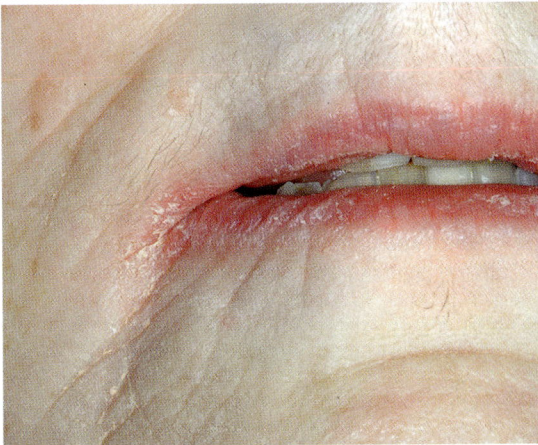

Figure 3.20 Salivary disease: Sjögren syndrome; candidosis (angular stomatitis).

Salivary gland disease (continued)

(Figures 3.21, 3.22). There may be conjunctival dryness and redness (termed injection) (Figure 3.23) and rheumatoid disease (Figure 3.24).

Aetiopathogenesis: autoimmune inflammatory exocrinopathy.

Gender predominance: women.

Age predominance: middle age or older.

Extraoral possible lesions: dry eyes (keratoconjunctivitis sicca): initially asymptomatic, later gritty sensation, itching, soreness or inability to cry. Swollen lachrymal glands. Extraglandular disease may precede exocrine problems by years, and includes fatiguability, fever and Raynaud phenomenon. Late complications include:

- glomerulonephritis
- lymphoma.

Main associated conditions: there is no connective tissue disease in primary (SS-1, sometimes termed sicca syndrome) but, in secondary Sjögren syndrome (SS-2) there is typically rheumatoid arthritis or less frequently primary biliary cirrhosis, and occasionally other autoimmune disorders. Sjögren syndrome predisposes especially to B cell non-Hodgkin lymphoma (NHL) – a mucosa-associated lymphoid tissue (MALT) malignancy. The risk is greatest in SS-1; affects up to 5% of patients and is seen mainly in mucosal extranodal sites (salivary glands – especially the parotids, mouth, skin, nodes, stomach, lung). Lymphoma is a high risk in those with persistent salivary gland swelling, splenomegaly or lymphadenopathy. Diagnosis of lymphoma is best by:

- ultrasonography
- high-resolution CT
- MRI
- MRI contrast sialography (gadolinium MRI with fat subtraction)
- histology.

Most of these lymphomas are relatively low-grade and require either no treatment apart from regular follow-up or low-dose chemotherapy.

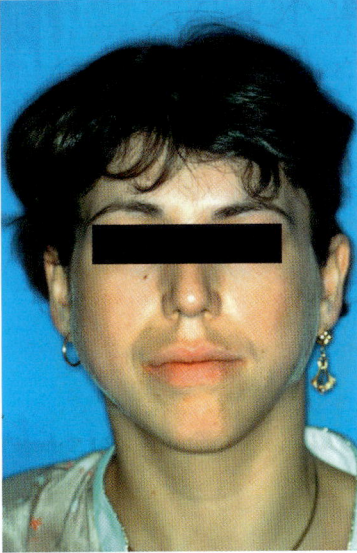

Figure 3.21 Salivary disease: Sjögren syndrome; salivary gland swelling and ocular involvement.

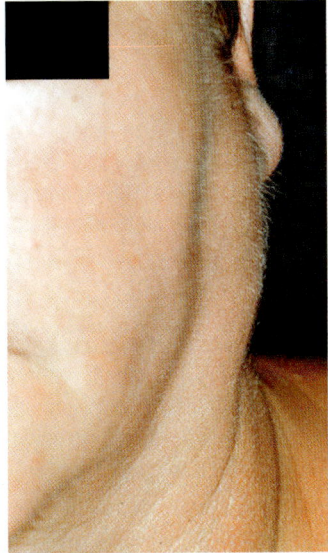

Figure 3.22 Salivary disease: Sjögren syndrome; salivary gland swelling.

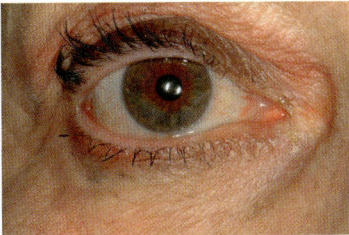

Figure 3.23 Salivary disease: Sjögren syndrome; dry eyes (keratoconjunctivitis sicca).

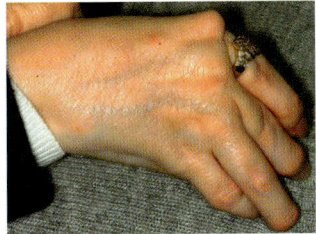

Figure 3.24 Salivary disease: Sjögren syndrome; rheumatoid arthritis showing finger ulnar deviations.

Salivary gland disease (continued)

Differential diagnosis: dry mouth can result from many other causes. Similar sicca syndromes may be seen in HCV or HIV disease, IgG_4 syndrome, or in graft-versus-host disease (GVHD).

Investigations: salivary flow rates (reduced); auto-antibodies, especially rheumatoid factor, Ro (SS-A) and La (SS-B) antibodies; serum IgG_4 levels, and ultrasound. Labial salivary gland biopsy is carried out in some centres and this and IgG_4 levels are most helpful in Ro/La negative patients. Sialography and/or scintigraphy are occasionally employed but are largely superseded by ultrasound.

Main diagnostic criteria: clinical features plus Ro (SS-A) and La (SS-B) antibodies, and ultrasound; occasionally labial salivary gland biopsy.

Main treatments: control underlying disease if possible (e.g. ciclosporin, azathioprine, hydroxychloroquine and anti-B cell monoclonals such as the anti-CD20 rituximab)

- dry eyes – methylcellulose eye drops or rarely ligation or cautery of nasolacrimal duct
- dry mouth:
  - saliva substitutes (mouth-wetting agents)
  - saliva stimulants (sialogogues); sugar-free chewing gum, or drugs (pilocarpine, cevimeline, anetholetrithione or bethanecol) may be used to stimulate salivation
  - interferon-alpha
  - preventive dental care (oral hygiene, limitation of sucrose and other sugar intake, use of fluorides, amorphous calcium phosphate, chlorhexidine)
  - treat infections.

IgG_4 syndrome

IgG_4 syndrome ('IgG_4 related systemic sclerosing disease', 'IgG_4-related autoimmune disease', 'IgG_4-related systemic disease', 'IgG_4-positive multi-organ lymphoproliferative syndrome') often manifests with enlarged salivary glands (previously called Mikulicz disease or Kuttner tumour [sclerosing sialadenitis]) and one-third also suffer from dry eyes and dry mouth and arthralgias, so for many years this was considered a subgroup of Sjögren syndrome.

IgG$_4$ syndrome affects mainly middle-aged men. Many other organs and tissues are also involved, including pancreas (the most commonly affected tissue), gall bladder, bile duct, retroperitoneum, kidneys, lung, prostate, lymph nodes, breast, and thyroid and pituitary glands.

Patients have neither anti-Ro/SS-A nor anti-La/SS-B autoantibodies but they have low titres of rheumatoid factor (RF), antinuclear autoantibodies (ANA), and decreased serum complement. Treatment includes systemic corticosteroids or anti-CD20 therapy (rituximab).

Lip lesions

Keypoints

- Lip lesions affecting the vermilion are often termed cheilitis.
- Cheilitis can have a wide range of causes.
- Common forms of cheilitis are traumatic, infective or follow exposure to UV radiation, low humidity, or temperature extremes (cold and heat).
- Blistering of the vermilion is commonly caused by a burn or herpes labialis ('cold sores').
- Blistering of the labial mucosa is commonly caused by mucoceles.
- Coloured lesions of the lips are usually brown (labial melanotic macules), red (telangiectasia) or purple/blue (angiomas).
- Bleeding from the lip may be from trauma or a fissure or vesiculobullous disorder such as erythema multiforme or pemphigus.
- Soreness of the lips may be seen in any type of cheilitis, especially factitious, allergic or infective varieties.
- White lesions of the lips are seen in actinic cheilitis, leukoplakia, candidosis and lichen planus.
- Ulceration of the lips can have many causes – systemic, malignant, local irritation, aphthae or drugs, but cancer and pemphigus are the most serious.
- Lumps/swelling of the lips can be seen after trauma, in allergies, in granulomatous disorders, neoplasms and from foreign bodies.

Lip lesions (continued)

Actinic burns and cheilitis

Mainly seen in fair-skinned individuals exposed in sunny climes or at high altitude.

Typical orofacial symptoms and signs: erythema, oedema, vesiculation and occasionally haemorrhage typify burns (Figures 3.25, 3.26); later whitish lesions or keratosis characterize actinic cheilitis – which is potentially malignant.

Main oral sites affected: lower lip.

Aetiopathogenesis: shortwave ultraviolet (UV) light (sunlight may also trigger herpes labialis and lupus erythematosus).

Gender predominance: male.

Age predominance: old age.

Extraoral possible lesions: cutaneous cancers on other areas of the face and exposed skin.

Differential diagnosis: from other causes of burns (e.g. friction and heat).

Investigations: biopsy.

Main diagnostic criteria: history and clinical features; biopsy persistent lesions.

Main treatments: prophylaxis – reduce sun exposure; bland or barrier creams (Uvistat); topical bleomycin, or lip shave.

Allergic angioedema

Uncommon: mainly seen in those with allergic (atopic) tendency.

Typical orofacial symptoms and signs: rapid development of oedematous swelling (Figure 3.27).

Main oral sites affected: lip(s) and tongue; oedema may spread to involve the neck and hazard the airway.

Aetiopathogenesis: type 1 allergic response.

Gender predominance: none.

Age predominance: none.

Extraoral possible lesions: atopy (allergic rhinitis, hayfever or eczema).

Main associated conditions: as above.

Differential diagnosis: from hereditary angioedema (C1 esterase inhibitor deficiency), and other causes of diffuse facial swelling including: oedema

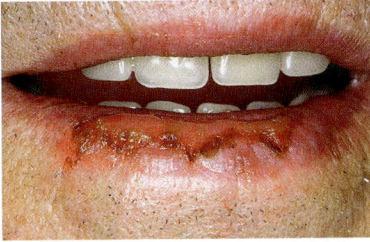

Figure 3.25 Lip lesion: actinic cheilitis from severe acute sun-exposure.

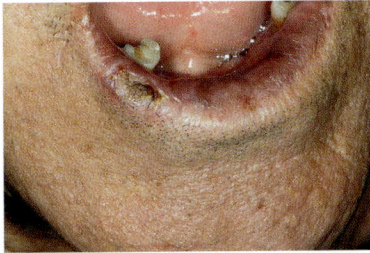

Figure 3.26 Lip lesion: actinic cheilitis (solar elastosis) with early carcinoma on the right.

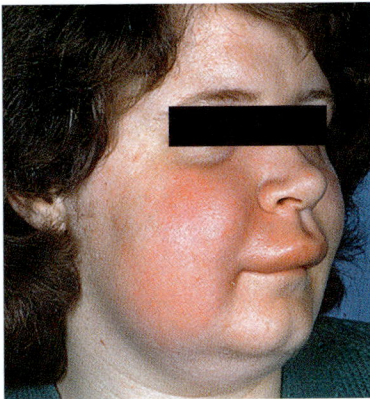

Figure 3.27 Lip lesion: angioedema causing facial and labial swelling.

Lip lesions (continued)

from trauma, infection or insect bite; surgical emphysema; Crohn disease, orofacial granulomatosis; sarcoidosis; cheilitis glandularis; lymphangioma; haemangioma.

Investigations: allergy testing, C1 esterase inhibitor levels.

Main diagnostic criteria: history of atopic disease and/or exposure to allergen; allergy testing (prick test).

Main treatments: mild angioedema – antihistamines; severe angioedema – intramuscular adrenaline, and intravenous corticosteroids.

Angioma (haemangioma)

These are fairly common oral lesions.

Typical orofacial symptoms and signs: a painless reddish, bluish or purplish soft vascular lesion which blanches on pressure (diascopy) (Figures 3.28, 3.29).

Main oral sites affected: most common on the lip, tongue, or buccal mucosa as painless reddish, or often bluish or purplish soft lesions which usually blanch on pressure, are fluctuant to palpation, are level with the mucosa or have a lobulated or raised surface. Haemangiomas are at risk from trauma and prone to excessive bleeding if damaged (e.g. during tooth extraction). Occasionally, oral haemangiomas calcify (phlebolithiasis).

Aetiopathogenesis: haemangiomas represent hamartomas or vascular anomalies. In children, they are usually congenital and developmental in origin. In adults, they may be acquired.

Gender predominance: female.

Age predominance: many haemangiomas appear in infancy, most by the age of 2 years, grow slowly and, by age 10, the majority have involuted (resolved). In adults, however, haemangiomas rarely involute spontaneously; rather they remain static or slowly enlarge.

Extraoral possible lesions: haemangiomas are typically seen in isolation but a few may be multiple and/or part of a wider syndrome such as:

- Sturge–Weber syndrome (angioma that extends deeply and rarely involves the ipsilateral meninges, producing a facial angioma and seizure disorder, sometimes with learning impairment)

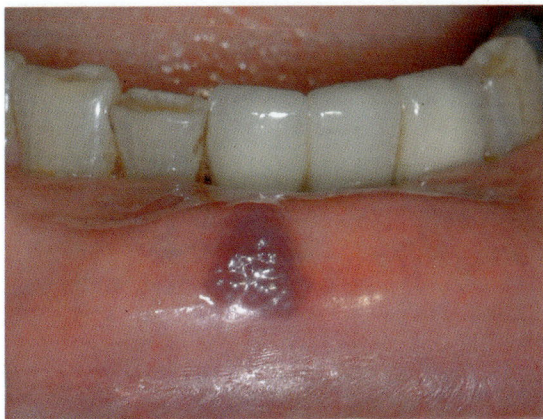

Figure 3.28 Lip lesion: haemangioma.

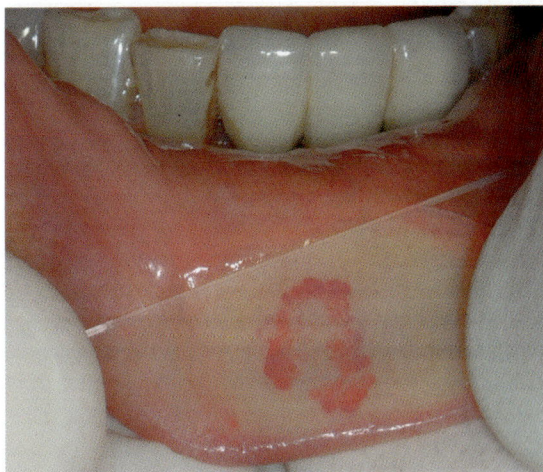

Figure 3.29 Lip lesion: haemangioma as in Figure 3.28 after diascopy.

Lip lesions (continued)

- blue rubber bleb naevus syndrome (BRBNS) – multiple cutaneous venous malformations in association with visceral lesions, most commonly affecting the GI tract
- Maffucci syndrome – multiple angiomas with enchondromas
- Dandy–Walker syndrome – a congenital brain malformation involving the cerebellum, or other posterior cranial fossa malformations.

Main associated conditions: as above.

Differential diagnosis: varicosities, pyogenic granuloma, lymphangioma, Kaposi sarcoma and epithelioid angiomatosis.

Investigations: for large angiomas, angiography may be needed rather than biopsy. After intravenous administration of contrast medium, enhancement is observed in haemangiomas in areas corresponding to those with high signal on T2-weighted MRI.

Main diagnostic criteria: angiomas blanch on pressure (diascopy), or contain blood on aspiration with a needle and syringe.

Main treatments: most angiomas are small, of no consequence and need no treatment but if they do for aesthetic or functional reasons or because of previous episodes of significant bleeding, they respond well to cryosurgery, laser ablation or intralesional injections of corticosteroids, sclerosing agents, interferon alpha, or systemic corticosteroids or propranolol. Very large haemangiomas may need to be treated with ligation or embolization – mainly for cosmetic reasons or if bleeding is troublesome.

Carcinoma

Uncommon in England and Wales (600 cases/year) and declining: much more common nearer the Equator, especially in white-skinned people.

Typical orofacial symptoms and signs: thickening, induration, crusting or ulceration, usually at vermilion border of lower lip just to one side of midline (Figures 3.30, 3.31). There is late involvement of the submental and other lymph nodes.

Main oral sites affected: lower lip.

Aetiopathogenesis: predisposing factors include UV irradiation (sun), immunosuppression and tobacco.

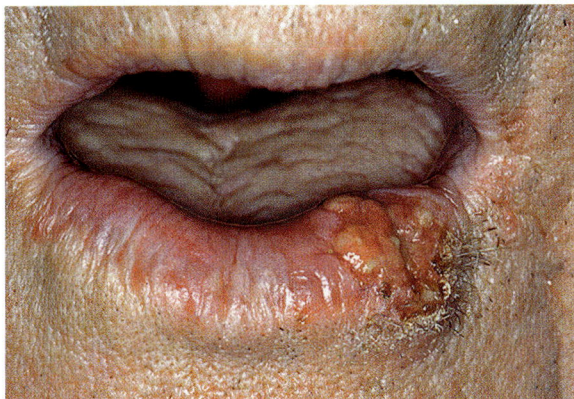

Figure 3.30 Lip lesion: carcinoma. This is a typical location and seen mainly in sun-exposed, older male Caucasian smokers.

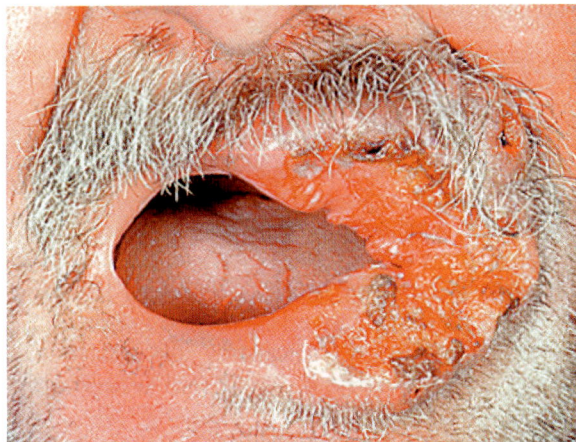

Figure 3.31 Lip lesion: advanced carcinoma.

Lip lesions (continued)

Gender predominance: male.

Age predominance: old age.

Extraoral possible lesions: cutaneous cancers on face and other sun-exposed skin.

Main associated conditions: xeroderma pigmentosum and discoid lupus erythematosus predisposed.

Differential diagnosis: from herpes labialis, keratoacanthoma, and (rarely) basal cell carcinoma (on skin), molluscum contagiosum.

Investigations: biopsy. Fibreoptic pharyngolaryngoscopy with autofluorescence (symptom-directed bronchoscopy/oesophagoscopy); ultrasound-guided fine needle aspiration biopsy of any neck mass; staging – supported by MRI (or CT) from skull base to sternoclavicular joints (plus USgFNA and/or FDG-PET if anything equivocal); CT thorax.

Main diagnostic criteria: biopsy is confirmatory.

Main treatments: surgery (wedge resection or lip shave) or irradiation. The prognosis is good: 70% 5-year survival.

Discoid lupus erythematosus (DLE)

Rare. DLE may be categorized as:

- Localized DLE – the head and neck only are involved.
- Widespread DLE – other areas are affected, even if the head and neck are also involved. People with widespread disease may have abnormalities of blood or positive serology, and are more likely to develop SLE (systemic lupus erythematosus).

Typical orofacial symptoms and signs: lesions on vermilion border are scaly and crusting. Intraoral lesions have central atrophic and often indurated red area with border of radiating white striae, and peripheral telangiectasia (Figure 3.32). There is a small predisposition to carcinoma of the lip.

Main oral sites affected: buccal mucosa, palate/alveolar ridges and lips (almost always the lower lip).

Aetiopathogenesis: unclear: drugs, hormones and viruses may contribute in genetically predisposed persons.

Gender predominance: females.

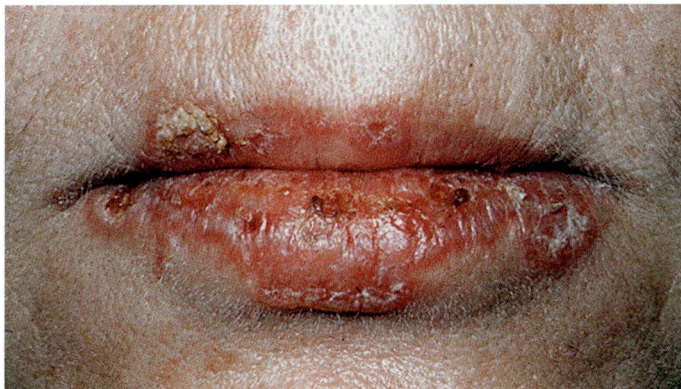

Figure 3.32 Lip lesion: discoid lupus erythematosus. Lesions can mimic lichen planus and can be potentially malignant.

Age predominance: adults.

Extraoral possible lesions: the discoid rash is usually on the face with red patches that are thick and often scaly, appearing red with a whitish, or at least, lighter-coloured, scaly rim. As the patches heal they tend to scar. If discoid lupus occurs on the scalp the hair will be lost, leaving permanent bald areas.

Main associated conditions: none; discoid lupus is a type of lupus that tends to be confined to the skin and mucosa and other organs in the body are not involved.

Differential diagnosis: systemic lupus erythematosus, lichen planus, leukoplakia (keratosis), lichenoid white lesions and carcinoma.

Investigations: biopsy; serology to exclude SLE.

Main diagnostic criteria: histology.

Main treatments: topical corticosteroids (e.g. betamethasone valerate 0.1% or clobetasol cream) or tacrolimus; cryosurgery or excision of localized lesions; follow-up because of increased risk for malignant transformation.

Lip lesions (continued)

Erythema multiforme

Uncommon.

Typical orofacial symptoms and signs: serosanguinous exudate on ulcerated swollen lips, and ulcers (Figures 3.33, 3.34).

Main oral sites affected: lips and oral mucosa.

Aetiopathogenesis: putative reaction to microorganisms (herpes simplex, mycoplasma), to drugs (e.g. NSAIDs, antimicrobials, sulphonamides, beta blockers, dapsone, salicylates, tetracyclines) or to other factors.

Gender predominance: males.

Age predominance: young adult.

Extraoral possible lesions: may affect mouth alone, or skin and/or other mucosa. The minor form affects only one or two mucosal sites and/or the skin. The major form (Stevens–Johnson syndrome) affects more than two mucosal sites and is widespread, with skin rashes, fever and toxicity. Rashes are various but typically 'target' lesions or bullae. The most severe form is toxic epidermal necrolysis (TEN) when the lesions affect most of the body surface and the condition is life-threatening.

Main associated conditions: as above.

Differential diagnosis: from other lip lesions, and other causes of mouth ulcers – particularly primary herpes stomatitis and pemphigus.

Investigations: history of exposure to agents and biopsy.

Main diagnostic criteria: clinical picture; biopsy sometimes helpful.

Main treatments: minor form – symptomatic treatment and systemic corticosteroids; major form – systemic corticosteroids or other immunomodulatory drugs.

Exfoliative cheilitis (factitious cheilitis, le tic de lèvres)

An uncommon chronic superficial inflammatory disorder characterized by hyperkeratosis and desquamation of the vermilion epithelium.

Typical orofacial symptoms and signs: persistent scaling of the lips.

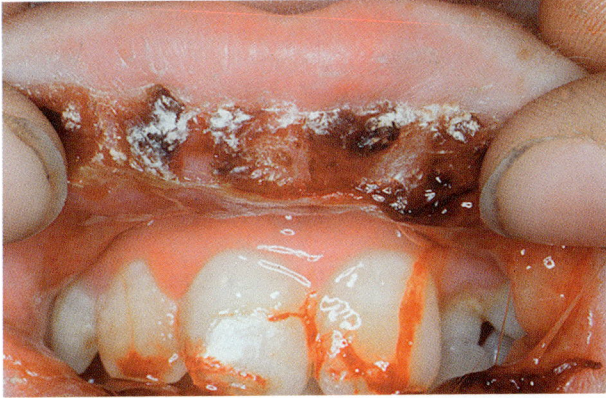

Figure 3.33 Lip lesion: erythema multiforme (patient's fingers).

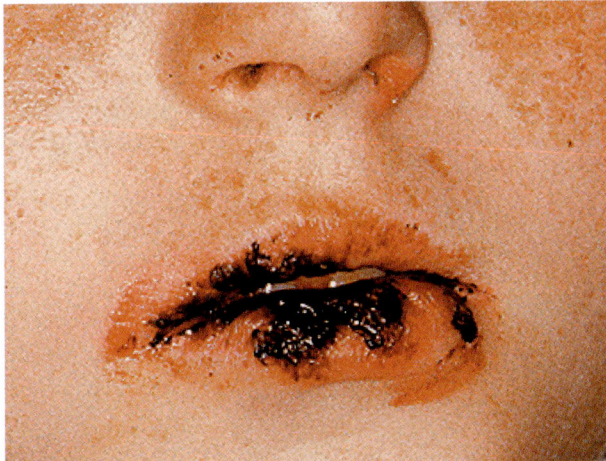

Figure 3.34 Lip lesion: erythema multiforme in a young boy showing blood-encrusted swollen lips.

Lip lesions (continued)

Main oral sites affected: often starts in the centre of the lower lip (Figures 3.35–3.38) and spreads to involve the whole of the lower or of both lips. The patient may complain of irritation or burning and can be observed frequently biting or sucking the lips. Lip scaling and crusting is more or less confined to the vermilion border, persisting in varying severity for months or years. There may be bizarre yellow hyperkeratotic or thick haemorrhagic crusts.

Aetiopathogenesis: most patients seem to have a personality disorder. A preoccupation with the lips is prevalent in some individuals. In some cases it appears to start with chapping or with atopic eczema, and develops into a habit tic. Many cases are thus thought to be factitious, caused by repeated self-induced trauma such as repetitive biting, picking, lip sucking, chewing or other manipulation of the lips. Exacerbations have been associated with stress.

Gender predominance: female.

Age predominance: children and young adults.

Extraoral possible lesions: none.

Main associated conditions: none.

Differential diagnosis: actinic cheilitis, contact cheilitis, glandular cheilitis, lupus erythematosus, *Candida* infections (where it is sometimes termed cheilo-candidosis), and HIV infection.

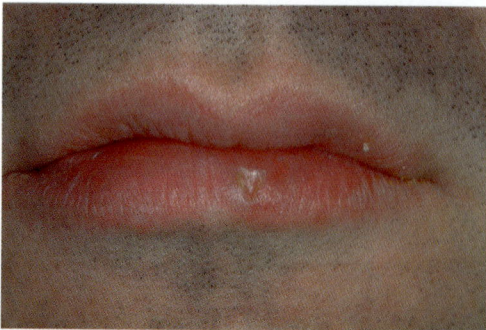

Figure 3.35 Lip lesion: chapping.

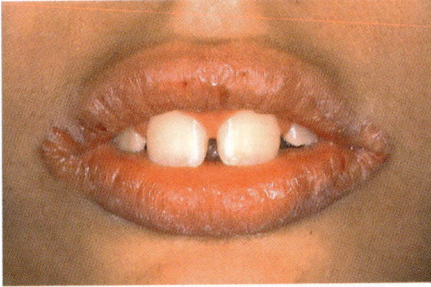

Figure 3.36 Lip lesion: cheilitis (factitious or artefactual- self-induced).

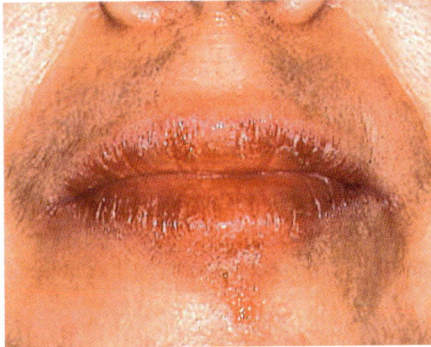

Figure 3.37 Lip lesion: cheilitis (the skin erythema beneath the lower lip is from licking).

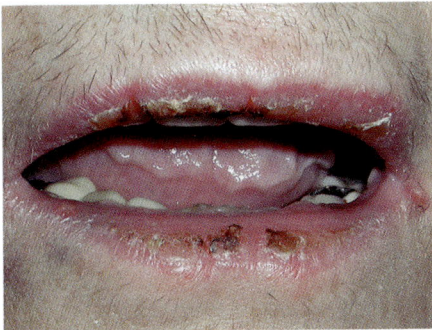

Figure 3.38 Lip lesion: cheilitis (exfoliative). Note also the crenated tongue, from pressing on the teeth.

Lip lesions (continued)

Investigations: biopsy is sometimes indicated and allergy testing for severe cases.

Main diagnostic criteria: diagnosis is restricted to those few patients whose cheilitis cannot be attributed to other causes, such as contact sensitization or UV light.

Main treatments: some cases resolve spontaneously or with improved oral hygiene. Reassurance and topical corticosteroids may be helpful but often exfoliative cheilitis is refractory to treatment. When a factitial cause is suspected, a psychiatric consultation and care may be beneficial; some improve with psychotherapy and antianxiolytic or antidepressant treatment.

Hereditary angioedema

Rare.

Typical orofacial symptoms and signs: as in allergic angioedema (above) but precipitated by trauma, e.g. dental treatment. There is high mortality in some families.

Main oral sites affected: lips and tongue.

Aetiopathogenesis: genetic defect of the inhibitor of activated first component of complement C1 (C1 esterase inhibitor); autosomal dominant inheritance generally.

Gender predominance: none.

Age predominance: none.

Extraoral possible lesions: sometimes abdominal pain and there may be swelling of the extremities.

Main associated conditions: rarely this condition is acquired in lymphoproliferative disorders.

Differential diagnosis: acute allergic angioedema and other causes of facial swelling.

Investigations: serum C1 esterase inhibitor and C4 levels.

Main diagnostic criteria: family history. C1 esterase inhibitor and C4 serum levels are reduced.

Main treatments: recombinant C1 esterase inhibitor; androgenic steroids (danazol; oxandrolone) kallikrein inhibitors (ecallantide) and bradykinin receptor antagonists (icatibant).

Herpes labialis

Common, especially in immunocompromised patients.

Typical orofacial symptoms and signs: prodromal paraesthesia or irritation. Erythema, then vesicles at/near mucocutaneous junction of the lip (sometimes termed 'cold sores' or 'fever blisters': Figures 3.39–3.42). Heals in 7–10 days.

Main oral sites affected: mucocutaneous junction of the lip.

Aetiopathogenesis: herpes simplex virus (HSV), usually type 1. HSV latent in trigeminal ganglion after primary infection is reactivated as herpes labialis ('cold sores'). It is precipitated by sun, trauma, menstruation, fever, HIV disease, immunosuppression etc.

Gender predominance: none.

Age predominance: none.

Extraoral possible lesions: none.

Main associated conditions: none.

Differential diagnosis: zoster, impetigo.

Main diagnostic criteria: clinical.

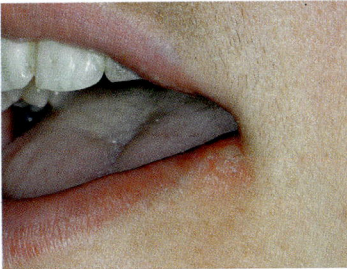

Figure 3.39 Lip lesion: herpes labialis – early vesicles.

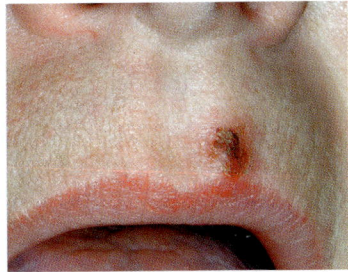

Figure 3.40 Lip lesion: herpes labialis – later scabbed lesion.

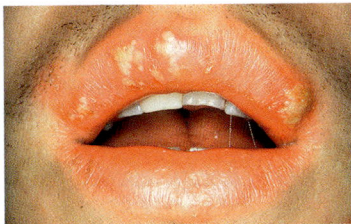

Figure 3.41 Lip lesion: herpes labialis showing multiple pustules.

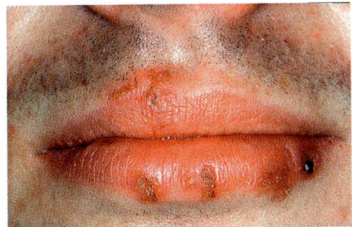

Figure 3.42 Lip lesion: herpes labialis on another occasion in the same patient shown in Figure 3.41.

Lip lesions (continued)

Main treatments: aciclovir, or penciclovir cream applied in prodrome. Oral aciclovir, valaciclovir, or famciclovir for frequent recurrences or immuno-compromised; i.v. antivirals may be needed for severely immunocompro-mised patients.

Herpes zoster ('shingles')

Typical orofacial symptoms and signs: pain and rash in a trigeminal der-matome (Figure 3.43) followed by ipsilateral oral vesicles, then mouth ulcers.

Main oral sites affected: any trigeminal nerve division.

Aetiopathogenesis: varicella-zoster virus (VZV), latent in the sensory ganglion after chickenpox (varicella) is reactivated mainly in older, or immunocom-promised people, such as in HIV infection.

Gender predominance: none.

Age predominance: older adults (immunocompetent). Any age in immunocompromised.

Extraoral possible lesions: see above.

Main associated conditions: none.

Differential diagnosis: pain – may simulate toothache; rash – differentiate from HSV infection. Mouth ulcers.

Investigations: there is no immunological test of value. Smears show viral damaged cells.

Main diagnostic criteria: clinical features.

Main treatments: analgesics; aciclovir or penciclovir cream to rash; for immunocompromised patients consider using famciclovir' valaciclovir tablets or aciclovir tablets, or intravenous aciclovir/foscarnet.

Labial melanotic macule

Typical orofacial symptoms and signs: asymptomatic smooth brown pig-mented macule <1 cm in diameter (Figure 3.44).

Main oral sites affected: lower lip vermilion.

Aetiopathogenesis: congenital or acquired lesions derived from melanoblasts.

Gender predominance: none.

Age predominance: adult.

Extraoral possible lesions: none.

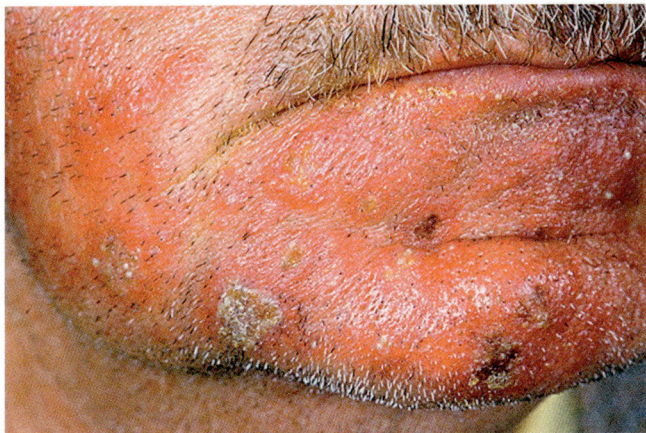

Figure 3.43 Lip lesion: zoster (shingles) – intact vesicles and crusted lesions. There is typically also, severe pain in the area.

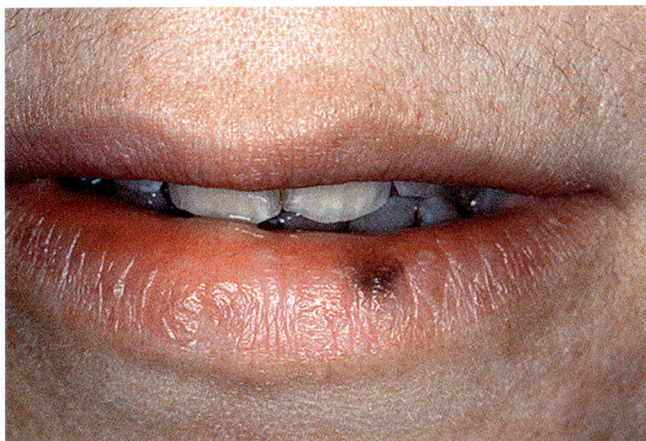

Figure 3.44 Lip lesion: melanotic macule.

Lip lesions (continued)

Main associated conditions: none.

Differential diagnosis: racial pigmentation, amalgam tattoo, drug-induced hyperpigmentation, pigmented naevus, malignant melanoma, Peutz–Jeghers, Laugier–Hunziker and other syndromes.

Investigations: biopsy is essential to exclude malignant melanoma.

Main diagnostic criteria: clinical supported by histology.

Main treatments: excision biopsy if concerned.

Mucocele

See Figure 3.45.

Orofacial granulomatosis (OFG; see also Crohn disease, pages 224 and 398)

An uncommon but increasing condition. The cause of OFG is unknown but it may be immunological; it is not thought to be inherited and it is not thought to be infectious. It appears related to conditions such as Crohn disease, which may affect the gut and other tissues. Some patients with OFG have food or food additive intolerance or allergy: most commonly this is to cinnamaldehyde, carnosine, monosodium glutamate, cocoa, carbone, or sunset yellow.

Typical orofacial symptoms and signs:

- facial and/or labial swelling (Figure 3.46)
- angular stomatitis and/or cracked or fissured lips
- ulcers
- mucosal tags and/or cobblestoning
- gingival hyperplasia
- cervical lymphadenopathy.

Sometimes effects of malabsorption. Variants include:

- Miescher cheilitis (cheilitis granulomatosa) – where lip swelling is seen in isolation.
- Melkersson–Rosenthal syndrome – facial swelling with fissured tongue and facial palsy: however, features can appear at different times or only two out of three being.

Main oral sites affected: lips.

Aetiopathogenesis: unknown. Some have gastrointestinal Crohn disease or sarcoidosis; others a postulated reaction to food or other antigens (e.g. cinnamaldehyde or benzoates.

Figure 3.45 Lip lesion: mucocele (excise and histopathologically examine but it may recur).

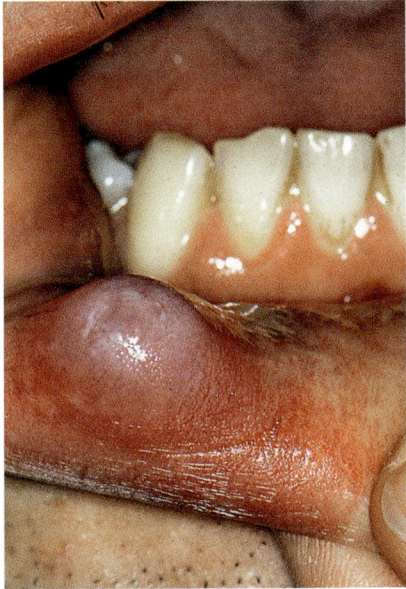

Figure 3.46 Lip lesion: granulomatous cheilitis – persistent painless swelling.

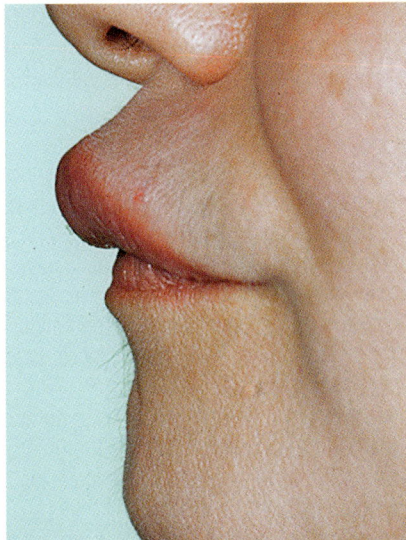

Lip lesions (continued)

Gender predominance: male.

Age predominance: young adults.

Extraoral possible lesions: see above; many ultimately manifest Crohn disease elsewhere.

Main associated conditions: see above.

Differential diagnosis: Crohn disease or sarcoidosis, tuberculosis and foreign body reactions, especially to cosmetic enlargement.

Investigations: blood tests, radiology, endoscopy and biopsy to exclude Crohn disease, sarcoidosis, or tuberculosis.

Main diagnostic criteria: diagnosis is confirmed by lesional biopsy.

Main treatments: control by avoiding allergens, or by using medicines – topical or intralesional corticosteroids; topical tacrolimus; occasionally systemic steroids, sulfasalazine or clofazimine.

Peutz–Jeghers syndrome

Rare; 'circumoral melanosis with intestinal polyposis'.

Typical orofacial symptoms and signs: multiple hyperpigmented brown macules.

Main oral sites affected: perioral and on labial (lower lip mainly) and/or buccal mucosa and gingivae (Figures 3.47, 3.48).

Aetiopathogenesis: autosomal dominant disorder.

Gender predominance: none.

Age predominance: none.

Extraoral possible lesions: hyperpigmented brown macules around nose and eyes and rarely on trunk and on the hands and feet. Gastrointestinal polyps – usually benign and in small intestine, predisposing to intussusceptions and sometimes malignancy (mainly gastrointestinal and pancreatic but also liver, lungs, breast, ovaries, uterus, testicles and other organs).

Differential diagnosis: racial pigmentation, Addison disease, freckles (ephelides) and Laugier–Hunziker syndrome (similar features but also with nail hyperpigmentation).

Investigations: gastrointestinal imaging and biopsy.

Main diagnostic criteria: clinical features pathognomonic.

Main treatments: reassure or excise for histological confirmation. Genetic consultation and counseling. Molecular genetic testing of *STK11 (LKB1)* reveals disease-causing mutations in nearly all individuals who have a

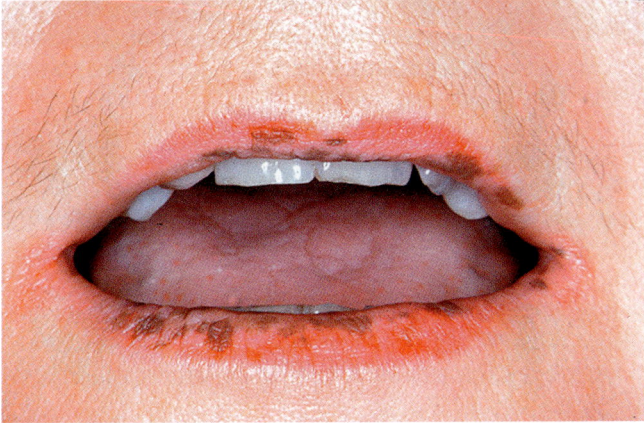

Figure 3.47 Lip lesions: Peutz–Jegher syndrome – multiple pigmented macules.

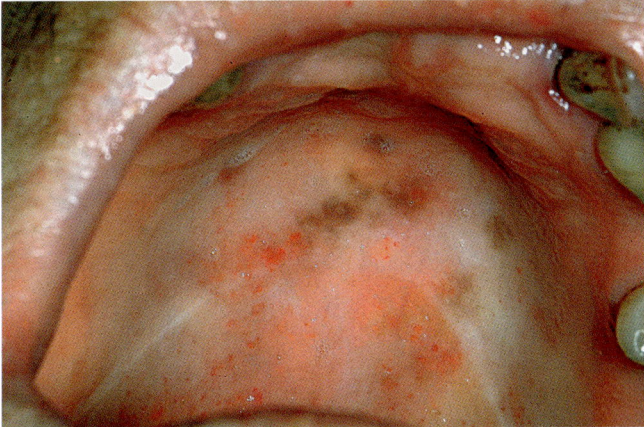

Figure 3.48 Lip and palatal lesions: Peutz–Jegher syndrome.

Lip lesions (continued)

positive family history and approximately 90% of individuals who have no family history. Cancer screening.

Pyogenic granuloma
Uncommon.

Typical orofacial symptoms and signs: small (<1 cm), red, painless mass that bleeds easily, ulcerates and grows rapidly – especially in pregnancy.

Main oral sites affected: gingival margin, tongue, or rarely the lip (Figures 3.49, 3.50).

Aetiopathogenesis: possibly reactive vascular lesion. Inflammatory infiltrate is superimposed.

Gender predominance: none.

Age predominance: children and young adults.

Extraoral possible lesions: none.

Main associated conditions: none.

Differential diagnosis: fibrous epulis, angiomatous proliferation, giant cell lesion, chancre, carcinoma, Kaposi sarcoma.

Investigations: biopsy.

Main diagnostic criteria: histopathology.

Main treatments: excision.

Intraoral lesions

Keypoints

- Coloured lesions if red are usually vascular, inflammatory or atrophic. Brown lesions are usually naevi; black lesions are usually due to amalgam tattoo.
- Soreness or ulceration is usually due to local causes or aphthae but other causes, especially malignant or systemic diseases, must be excluded.
- White lesions that wipe off with gauze are usually due to debris or candidosis; others to lichen planus or keratosis.
- Lumps/swelling can have a range of causes but neoplasms are amongst the most important.

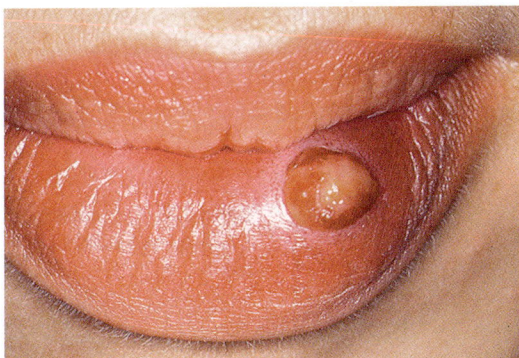

Figure 3.49 Lip lesion: pyogenic granuloma (excise and histopathologically examine but it may recur).

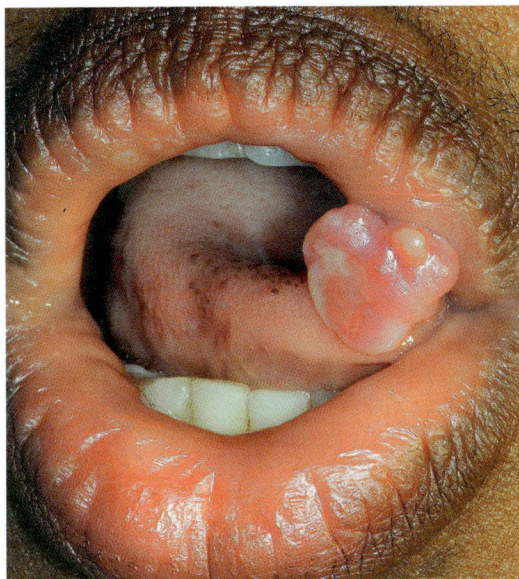

Figure 3.50 Lip lesion: pyogenic granuloma (excise and histopathologically examine but it may recur).

Coloured lesions: red

Erythematous candidosis

Typical orofacial symptoms and signs: sore red mouth (Figures 3.51, 3.52).
Main oral sites affected: tongue, palate.

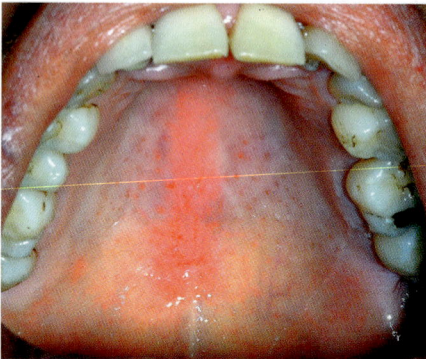

Figure 3.51 Intraoral lesion: candidosis presenting as red lesion.

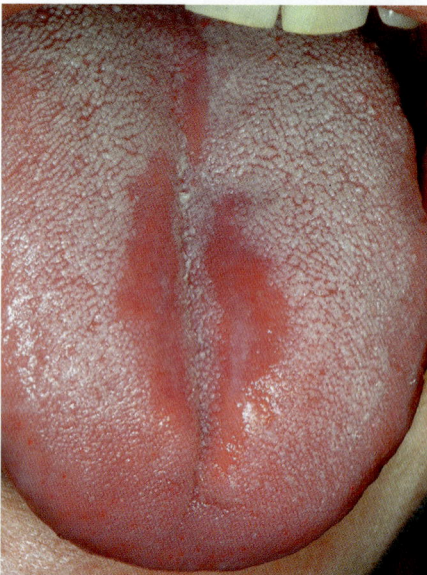

Figure 3.52 Intraoral lesion: candidosis on tongue (same patient shown in Figure 3.51 – a 'kissing lesion'.

Aetiopathogenesis: candidosis may cause sore red mouth, especially in patients on broad spectrum antimicrobials. Erythematous candidosis, especially on the palate or tongue, may also be a feature of HIV disease.

Gender predominance: none.

Age predominance: none.

Extraoral possible lesions: see above.

Main associated conditions: see above.

Differential diagnosis: other causes of glossitis.

Investigations: swab and culture; blood tests.

Main diagnostic criteria: clinical and microbiology.

Main treatments: antifungals.

Erythroplasia (erythroplakia)

Much less common than leukoplakia, but far more likely to be dysplastic or malignant.

Typical orofacial symptoms and signs: red velvety patch of variable configuration, usually level with or depressed below surrounding mucosa (Figures 3.53–3.56) .

Main oral sites affected: soft palate or floor or mouth.

Aetiopathogenesis: tobacco, alcohol and betel use predispose.

Gender predominance: males.

Age predominance: older.

Extraoral possible lesions: none.

Main associated conditions: in some may be cancer in the upper aerodigestive tract (nasal, pharyngeal, laryngeal, bronchial, oesophageal).

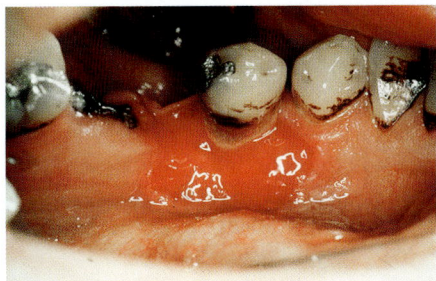

Figure 3.53 Intraoral lesion; erythroplakia (erythroplasia).

Coloured lesions: red (continued)

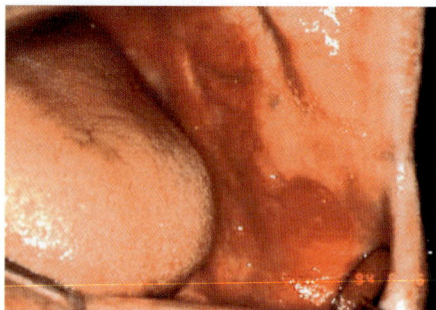

Figure 3.54 Intraoral lesion: erythroplakia.

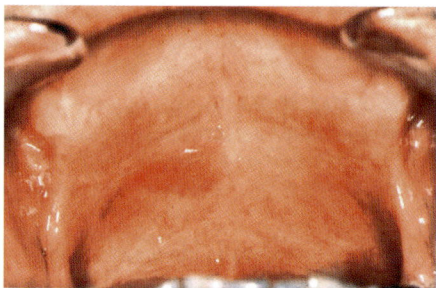

Figure 3.55 Intraoral lesion: erythroplakia.

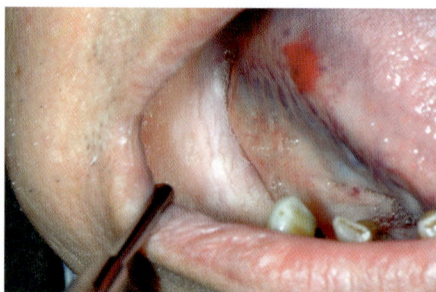

Figure 3.56 Intraoral lesion: erythroplakia on tongue.

Differential diagnosis: inflammatory and atrophic lesions, e.g. in deficiency anaemias, geographic tongue (erythema migrans), lichen planus, erythematous candidosis, contact allergy.

Investigations: biopsy for epithelial dysplasia and carcinoma.

Main diagnostic criteria: clinical and microscopic.

Main treatments: excise, but the prognosis is often poor.

Hereditary haemorrhagic telangiectasia (HHT; Osler–Rendu–Weber syndrome)

Rare.

Typical orofacial symptoms and signs: telangiectases are present orally and periorally (Figure 3.57) and may bleed, resulting in iron deficiency anaemia.

Main oral sites affected: palate, tongue, lips.

Aetiopathogenesis: autosomal dominant inheritance but family history may be negative.

Gender predominance: none.

Age predominance: from birth.

Extraoral possible lesions: nose, gastrointestinal tract and occasionally on palms or fingers.

Main associated conditions: iron deficiency anaemia. Predisposes to cerebral emboli.

Differential diagnosis: scleroderma, chronic liver disease and post-irradiation telangiectasia.

Investigations: clinical features; blood picture.

Figure 3.57 Intraoral lesions: multiple telangiectasia in hereditary haemorrhagic telangiectasia.

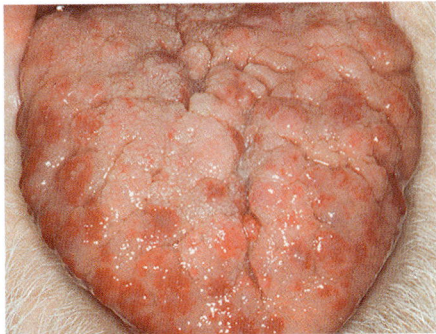

Coloured lesions: red (continued)

Main diagnostic criteria: clinical.

Main treatments: cryosurgery or laser if bleeding is troublesome; treat anaemia.

Scleroderma

Typical orofacial symptoms and signs: oral opening restricted with microstomia and pale fibrotic 'chicken' tongue; widened periodontal space on radiography in a few, but teeth not mobile. Occasionally: telangiectasia (Figures 3.58–3.60); secondary Sjögren syndrome; bone lesions.

Rare variant: CREST syndrome (calcinosis, Raynaud disease, esophageal strictures, sclerodactyly, telangiectasia).

Main oral sites affected: lips, tongue, palate.

Aetiopathogenesis: autoimmune.

Gender predominance: female.

Age predominance: middle age.

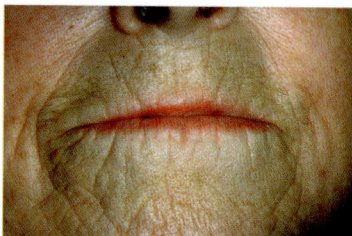

Figure 3.58 Lip tightening in scleroderma.

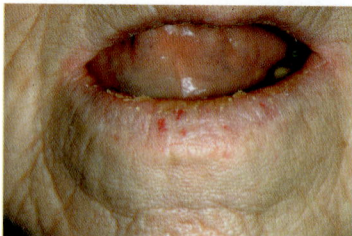

Figure 3.59 Lip lesion in same patient shown in Figure 3.58: telangiectasia.

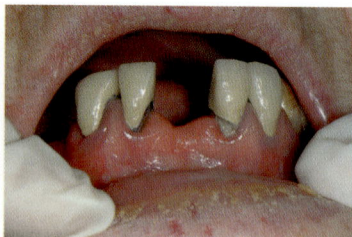

Figure 3.60 Intraoral lesion in same patient shown in Figure 3.59: dry mouth and caries in associated Sjögren syndrome.

Extraoral possible lesions: oesophagus, skin – tight and waxy, and on extremities.

Main associated conditions: Raynaud disease, Sjögren syndrome.

Differential diagnosis: from oral submucous fibrosis, telangiectasia (e.g. HHT, see below) and secondary Sjögren syndrome.

Investigations: serum autoantibodies (ANF and Scl 70 especially).

Main diagnostic criteria: clinical features; histopathology; auto-antibodies.

Main treatments: penicillamine, iloprost, cyclophosphamide.

Coloured lesions: brown

Addison disease (hypoadrenocorticism)

Rare.

Typical orofacial symptoms and signs: symptomless brown hyperpigmentation especially in sites usually pigmented or traumatized (Figure 3.61).

Main oral sites affected: gingiva, occlusal line.

Aetiopathogenesis: adrenocortical destruction from autoimmune hypoadrenalism and, rarely, tuberculosis, histoplasmosis (sometimes in HIV/AIDS) and carcinomatosis. Nelson syndrome is similar but iatrogenic, resulting from adrenalectomy in the management of breast cancer.

Gender predominance: females.

Age predominance: young or middle age.

Extraoral possible lesions: hyperpigmentation, especially in sites usually pigmented (breast areolae, and genitals), or traumatized (skin flexures).

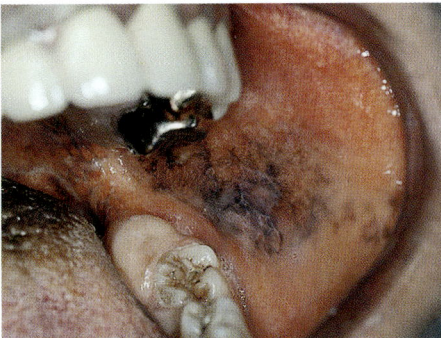

Figure 3.61 Intraoral lesion; pigmentation in Addison disease.

Coloured lesions: brown (continued)

Main associated conditions: rarely associated with HIV/AIDS, other autoimmune glandular disease; or candidosis-endocrinopathy syndrome.

Differential diagnosis: other causes of pigmentation, especially racial and drugs.

Investigations: blood pressure; plasma electrolyte and cortisol levels and response to ACTH (Synacthen test).

Main diagnostic criteria: clinical, hypotension, low cortisol.

Main treatments: idiopathic (autoimmune) Addison disease – replacement therapy (fludrocortisone and corticosteroids). Other causes: treat cause, give replacement therapy.

Amalgam tattoo

Common.

Typical orofacial symptoms and signs: asymptomatic black or bluish-black (usually), solitary, small pigmented area beneath normal mucosa (Figures 3.62, 3.63).

Main oral sites affected: lower ridge or buccal vestibule, or floor of mouth.

Aetiopathogenesis: amalgam particles or dust can become incorporated in healing wounds after tooth extraction or apicectomy or beneath mucosa.

Gender predominance: none.

Age predominance: adults.

Extraoral possible lesions: none.

Main associated conditions: none.

Differential diagnosis: other causes of pigmentation, especially naevi and melanoma.

Investigations: imaging (may rarely be radioopaque). In uncertain cases excision biopsy can be performed.

Main diagnostic criteria: clinical, imaging.

Main treatments: excision biopsy may be necessary if the lesion is not radioopaque, in order to distinguish from naevus or melanoma.

Malignant melanoma

Typical orofacial symptoms and signs: heavily black pigmented macule usually (occasionally non-pigmented), or later, nodules and ulceration (Figure 3.64). It may spread across several centimetres and metastasize to cervical lymph nodes and then the bloodstream. Worrying features in a

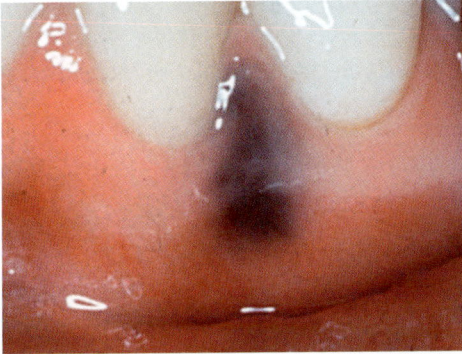

Figure 3.62 Intraoral lesion: pigmentation from an amalgam tattoo.

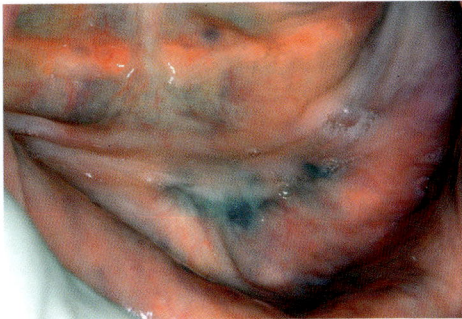

Figure 3.63 Intraoral lesion: extensive pigmentation from an amalgam tattoo.

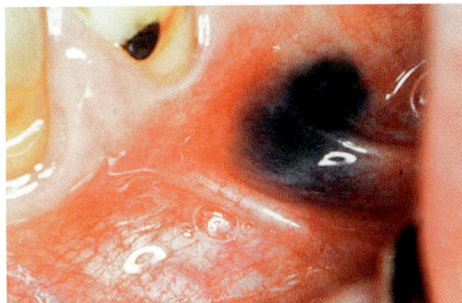

Figure 3.64 Intraoral lesion: pigmentation from a melanoma.

Coloured lesions: brown (continued)

pigmented lesion are rapid growth, irregular edge, nodularity or uneven or changing colour.

Main oral sites affected: palate.

Aetiopathogenesis: malignant tumour of melanocytes.

Gender predominance: male.

Age predominance: older.

Extraoral possible lesions: regional lymph node involvement.

Main associated conditions: none.

Differential diagnosis: naevi and other pigmented lesions.

Investigations: biopsy.

Main diagnostic criteria: clinical, supported by histology.

Main treatments: wide excision biopsy, assessment of invasion depth. Prognosis is poor unless treatment is exceptionally early – hence the need to biopsy small pigmented lesions.

Naevi

Common.

Typical orofacial symptoms and signs: asymptomatic brownish or bluish macules, usually <1 cm across (Figure 3.65).

Main oral sites affected: gingivae and hard palate.

Aetiopathogenesis: congenital.

Gender predominance: none.

Age predominance: adults.

Extraoral possible lesions: none.

Main associated conditions: none.

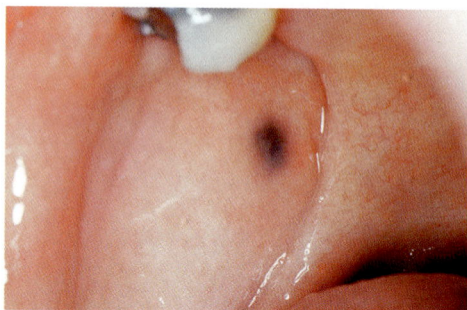

Figure 3.65 Intraoral lesion: pigmented naevus.

Differential diagnosis: other causes of pigmentation, especially amalgam tattoo, melanotic macule or melanoma.

Investigations: biopsy.

Main diagnostic criteria: clinical, supported by histology.

Main treatments: excision to exclude malignant melanoma.

Soreness/ulcers

Causes may be systemic or infectious.

Systemic causes

Blood (haematological) disorders (see page 356)

Anaemia, leucopenia and leukaemia may present with ulceration.

Infectious causes

Hand, foot and mouth disease

Very common. It usually occurs in small epidemics, in children.

Typical orofacial symptoms and signs: red papules that evolve to superficial vesicles and ulcers, resembling herpetic stomatitis but with no gingivitis (Figure 3.66).

Main oral sites affected: labial and buccal mucosa.

Aetiopathogenesis: Coxsackie viruses (usually A16; rarely A5 or 10).

Gender predominance: none.

Age predominance: young children.

Extraoral possible lesions: palmoplantar involvement with erythematous papules and a few vesicles with perilesional erythema, mild fever, malaise and anorexia.

Figure 3.66 Intraoral lesion: ulceration in hand, foot and mouth disease.

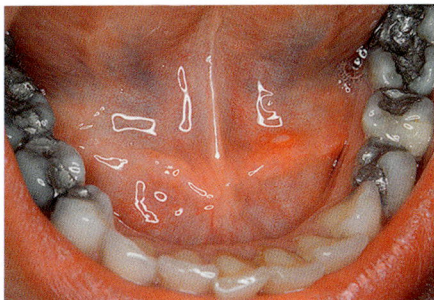

Soreness/ulcers (continued)

Main associated conditions: rash – in a few days, found mainly on palms and soles.

Differential diagnosis: herpetic stomatitis, chickenpox.

Investigations: none.

Main diagnostic criteria: clinical features. Serology is confirmatory but rarely required.

Main treatments: symptomatic (soft diet; analgesics; reduce fever).

Herpangina

Uncommon. Small outbreaks are seen, usually among young children.

Typical orofacial symptoms and signs: pharyngeal ulcers, usually resembling herpetic ulcers but affecting posterior mouth alone (soft palate and uvula) and causing sore throat; no gingivitis.

Main oral sites affected: soft palate and uvula (Figures 3.67, 3.68).

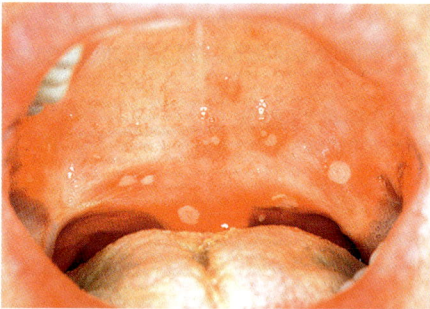

Figure 3.67 Intraoral lesions: ulceration in herpangina. Lesions are mainly on the palate.

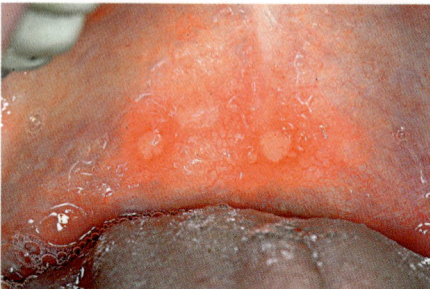

Figure 3.68 Intraoral lesions: ulceration in herpangina.

Aetiopathogenesis: Coxsackie viruses usually (A7, 9, 16; B1, 2, 3, 4 or 5); ECHO viruses (9 or 17).

Gender predominance: none.

Age predominance: young children.

Extraoral possible lesions: cervical lymphadenitis (moderate); fever; malaise; irritability, anorexia, vomiting.

Main associated conditions: none usually.

Differential diagnosis: herpetic stomatitis, hand, foot and mouth disease, chickenpox.

Investigations: none.

Main diagnostic criteria: clinical features. Serology (theoretically) is confirmatory.

Main treatments: symptomatic (see above).

Herpetic stomatitis

Common.

Typical orofacial symptoms and signs: multiple vesicles and round scattered ulcers with yellow slough and erythematous halo; ulcers fuse to produce irregular lesions (Figures 3.69–3.72). Gingivitis: diffuse erythema and oedema, occasionally haemorrhagic.

Main oral sites affected: any.

Aetiopathogenesis: herpes simplex virus (HSV), usually type 1 in young children. Type 2 often in older age groups.

Gender predominance: none.

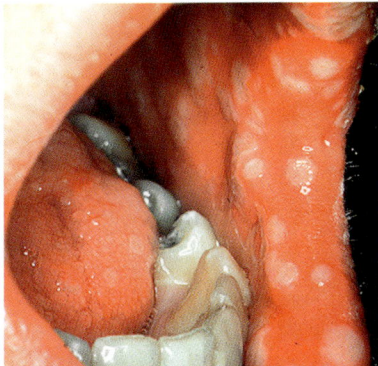

Figure 3.69 Intraoral lesions: ulceration in herpetic stomatitis.

Soreness/ulcers (continued)

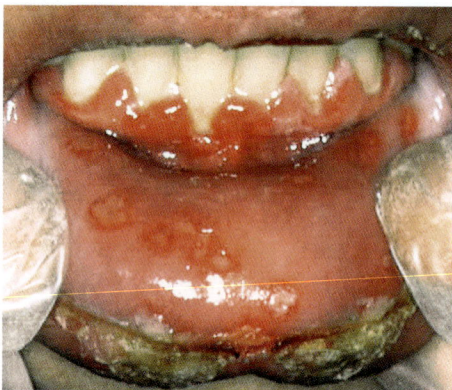

Figure 3.70 Intraoral lesions: ulceration in herpetic stomatitis, with gingival swelling and erythema.

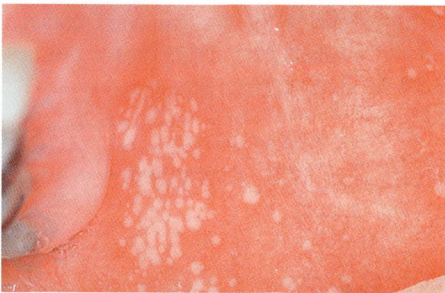

Figure 3.71 Intraoral lesions: ulceration in herpetic stomatitis.

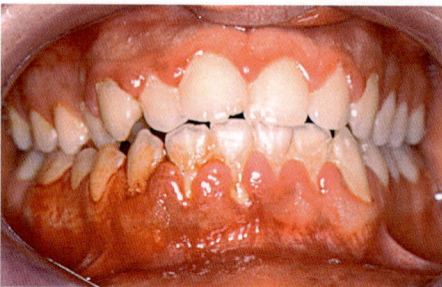

Figure 3.72 Intraoral lesions: ulceration in herpetic stomatitis, with gingival swelling and erythema.

Age predominance: children and adolescents. It is also seen in adults, especially in more affluent communities or among those who work with children.

Extraoral possible lesions: cervical lymphadenitis (moderate); fever; malaise; irritability, anorexia, vomiting.

Main associated conditions: rarely: skin lesions, ocular or CNS involvement.

Differential diagnosis: other causes of mouth ulcers, especially hand, foot and mouth disease, chickenpox and shingles, herpangina, erythema multiforme and leukaemia.

Investigations: none usually. Viral immunostaining, or DNA studies. Culture or electron microscopy used occasionally. A rising titre of antibodies is confirmatory.

Main diagnostic criteria: clinical.

Main treatments: symptomatic (soft diet and adequate fluid intake; antipyretics/analgesics [paracetamol elixir]; local antiseptics; aqueous chlorhexidine mouthwashes); aciclovir orally or suspension or tablets parenterally in severe cases or immunocompromised patients.

Recurrences usually present as herpes labialis or unilateral palatal or gingival lesions (Figure 3.73). In immunocompromised patients extensive oral and cutaneous lesions can be seen (eczema herpeticum). HSV infection may rarely precipitate erythema multiforme.

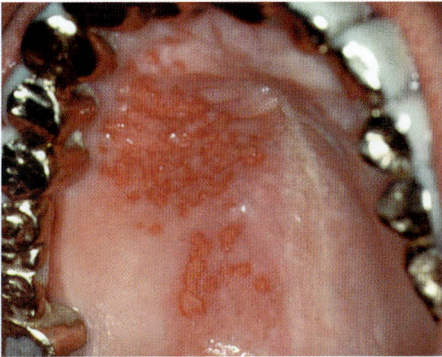

Figure 3.73 Intraoral lesions: ulceration in recurrent herpes simplex can mimic zoster.

Soreness/ulcers (continued)

Herpes varicella-zoster virus (chickenpox; varicella)

Common childhood exanthema (viral rash).

Typical orofacial symptoms and signs: ulcers: indistinguishable from HSV, but no associated gingivitis (Figure 3.74).

Main oral sites affected: any.

Aetiopathogenesis: herpes varicella-zoster virus (VZV).

Gender predominance: none.

Age predominance: children.

Extraoral possible lesions: fever; rash — mainly on face and trunk (papules then vesicles, pustules and scabs, in crops). Malaise, irritability, anorexia. Cervical lymphadenitis. Rarely: pneumonia or encephalitis.

Main associated conditions: none.

Differential diagnosis: from other mouth ulcers, especially HSV and other viral infections.

Investigations: none; cytology may help.

Main diagnostic criteria: clinical. Rising antibody titre is confirmatory.

Main treatments: symptomatic; immunoglobulin or aciclovir in immunocompromised patients. Immunize to prevent.

Shingles (herpes zoster)

Uncommon.

Typical orofacial symptoms and signs:

- pain — before, with and after rash
- rash: unilateral vesiculating, then scabbing in dermatome
- mouth ulcers: sheets of vesicles that rupture and coalesce to form painful irregular ulcers that stop at the midline (Figure 3.75)
- main oral sites affected: mandibular zoster — ipsilateral on buccal and lingual mucosa; maxillary — ipsilateral on palate and vestibule
- rarely: geniculate zoster (rash in ear, facial palsy and ulcers on ipsilateral soft palate) — Ramsay Hunt syndrome.

Aetiopathogenesis: reactivation of VZV latent in sensory ganglia, often because of immune defects.

Gender predominance: none.

Age predominance: older adults.

Extraoral possible lesions: fever; pain and rash in dermatome.

Main associated conditions: any immune defect (e.g. HIV/AIDS).

Figure 3.74
Intraoral lesion: ulceration in herpes varicella-zoster virus primary infection (chickenpox).

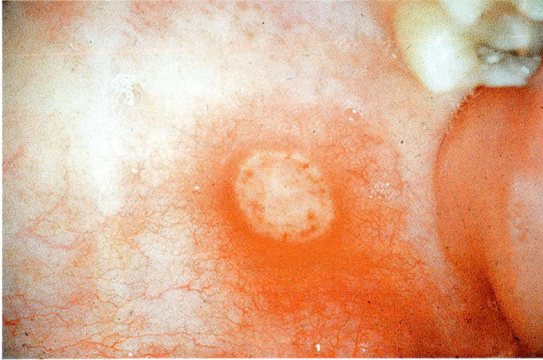

Figure 3.75
Intraoral lesions: unilateral ulceration in herpes varicella-zoster virus recurrence (zoster or shingles). There is also an ipsilateral rash, and pain.

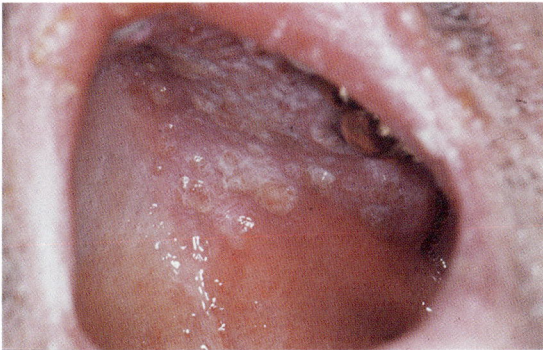

Differential diagnosis: toothache and other causes of ulcers, especially HSV.

Investigations: cytologic smear from fresh lesion for immunostaining or DNA studies.

Main diagnostic criteria: clinical features.

Main treatments: antiviral therapy (aciclovir, famciclovir, valaciclovir in high dose, orally or parenterally, especially in the immunocompromised) and corticosteroids shorten the acute illness period; opioids and anticonvulsants can reduce acute pain; tricyclic antidepressants, opioids and carbamazepine can help relieve chronic pain; symptomatic treatment of ulcers. *Ophthalmic zoster:* ophthalmological opinion.

Soreness/ulcers (continued)

Infectious mononucleosis (glandular fever)

Common.

Typical orofacial symptoms and signs: sore throat, faucial swelling and ulceration with creamy exudate and palatal petechia; occasional mouth ulcers; cervical lymph node enlargement (Figures 3.76–3.78).

Main oral sites affected: fauces.

Aetiopathogenesis: Epstein–Barr virus (EBV).

Gender predominance: none.

Age predominance: adolescents.

Extraoral possible lesions: generalized tender lymphadenopathy; fever, malaise, anorexia and lassitude.

Main associated conditions: macular rash, splenomegaly.

Differential diagnosis: streptococcal pharyngitis, diphtheria, *Toxoplasma gondii* infection and other viral glandular-like fever syndromes (e.g. HIV infection, HHV-6, cytomegalovirus) infection.

Investigations: Paul–Bunnell test for heterophil antibodies.

Main diagnostic criteria: clinical features; blood picture; serology.

Main treatments: symptomatic; metronidazole may improve sore throat.

Syphilis

Predominantly an infection of the sexually promiscuous (prostitutes, male homosexuals, travellers, armed forces). Oral lesions uncommon. Non-venereal treponematoses, including yaws, bejel and pinta, are rare in the UK/USA.

Typical orofacial symptoms and signs:

- congenital syphilis: head and neck – frontal bossing, saddle nose, Hutchinsonian incisors, Moon or mulberry molars and rhagades (circumoral scars); others – learning impairment, interstitial keratitis (blindness), deafness, sabre tibiae and Clutton joints

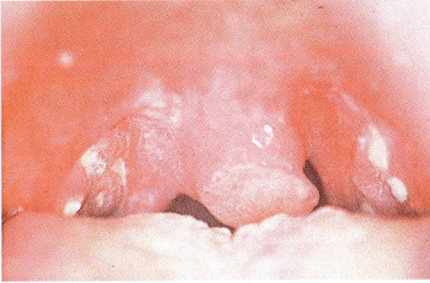

Figure 3.76 Intraoral lesion: ulceration and candidosis; infectious mononucleosis (glandular fever).

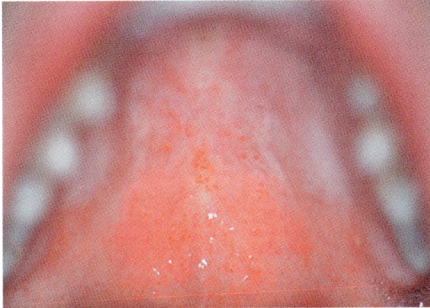

Figure 3.77 Intraoral lesion: infectious mononucleosis with palatal petechiae.

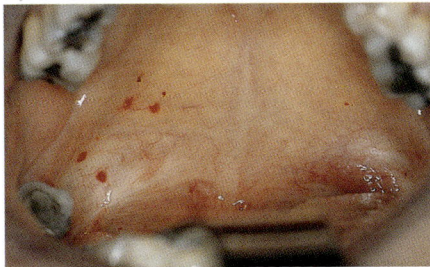

Figure 3.78 Intraoral lesion: infectious mononucleosis with palatal petechiae.

Soreness/ulcers (continued)

- acquired syphilis: oral lesions may be seen in all three stages:
  - a primary syphilis – a Hunterian or hard chancre is a small papule that develops into large painless indurated ulcer (Figure 3.79), with regional lymphadenitis. Chancre is highly infectious, and though usually on genitals, breast or perianally may appear on lip, tongue or palate; heals spontaneously in 1–2 months.
  - b secondary syphilis – oral lesions are highly infectious and include: mucous patches, split papules or snail-track ulcers (Figure 3.80). Rash (coppery coloured, typically on palms

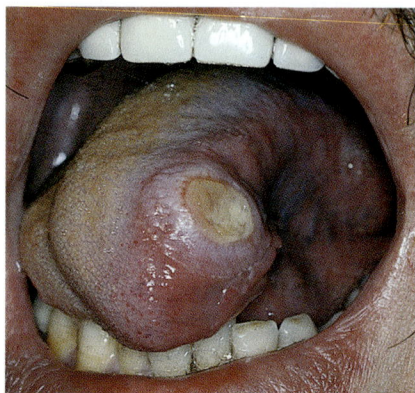

Figure 3.79 Intraoral lesion: ulceration of a hard (Hunterian) chancre in primary syphilis.

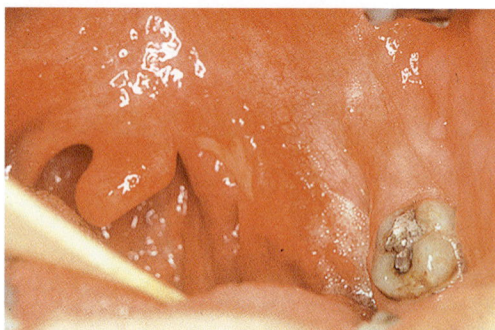

Figure 3.80 Intraoral lesion: ulceration in secondary syphilis. Ulcers sometimes have a 'snailtrack' appearance.

and soles), condylomata lata and generalized lymph node enlargement can also be present.

c tertiary syphilis – oral lesions are non-infectious and include glossitis (leukoplakia) and gumma (Figure 3.81). These may be associated with cardiovascular complications (aortic aneurysm) or neurosyphilis (tabes dorsalis; general paralysis of the insane; Argyll Robinson pupils [react to focus but not to light]).

Main oral sites affected: chancre; on lip (upper) or intraorally – usually tongue. Lesions of secondary syphilis – any site. Lesions of tertiary syphilis – usually midline in palate, or dorsum of tongue.

Aetiopathogenesis: Treponema pallidum – sexually shared.

Gender predominance: none.

Age predominance: adults.

Extraoral possible lesions: as above.

Main associated conditions: HIV and other sexually shared infections.

Differential diagnosis: trauma, herpes labialis, pyogenic granuloma, carcinoma. Very rarely: non-venereal treponematoses.

Investigations: T. pallidum in direct smear (darkfield examination) of primary- and secondary-stage lesions. Serology positive from late in primary stage.

Main diagnostic criteria: serology.

Main treatments: penicillin (depot injection); if allergic to penicillin, use erythromycin, clarithromycin or tetracycline. Contact tracing.

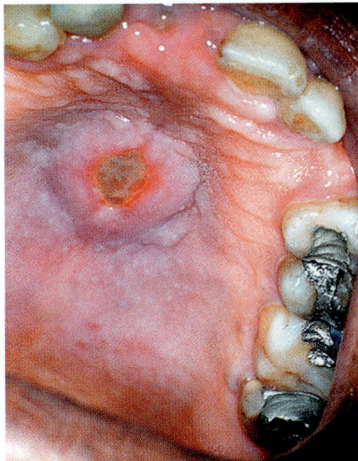

Figure 3.81 Intraoral lesion: ulceration of a gumma in tertiary syphilis.

Soreness/ulcers (continued)

Tuberculosis

Uncommon generally; but seen mainly in alcoholics, diabetics, patients with immune defects (including HIV infection), and particularly in groups from the developing world (e.g. Asian, African). One-third of the world population is infected.

Typical orofacial symptoms and signs: ulceration or lump – usually single chronic ulcer on dorsum of tongue associated with (post-primary) pulmonary infection (Figure 3.82).

Main oral sites affected: tongue, palate, gingivae.

Aetiopathogenesis: mycobacteria: usually *M. tuberculosis*, but rarely atypical mycobacteria (non-tuberculous mycobacteria), e.g. *M. avium-intracellulare*, *M. scrofulaceum*, *M. kansasii*, especially in HIV infection.

Gender predominance: none.

Age predominance: adult.

Extraoral possible lesions: cervical nodes, pulmonary.

Main associated conditions: HIV/AIDS patients commonly infected, especially if from developing world.

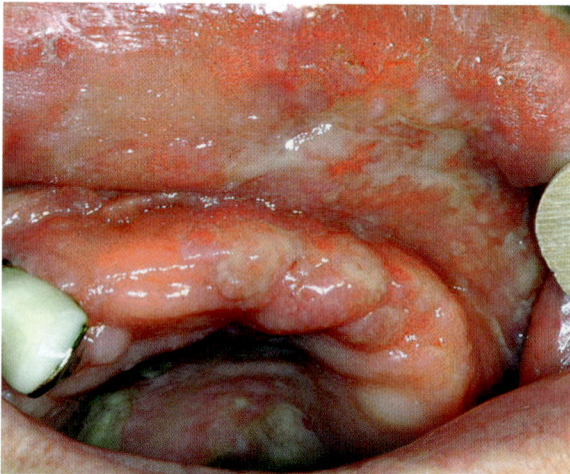

Figure 3.82 Intraoral lesion: extensive tuberculous ulceration.

Differential diagnosis: other causes of mouth ulcers, especially syphilis and carcinoma.

Investigations: lesional biopsy; sputum culture; chest radiography.

Main diagnostic criteria: clinical, imaging, histology.

Main treatments: combination antimicrobial chemotherapy. TB may be multi-drug resistant (MDR-TB) or have extended drug resistance (XDR-TB).

Gastrointestinal disorders

Oral lesions may affect people with coeliac disease, or inflammatory bowel disease (IBD) – a collective term for diseases that cause inflammation in the intestines and which encompasses the spectrum of disease seen in Crohn disease and ulcerative colitis (UC).

Coeliac disease (CD: gluten-sensitive enteropathy; coeliac sprue, nontropical sprue)

Most common genetic disease in Europe; approaches 1% in some populations.

Typical orofacial symptoms and signs: variably ulceration, glossitis, angular stomatitis, enamel hypoplasia (Figure 3.83).

Main oral sites affected: any.

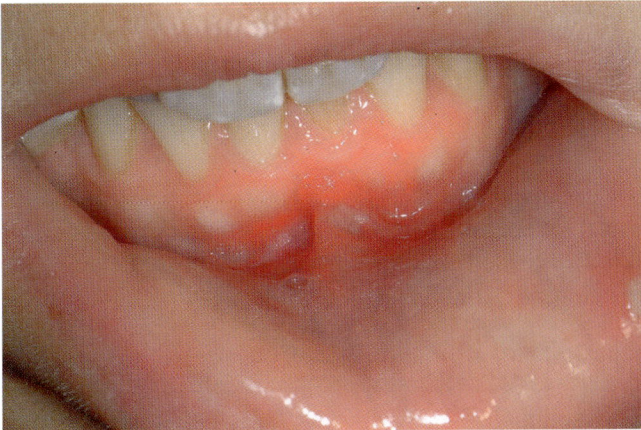

Figure 3.83 Intraoral lesion: aphthous-like ulceration in coeliac disease (gluten-sensitive enteropathy).

Soreness/ulcers (continued)

Aetiopathogenesis: genetic background of HLA-DQw2 or DRw3; a hypersensitivity or toxic reaction of the small intestine mucosa to the gliadin component of gluten (prolamine), a group of proteins found in all forms of wheat and related grains (rye, barley, triticale) causing destruction of jejunal villi (villous atrophy) and inflammation, leading to malabsorption.

Gender predominance: none.

Age predominance: none, but severe cases present at weaning.

Extraoral possible lesions: one of the great mimics in medicine, coeliac disease may present at any age with malabsorption (leading to growth retardation, vitamin and mineral deficiencies that may result in anaemia, osteomalacia, bleeding tendencies and neurological disorders), abdominal pain, steatorrhoea and behavioural changes. Intestinal lymphomas arise in about 6% of individuals.

Main associated conditions: other autoimmune disorders including Sjögren syndrome, food sensitivities, or lactose intolerance.

Differential diagnosis: other causes of ulcers, angular stomatitis and glossitis.

Investigations: serum antibody screening – transglutaminase; full blood count (ferritin, vitamin B_{12} and folate levels); stool examination; digestion/absorption tests include lactose tolerance and D-xylose tests. Endoscopic biopsy of jejunal mucosa.

Main diagnostic criteria: serum transglutaminase, and jejunal histology.

Main treatments: rectify nutritional deficiencies, and a gluten-free diet for life.

Crohn disease (see also Orofacial granulomatosis, page 196)
Uncommon.

Typical orofacial symptoms and signs: lip or facial persistent painless swelling; mucosal cobblestoning or tags, gingival swelling, or ulcers – typically solitary, persistent and ragged with hyperplastic margins (Figures 3.84-3.87). Mouth ulcers can be due to Crohn disease itself, secondary to folate or other deficiency, or coincidentally associated.

Main oral sites affected: lips, buccal mucosa, gingivae.

Aetiopathogenesis: susceptibility related to the *CARD 15* gene, or autophagy gene *ATG16L1*, which may hinder the ability to resist bacteria. Possible microorganisms involved include *Mycobacterium avium* subspecies *paratuberculosis*, or *Escherichia coli* strains.

Figure 3.84 Intraoral lesions: Crohn disease showing mucosal tags.

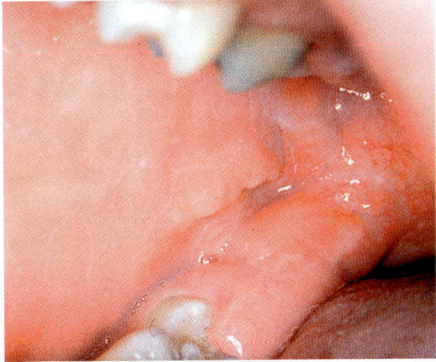

Figure 3.85 Intraoral lesions: Crohn disease showing mucosal tags and ulceration.

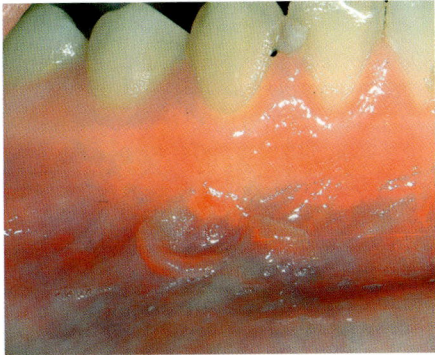

Figure 3.86 Intraoral lesions: Crohn disease showing gingival erythema and swelling.

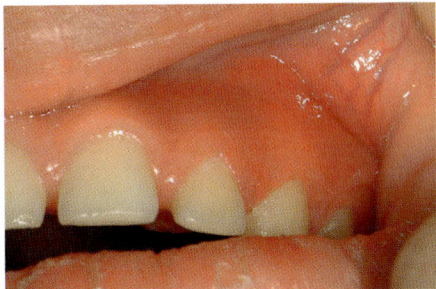

Soreness/ulcers (continued)

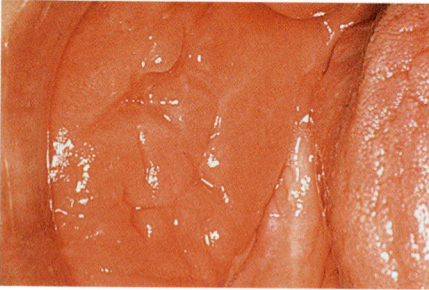

Figure 3.87 Intraoral lesions: Crohn disease showing mucosal 'cobblestoning'.

Gender predominance: none.

Age predominance: young adults.

Extraoral possible lesions: can affect any part of gastrointestinal tract from top to tail (mouth to anus) but especially the ileocaecal region, typically with ulceration, fissuring and fibrosis of the wall. Complications include weight loss, gastrointestinal obstruction, fistulas, perianal fissures, abscesses, arthralgia, sclerosing cholangitis, renal stones or infections and a predisposition to large bowel carcinoma comparable with that in ulcerative colitis, and a slight predisposition to small bowel carcinoma.

Main associated conditions: as above.

Differential diagnosis: other causes of mouth ulcers, especially malignant lesions or chronic bacterial infections. Also from ulcerative colitis, tuberculosis, ischaemic colitis, infections, infestations such as giardiasis, and lymphoma.

Investigations: blood count; serum potassium, zinc and albumin (usually depressed); erythrocyte sedimentation rate (raised), C-reactive protein (raised) and seromucoid; faecal calprotectin; white cell scan; abdominal plain-film and contrast radiography; ultrasound and MRI; and endoscopy (sigmoidoscopy, colonoscopy) with biopsy.

Main diagnostic criteria: biopsy; blood picture; gastrointestinal results.

Main treatments: topical or intralesional corticosteroids; systemic or possibly topical sulfasalazine, biological response modifiers such as infliximab.

At least some cases of OFG represent latent Crohn disease.

Ulcerative colitis

Uncommon.

Typical orofacial symptoms and signs: mucosal pustules (pyostomatitis vegetans) or irregular chronic ulcers (Figure 3.88) can be associated with ulcerative colitis, or may be secondary to anaemia due to chronic bowel haemorrhage.

Main oral sites affected: any.

Aetiopathogenesis: unknown but autoimmunity, diet, sulphate-reducing bacteria, drugs such as isotretinoin, and a genetic basis have been suggested.

Gender predominance: none.

Age predominance: adults.

Extraoral possible lesions: persistent diarrhoea, frequently painless with blood and mucus. In severe cases: iron deficiency anaemia, weight loss, arthralgia, conjunctivitis, uveitis, iritis, finger clubbing, sacroileitis, erythema nodosum, pyoderma gangrenosum, primary sclerosing cholangitis, gallstones, renal calculi and thromboembolism.

Main associated conditions: predisposition to colorectal carcinoma.

Differential diagnosis: other causes of mouth ulcers, particularly Crohn disease.

Investigations: biopsy; full blood picture; erythrocyte sedimentation rate/C-reactive protein; sigmoidoscopy; colonoscopy; barium enema.

Main diagnostic criteria: raised erythrocyte sedimentation rate/C-reactive protein, imaging and histology.

Main treatments: haematinics for any secondary deficiencies; topical corticosteroids (corticosteroid enemas) may be helpful; sulfasalazine.

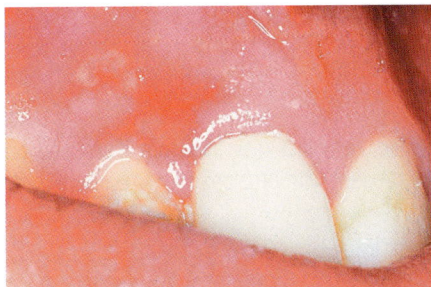

Figure 3.88 Intraoral lesion: ulceration in pyostomatitis vegetans in ulcerative colitis.

Soreness/ulcers (continued)

Skin disorders

Epidermolysis bullosa

Epidermolysis bullosa (EB) is a group of rare heritable mechanobullous disorders characterized by skin cutaneous basement membrane zone (BMZ) fragility.

Typical orofacial symptoms and signs: in EB simplex there are mainly skin blisters after trauma, which heal without scars and oral lesions are rare, but the junctional and dystrophic forms can present both skin and mouth bullae in neonates, which heal slowly and scar (Figures 3.89, 3.90). Some die; others improve slowly.

Main oral sites affected: any.

Aetiopathogenesis: genetic mostly, including various autosomal dominant (relatively benign) and recessive (more severe) forms. Inherited EB may be separated into three general types based upon the area of separation of the blister: (a) the simplex (epidermal); (b) the junctional (basement membrane zone); and (c) the dystrophic (dermal). Each type has many variants. An acquired form has also been described (EB acquisita).

Gender predominance: none.

Age predominance: from early age.

Extraoral possible lesions: skin blistering.

Main associated conditions: none.

Differential diagnosis: other vesiculobullous disorders.

Investigations: family history; biopsy to exclude other blistering diseases.

Main diagnostic criteria: family history; histology.

Main treatments: avoid trauma. Antibiotics for skin lesions. Phenytoin may benefit some. Corticosteroids are possibly helpful.

Erythema multiforme (see page 188)

Lichen planus

Lichen planus usually causes white lesions and is therefore discussed on page 243. However, it can often present with erosions.

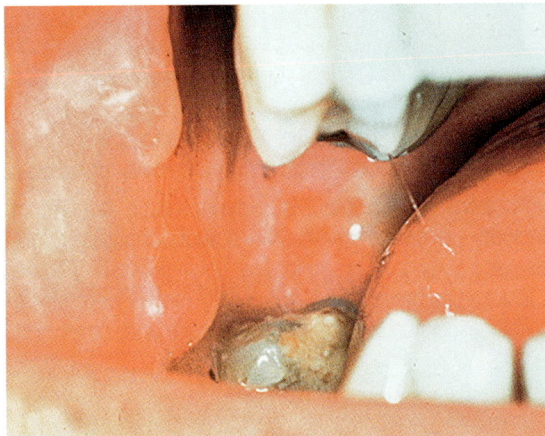

Figure 3.89 Intraoral lesions: blisters and ulceration in epidermolysis bullosa.

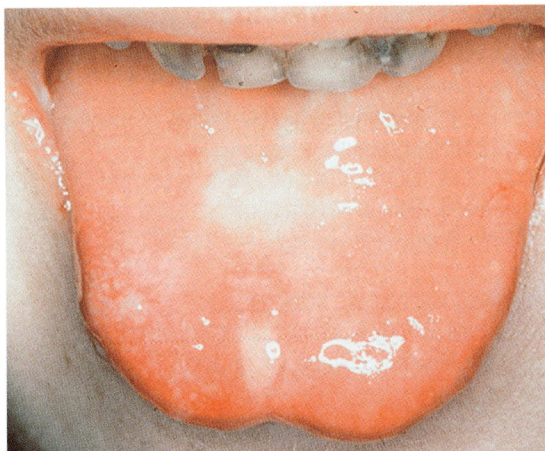

Figure 3.90 Intraoral lesions: scarring and depapillation from ulceration in epidermolysis bullosa.

Soreness/ulcers (continued)

Lupus erythematosus (see also Discoid lupus erythematosus, page 186)

Uncommon. Both discoid (DLE) and systemic (SLE) can affect the mouth, and oral lesions can precede other manifestations in a minority of patients.

Typical orofacial symptoms and signs: DLE: characteristic features of intraoral lesions include – central erythema, white spots or papules, radiating white striae at margins and peripheral telangiectasia (Figures 3.91–3.93). SLE: lesions like those in DLE but usually more severe ulceration. SLE may also be associated with Sjögren syndrome and, rarely, TMJ arthritis.

Main oral sites affected: any.

Aetiopathogenesis: unknown. Connective tissue disease (autoimmune).

Gender predominance: female.

Age predominance: adult.

Extraoral possible lesions: skin rash.

Main associated conditions: SLE is a multisystem disorder that is a great mimic of other disorders and can manifest in most tissues/organs, especially heart, joints, lungs, blood vessels, liver, kidney and CNS. Raynaud and Sjögren syndromes are often associated.

Differential diagnosis: DLE: differentiate from other causes of mouth ulcers, and especially from SLE, lichen planus and leukoplakia.

SLE: differentiate from other causes of mouth ulcers, especially DLE.

Investigations: biopsy; blood picture; autoantibodies, especially crithidial (double-stranded DNA). Antinuclear factors are present in SLE, not DLE.

Main diagnostic criteria: autoantibodies; histology.

Main treatments: DLE – topical corticosteroids (rarely systemic); SLE – systemic corticosteroids, azathioprine, chloroquine or gold.

Pemphigoid

There are several forms of pemphigoid but the forms that affect the mouth are termed mucous membrane pemphigoid. Not an uncommon condition; the cause is immunological, and not thought to be inherited or infectious. It occasionally affects the skin, eyes, genitals or other sites.

Figure 3.91 Skin lesion of lupus erythematosus.

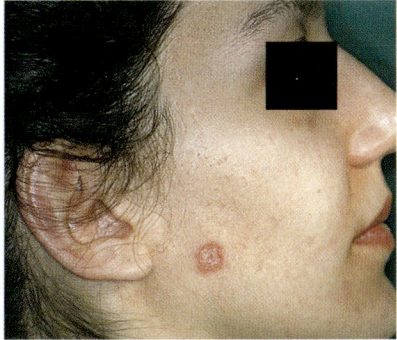

Figure 3.92 Intraoral lesion: white lesion and ulceration of lupus erythematosus.

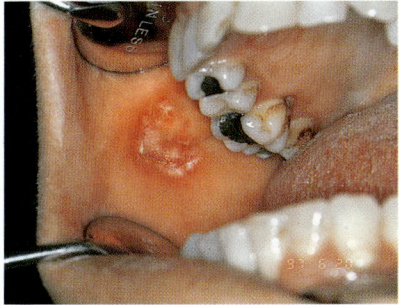

Figure 3.93 Intraoral lesion: white lesion of lupus erythematosus. Such lesions may mimic lichen planus.

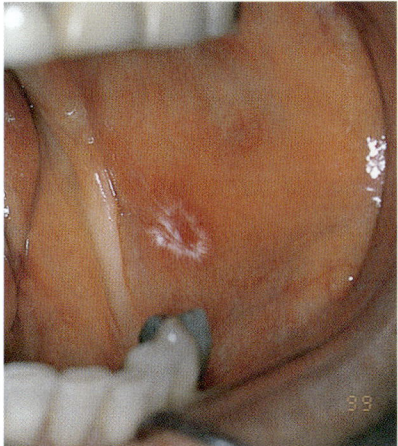

Soreness/ulcers (continued)

Pemphigoid must not be confused with the more serious *pemphigus*.

Typical orofacial symptoms and signs: blisters (sometimes blood-filled) can present anywhere, but especially at sites of trauma (Figures 3.94–3.99). Nikolsky sign may be positive (gentle trauma in an unaffected area causing blister formation). Ulcers: may heal with scarring. 'Desquamative gingivitis' is common.

Main oral sites affected: palate, gingivae.

Aetiopathogenesis: autoimmune. It is rarely caused by drugs (e.g. furosemide) or other agents.

Gender predominance: female.

Age predominance: middle age or older.

Extraoral possible lesions: conjunctival lesions – leading to impaired sight (entropion or symblepharon); laryngeal lesions – may lead to stenosis; skin lesions – blisters rarely (unlike bullous pemphigoid which rarely affects the mouth), eczematous-like lesions.

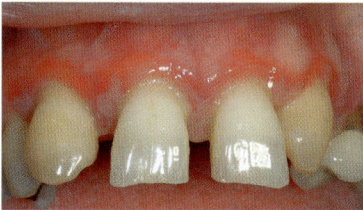

Figure 3.94 Intraoral lesion: desquamation, erosion and ulceration in pemphigoid.

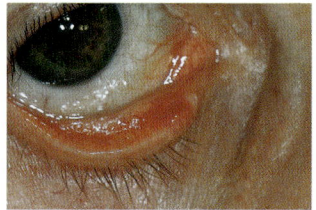

Figure 3.95 Conjunctival pemphigoid with shortening of fornix.

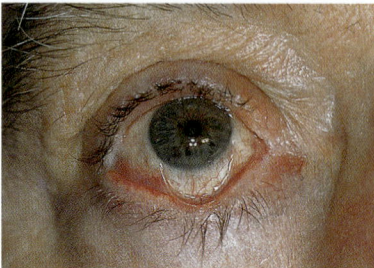

Figure 3.96 Conjunctival pemphigoid with symblepharon.

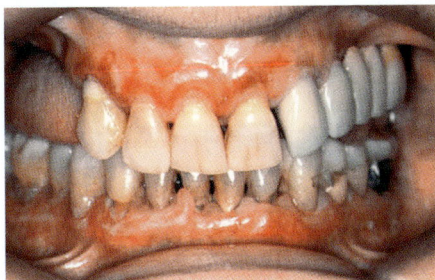

Figure 3.97 Intraoral lesion: pemphigoid; desquamative gingivitis the main cause of chronically sore gingivae.

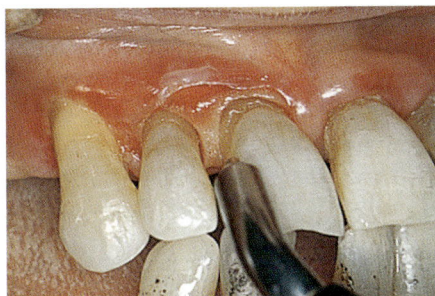

Figure 3.98 Intraoral lesion: pemphigoid; Nikolsky sign.

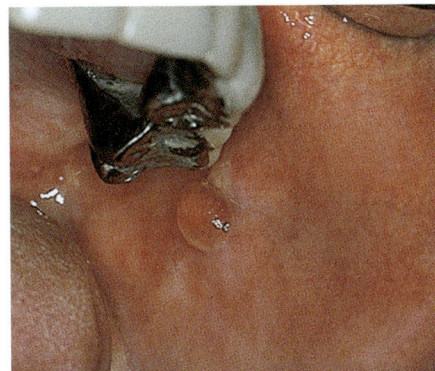

Figure 3.99 Intraoral lesion: pemphigoid; blister.

Soreness/ulcers (continued)

Main associated conditions: some subtypes (anti-laminin 332) are associated with internal malignant disease.

Differential diagnosis: other causes of mouth ulcers, especially pemphigus and localized oral purpura.

Investigations: biopsy.

Main diagnostic criteria: biopsy – subepithelial split, including immunostaining (C3 and IgG, IgA at basement membrane). Direct immunofluorescence (DIF) and salt-split skin indirect immunofluorescence (IIF).

Main treatments: potent topical corticosteroids or systemic corticosteroids with or without immunosuppressants or dapsone.

Pemphigus

Rare but potentially lethal. An immunological disease, the reaction damaging the skin and mucosae. It affects the mouth, skin and other sites. It is most commonly seen in persons from around the Mediterranean but is not usually inherited.

There are several variants, the most common being pemphigus vulgaris, which is mainly a disease of people from Asia or around the Mediterranean, and Ashkenazi Jews.

A rare pemphigus variant called paraneoplastic pemphigus is associated with malignant tumours (especially chronic lymphocytic leukaemia and non-Hodgkin lymphomas), typically causing extensive oral lesions with almost constant involvement of the lips with crusted lesions.

Typical orofacial symptoms and signs: oral lesions are most common in pemphigus vulgaris and often precede skin lesions. Blisters anywhere on the mucosa rupture rapidly to leave ragged red lesions followed by erosions and ulceration (Figures 3.100, 3.101). Nikolsky sign is positive.

Main oral sites affected: palate, gingivae or any traumatized area.

Aetiopathogenesis: autoimmune – circulating autoantibodies to desmoglein of epithelial intercellular substance. Antibodies to desmoglein 3 cause oral lesions and to desmoglein 1 cause skin lesions. Pemphigus is rarely caused by drugs (e.g. penicillamine) or other agents.

Gender predominance: female.

Age predominance: older adults.

Extraoral possible lesions: skin lesions are large flaccid blisters especially where there is trauma. Lesions may affect other mucosa.

Figure 3.100 Intraoral lesion: ulceration in pemphigus. There is a red lesion of early pemphigus surrounded by mucosa which is necrotic and appears whitish.

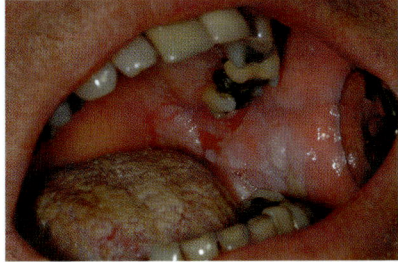

Figure 3.101 Intraoral lesion: ragged red lesions leading eventually to ulceration in pemphigus.

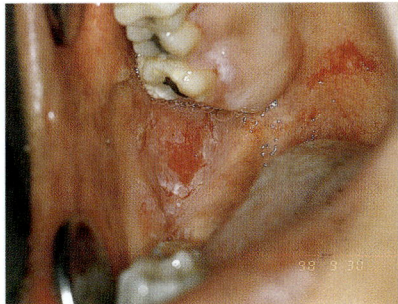

Main associated conditions: rarely, myasthenia gravis or thymoma.

Differential diagnosis: other causes of mouth ulcers, especially mucous membrane pemphigoid and erythema multiforme.

Investigations: biopsy and serology; DIF and IIF.

Main diagnostic criteria: histology to show acantholysis, including direct immunofluorescence to show IgG and C3 binding to intercellular attachments of epithelial cells. Serology (antibodies to epithelial intercellular substance), using enzyme-linked immunosorbent assay (ELISA) for anti-desmoglein 3 and 1.

Soreness/ulcers (continued)

Main treatments: largely based on systemic immunosuppression using systemic corticosteroids plus mycophenolate mofetil, or azathioprine or cyclophosphamide. In recalcitrant cases, intravenous immunoglobulins or rituximab.

Malignancy (see page 269)

Most malignant oral ulcers are squamous cell carcinomas but other primary tumours can be antral (rarely), or of salivary glands, lymphomas, Kaposi sarcoma or metastases.

Local causes

Ulcers of local cause are common but rarely present for care as they are usually self-limiting and the aetiology often quite obvious to the patient. Causes may include:

- Trauma, including from orthodontic appliances, dentures (Figures 3.102, 3.103) or interdental wiring, ulceration of lingual fraenum caused by repeated coughing or cunnilingus, and self-induced lesions due to cheek biting (a neurotic habit) and in some rare syndromes. Other causes to be considered include child abuse, or pterygoid ulcers of palate in neonates (Bednar's aphthae).
- Burns (from electrical injury, heat or cold, or chemicals) or radiation (mucositis).

Most ulcers of local cause resolve with use of antiseptics such as aqueous chlorhexidine. Failure to resolve within 3 weeks mandates biopsy.

Aphthae (recurrent aphthous stomatitis – RAS)

Common. Children *may* inherit ulcers from parents.

Aphthous ulcers are not thought to be infectious. The cause is not known but some follow use of toothpaste with sodium dodecyl sulphate, certain foods/drinks, or stopping smoking. Some vitamin or other deficiencies or conditions may predispose to ulcers. No long-term consequences are known.

Typical orofacial symptoms and signs: recurrent ulcers usually lasting from 1 week to 1 month. There are three distinct clinical patterns:

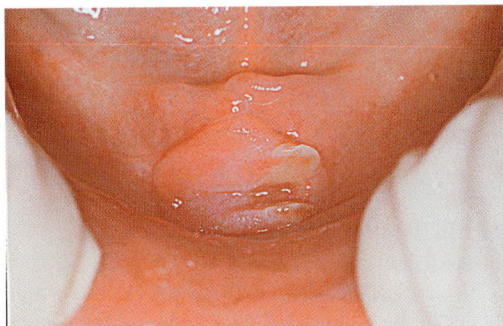

Figure 3.102 Intraoral lesion: ulceration from overextended denture flange.

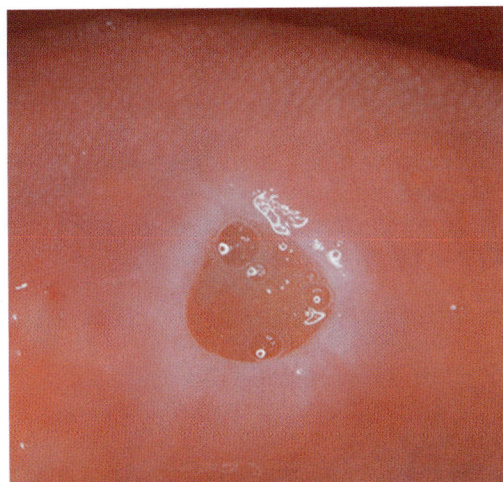

Figure 3.103 Intraoral lesion: ulceration from chronic trauma; note white border.

Soreness/ulcers (continued)

- Minor aphthae – small ulcers (<4 mm) on mobile mucosa, healing within 14 days, no scarring (Figure 3.104).
- Major aphthae – large ulcers (may >1 cm), any site including dorsum of tongue and hard palate, healing within 1–3 months, with scarring (Figure 3.105) .
- Herpetiform ulcers – multiple minute ulcers that coalesce to produce ragged ulcers (Figure 3.106).

Main oral sites affected: buccal vestibule, ventrum of tongue, floor of mouth.

Aetiopathogenesis: immunological changes are detectable but there is no reliable evidence of autoimmune disease or any classical immunological reactions. Aphthae may be due to changes in cell-mediated immune responses and cross-reactivity with *Streptococcus sanguinis*. Underlying predisposing factors are seen in a minority with aphthous-like ulcers: haematinic (iron, folate or vitamin B_{12}) deficiency in about 10%, relationship with luteal phase of menstruation (rarely), 'stress', food allergies (possibly) and smoking cessation.

Gender predominance: none.

Age predominance: onset usually in childhood or adolescence.

Extraoral possible lesions: none by definition.

Main associated conditions: none; if other manifestations are present, the ulcers are termed 'aphthous-like' ulcers.

Differential diagnosis: other causes of mouth ulcers, especially coeliac disease, Crohn disease, Behçet syndrome, autoinflammatory disorders or HIV/AIDS.

Investigations: full blood picture, haematinic assays, transglutaminase and erythrocyte sedimentation rate, to exclude systemic diseases.

Main diagnostic criteria: history of recurrences and clinical features. There is no immunological test of value.

Main treatments: treat any underlying predisposing factors. Treat aphthae with chlorhexidine 0.2% aqueous mouthwash or systemic vitamin B_{12}, or topical corticosteroids (hydrocortisone hemisuccinate oromucosal tablets or beclomethasone as a mouthwash or fluocinonide gel), or amlexanox. In adults only, tetracycline (doxycycline) rinses. Rarely, other potent topical corticosteroids (e.g. betamethasone, clobetasol) may be needed. Specialists may offer systemic immunomodulatory agents such as steroids, colchicine or thalidomide (not if there is any possibility of pregnancy).

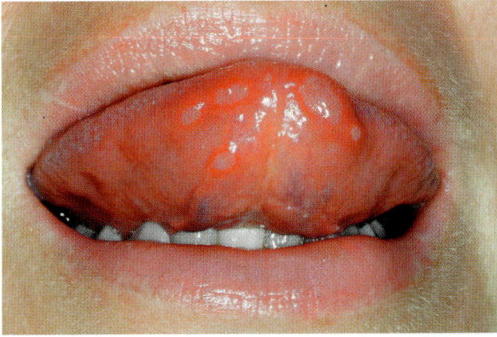

Figure 3.104 Intraoral lesion: ulceration of minor aphthae (small and of only a week or so duration).

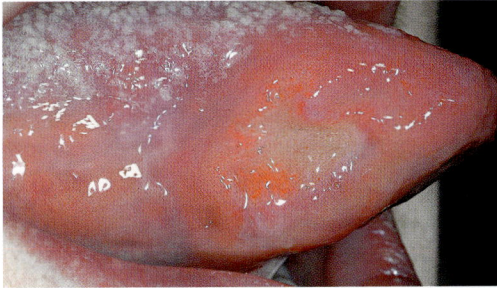

Figure 3.105 Intraoral lesion: ulceration of major aphthae (large and persistent for several weeks). These tend to heal with scarring.

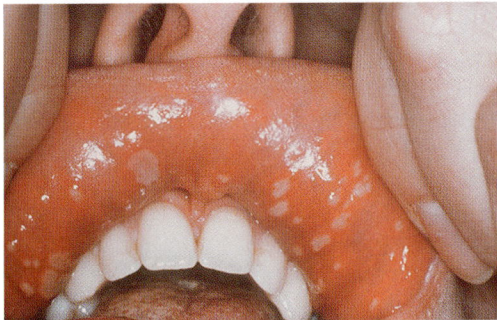

Figure 3.106 Intraoral lesion: ulceration of herpetiform ulcers (some ulcers have coalesced).

Soreness/ulcers (continued)

Aphthous-like ulcers

This term is applied to recurrent oral ulcers that may clinically mimic aphthae but are seen in patients with definable systemic immune diseases such as:

- Behçet syndrome (Figure 3.107).
- Gastrointestinal disorders; coeliac disease or Crohn disease (Figure 3.108).
- Autoinflammatory conditions.
- Immune defects such as HIV/AIDS and cyclic neutropenia.

Behçet syndrome

Rare: most common in peoples from around the area of the old Silk Road of Marco Polo, and particularly in people from Japan, Korea and Turkey.

Typical orofacial symptoms and signs: recurrent ulcers often mimicking major aphthae.

Main oral sites affected: palate.

Aetiopathogenesis: immunological changes resemble those in aphthae. Immune complexes, possibly with herpes simplex virus, may be implicated in persons with specific HLA associations (B5101).

Gender predominance: male.

Age predominance: adults.

Extraoral possible lesions: non-specific features which may precede mucosal ulceration include sore throats, myalgias, migratory erythralgias, malaise, anorexia, weight loss, weakness, headache, sweating, lymphadenopathy, large joint arthralgia and pain in substernal and temporal regions. Multi-system disorder may include:

- eye disease: reduced visual acuity, uveitis, retinal vasculitis
- skin disease: acneiform rashes; pustules at venepuncture sites (pathergy); pseudofolliculitis and erythema nodosum (tender red nodules over shins)
- joint disease: arthralgia of large joints
- neurological disease: headache, psychiatric, motor or sensory manifestations; meningoencephalitis, cerebral infarction (stroke), psychosis, cranial nerve palsies, cerebellar and spinal cord lesions
- others: genital ulcers, thromboses, colitis, renal disease, etc.

Main associated conditions: as above.

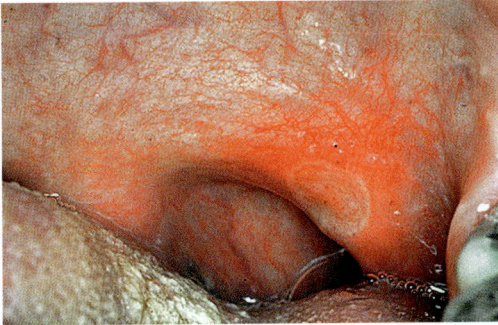

Figure 3.107 Intraoral lesion: aphthous-like ulceration in Behçet syndrome.

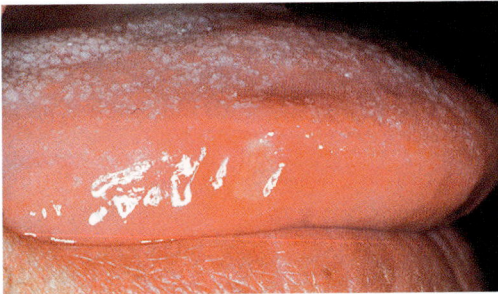

Figure 3.108 Intraoral lesion: aphthous-like ulceration in vitamin B_{12} deficiency.

Differential diagnosis: other oculomucocutaneous disorders, especially erythema multiforme, syphilis and Reiter syndrome (reactive arthritis), and inflammatory bowel disease.

Investigations: erythrocyte sedimentation rate, C-reactive protein, full blood picture, HLA typing.

Main diagnostic criteria: there is no immunological test of value. Clinical features – mouth ulcers (at least three episodes in a year) plus two or more of:

- genital ulcers
- ocular lesions
- CNS lesions
- skin lesions and pathergy.

Soreness/ulcers (continued)

Main treatments: oral ulcers: treat as for aphthae (above). Specialists may offer systemic immunosuppression using colchicine, corticosteroids, azathioprine, ciclosporin, dapsone or thalidomide (not if there is any possibility of pregnancy).

Drugs (see also pages 337)

Mouth ulcers can be caused by burns from drugs left in the mouth, or by various other mechanisms, but often the mechanism is unclear. Drugs that can cause ulceration (Figure 3.109) include those that are:

- cytotoxics – ulcers or mucositis can follow the use of any chemotherapeutic agent
- bone marrow suppressants e.g. drugs such as antithyroid agents
- drugs that cause lichenoid reactions – antimalarials, antihypertensives.

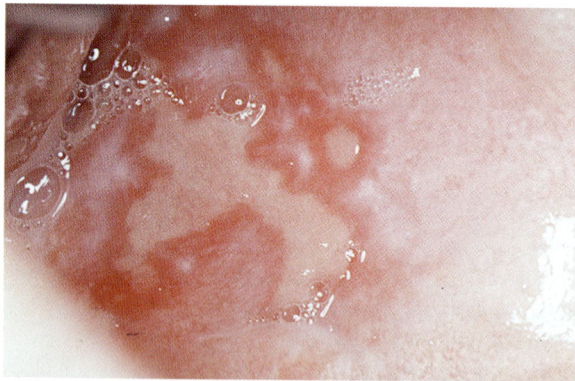

Figure 3.109 Intraoral lesion: erosions in the buccal mucosa caused by a drug reaction to penicillamine.

White lesions

Cancer

Keratinizing carcinomas may appear as oral white lesions *ab initio* or may occasionally arise in other oral white lesions, notably in some keratoses, dyskeratosis congenita, oral submucous fibrosis, or in lichen planus.

Candidosis

Thrush (acute pseudomembranous candidosis) Common but rare in healthy patients.

Typical orofacial symptoms and signs: white or creamy papules or plaques that can be wiped off to leave a red base (Figure 3.110).

Main oral sites affected: any.

Aetiopathogenesis: neonatal immature immune system; oral microflora disturbed by drugs (antibiotics, corticosteroids or those impairing salivation); hyposalivation; or immune defects, especially HIV/AIDS, immunosuppressive treatment, leukaemias, lymphomas and diabetes.

Gender predominance: none.

Age predominance: extremes of life.

Extraoral possible lesions: see aetiopathogenesis.

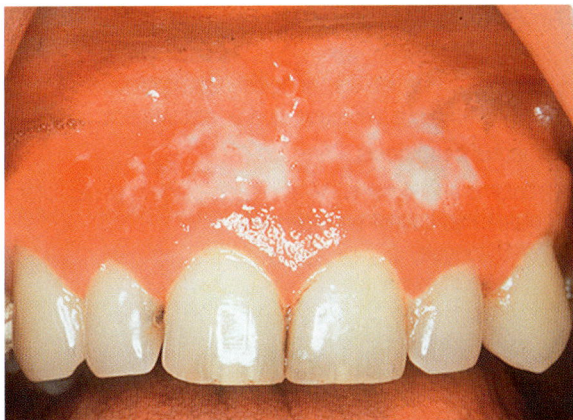

Figure 3.110 Intraoral lesion: white lesions of acute candidosis ('thrush') on erythematous background. These lesions will wipe off with a gauze swab.

White lesions (continued)

Main associated conditions: see aetiopathogenesis.

Differential diagnosis: mucosal sloughing, Koplik or Fordyce spots.

Investigations: cytologic smear with periodic acid Schiff (PAS) or Gram stain (hyphae); full blood picture.

Main diagnostic criteria: clinical.

Main treatments: treat predisposing cause. Antifungals: nystatin oral suspension or pastilles or miconazole gel or tablets or fluconazole tablets (in USA, clotrimazole troches).

Candidal leukoplakia (limited type) Common.

Typical orofacial symptoms and signs: leukoplakia, often speckled (Figures 3.111, 3.112). There is a higher malignant potential than many other leukoplakias.

Main oral sites affected: commissures and sometimes tongue.

Aetiopathogenesis: unclear – smoking predisposes.

Gender predominance: male.

Age predominance: adult.

Extraoral possible lesions: none.

Main associated conditions: none.

Differential diagnosis: lichen planus, leukoplakia, cheek biting.

Investigations: biopsy; blood picture.

Main diagnostic criteria: clinical and histology.

Main treatments: smoking cessation. Antifungals: nystatin oral suspension or pastilles; miconazole gel or tablets, or fluconazole tablets may help (in USA, clotrimazole troches). Remove (excision or cryosurgery).

Chronic mucocutaneous candidosis Rare.

Typical orofacial symptoms and signs: white or creamy plaques or persistent widespread leukoplakia that cannot be wiped off.

Main oral sites affected: tongue.

Aetiopathogenesis: genetic immune defect.

Gender predominance: none.

Age predominance: from infancy usually.

Extraoral possible lesions: cutaneous – nail and skin candidosis.

Main associated conditions: rarely familial multiple endocrinopathies, iron deficiency or thymoma.

Differential diagnosis: lichen planus, leukoplakia.

Figure 3.111 Intraoral lesion: white lesions of chronic candidosis (candidal leukoplakia).

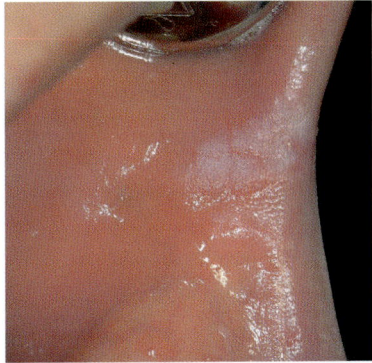

Figure 3.112 Intraoral lesion: white lesions of chronic candidosis (candidal leukoplakia).

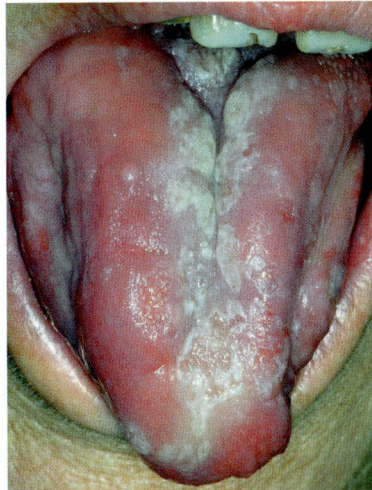

Investigations: family history; biopsy; blood picture; autoantibody; endocrine studies.

Main diagnostic criteria: clinical and histology.

Main treatments: treat predisposing cause. Smoking cessation. Antifungals: nystatin oral suspension or pastilles; miconazole gel or tablets, or fluconazole tablets may help (in USA, clotrimazole troches). Remove (excision or cryosurgery).

White lesions (continued)

Cheek biting (morsicatio buccarum)

Common.

Typical orofacial symptoms and signs: symptomless abrasion of superficial epithelium leaves whitish fragments on reddish background.

Main oral sites affected: invariably restricted to lower labial mucosa and/or buccal mucosa near occlusal line. The lesions may range from a linea alba on the buccal mucosae or/and lateral margins of tongue, through to definite cheek biting (Figures 3.113–3.117). May also be due to masseteric hypertrophy.

Aetiopathogenesis: anxious personality or anxiety neurosis (see also Frictional keratosis.

Gender predominance: female.

Age predominance: young adult.

Extraoral possible lesions: psychologically related disorders, e.g. temporomandibular pain-dysfunction syndrome. Rarely, self-mutilation is seen in psychiatric disorders, learning impairment or some rare syndromes.

Main associated conditions: none.

Differential diagnosis: other causes of white lesions, particularly cinnamon contact allergy and, rarely, white sponge naevus.

Investigations: none.

Main diagnostic criteria: clinical.

Main treatments: stop the habit if possible.

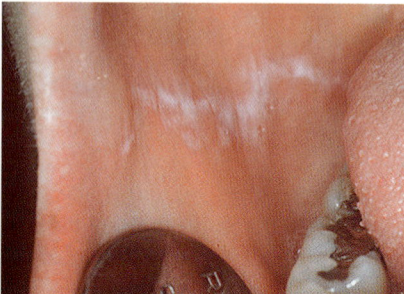

Figure 3.113 Intraoral lesion: white lesions from occlusal frictional trauma (linea alba).

Figure 3.114 Intraoral lesion: white lesions from cheek biting (morsicatio buccarum).

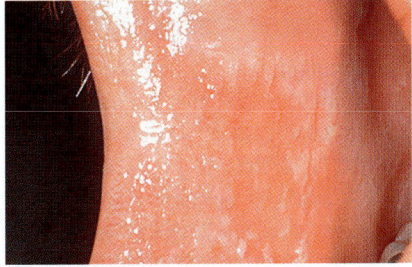

Figure 3.115 Intraoral lesion: white lesions from cheek biting can mimic white sponge naevus.

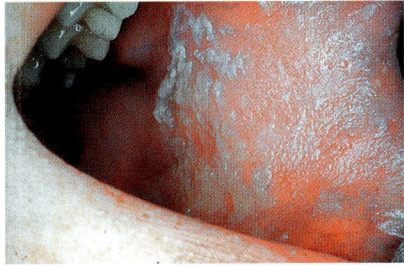

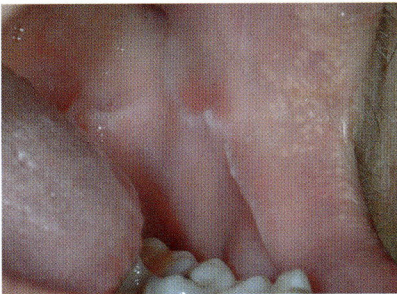

Figure 3.116 Intraoral lesion: white lesions from stress causing self-induced lesions (see also Figure 3.124). There are Fordyce spots at the commissure.

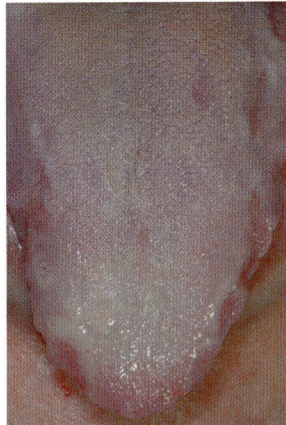

Figure 3.117 Intraoral lesion: white lesions from stress causing self-induced lesions.

White lesions (continued)

Leukoplakia

Hyperkeratotic white mucosal lesions of unknown cause. There are no specific histopathological connotations. Common. Leukoplakia is a potentially malignant disorder.

Typical orofacial symptoms and signs: symptomless white patches or plaques; most are smooth (homogeneous leukoplakias); some are warty (verrucous leukoplakia); some are mixed white and red lesions (speckled leukoplakias) (Figures 3.118–3.123). Malignant potential is:

- low in homogeneous leukoplakias
- higher in verrucous leukoplakias, and is
- highest in speckled leukoplakias.

The most important risk factors for malignant transformation are the site (location on the tongue and/or floor of the mouth) and presence of epithelial dysplasia.

Main oral sites affected: no special site predilection. Sulcus is mainly affected in presence of tobacco/betel quid chewing.

Aetiopathogenesis: most cases are idiopathic. Others are related to risk habits such as smoking, smokeless tobacco, alcohol, snuff-dipping, betel quid chewing.

Gender predominance: males.

Age predominance: older.

Extraoral possible lesions: see aetiopathogenesis.

Main associated conditions: those caused by lifestyle.

Differential diagnosis: other causes of white lesions.

Investigations: biopsy for epithelial dysplasia and carcinoma.

Main diagnostic criteria and treatments: in all, habits such as tobacco, alcohol and betel use should be stopped.

- *Idiopathic leukoplakias:* excision with scalpel or laser is recommended but this may not reduce transformation, and lesions may recur.
- *Frictional keratoses:* mainly affect occlusal line and on alveolar ridges, are homogeneous and resolve when irritation removed.
- *Snuff-dipping:* associated predominantly with verrucous keratoses which can progress to verrucous carcinoma. Excision is recommended.

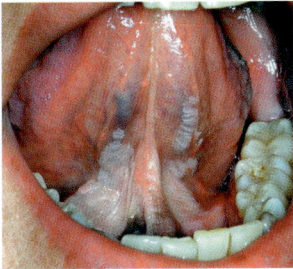

Figure 3.118 Intraoral lesion: white lesions of sublingual leukoplakia.

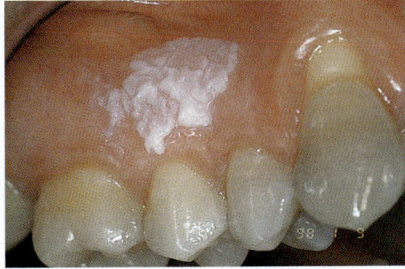

Figure 3.119 Intraoral lesion: white lesions of leukoplakia.

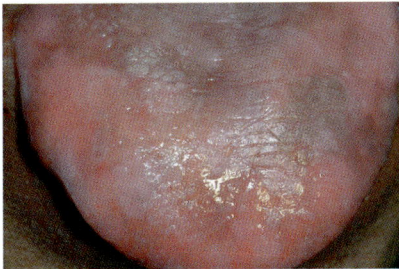

Figure 3.120 Intraoral lesion: white lesions of plaque-like lichen planus – difficult to distinguish from leukoplakia.

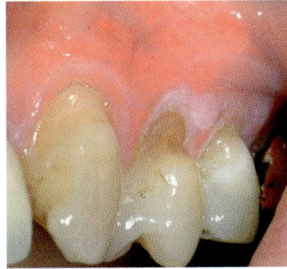

Figure 3.121 Intraoral lesion: white lesions of keratosis from friction of tooth-brushing (note abrasion).

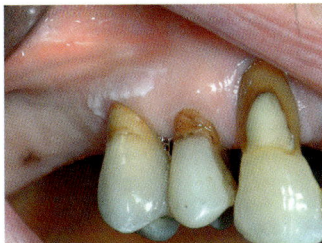

Figure 3.122 Intraoral lesion: white lesions of keratosis from friction of tooth-brushing (note abrasion).

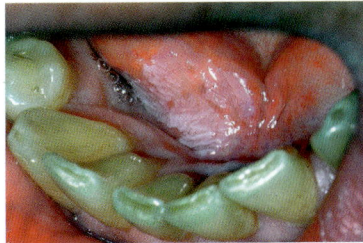

Figure 3.123 Intraoral lesion: white lesions of sublingual leukoplakia.

White lesions (continued)

- *Tobacco-related keratosis:* typically resolve on stopping the habit.
- *Candidal leukoplakia: C. albicans* can cause or colonize other keratoses, particularly in smokers, and is especially likely to form speckled leukoplakias at commissures. It may be dysplastic and have higher premalignant potential than some other keratoses. Candidal leukoplakias may respond to antifungals and stopping smoking.
- *Syphilitic leukoplakia:* especially on the dorsum of tongue, is a feature of tertiary syphilis but is rarely seen now. Malignant potential is high. Antimicrobials are indicated.
- *Hairy leukoplakia:* has a corrugated surface and mainly affects margins of the tongue almost exclusively. It is seen in the immunocompromised and is a complication of HIV infection and a predictor of those who will progress to full-blown AIDS. The condition appears to be benign, and self-limiting, or may respond to aciclovir.
- *Leukoplakia in chronic renal failure:* symmetrical soft keratosis may complicate chronic renal failure, but resolves after treatment by renal transplantation or dialysis.
- *Sublingual leukoplakia:* seen in the floor of the mouth/ventrum of tongue, they were formerly thought to be naevi (congenital) but, although of unknown aetiology, are now reported to have malignant transformation. Often homogeneous, there may be speckled areas. The surface has an 'ebbing tide' appearance. Opinions vary as to whether the lesion should be left undisturbed or removed surgically or by laser or cryoprobe.

Lichen planus (LP)

Common condition affecting stratified squamous epithelium (the mouth, skin, hair, nails or genitals) but the cause is unknown. Children do not usually inherit it from parents; it is not thought to be infectious but it is sometimes related to diabetes, drugs, dental fillings, or other conditions. Autoimmune conditions may occasionally be associated.

Typical orofacial symptoms and signs: lesions may be asymptomatic, especially if only white. Lesions tend to be bilateral and are occasionally hyperpigmented. They may include (Figures 3.124–3.135):

Figure 3.124 Intraoral lesions: white lesions and erosions of plaque-like lichen planus which mimics leukoplakia.

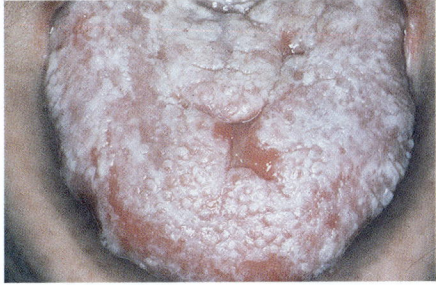

Figure 3.125 Skin lesions of lichen planus (purple, pruritic, papules).

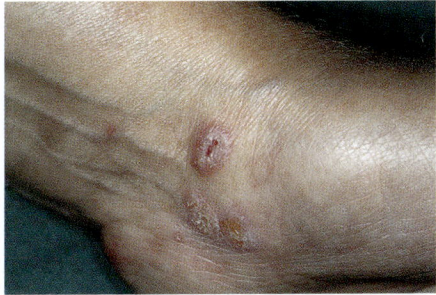

Figure 3.126 Intraoral lesions: white reticular lesions of lichen planus in the most common site affected.

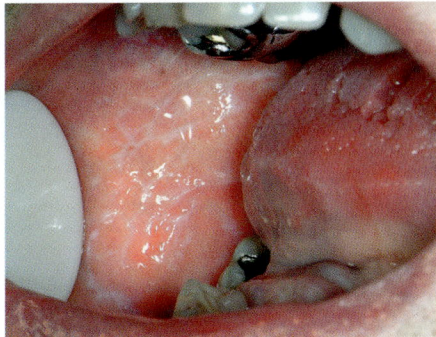

White lesions (continued)

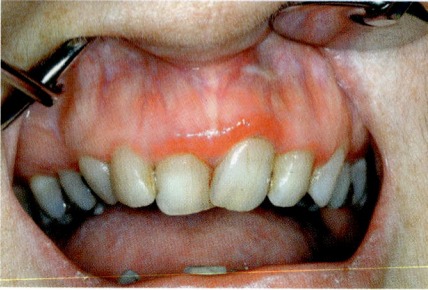

Figure 3.127 Intraoral lesions: white and red lesions and desquamative gingivitis of lichen planus.

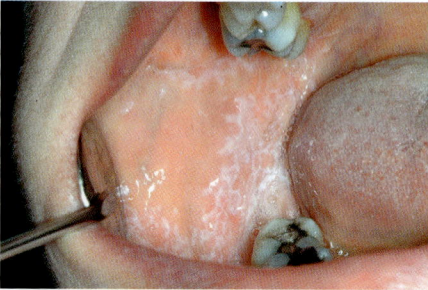

Figure 3.128 Intraoral lesions: white lesions of lichen planus.

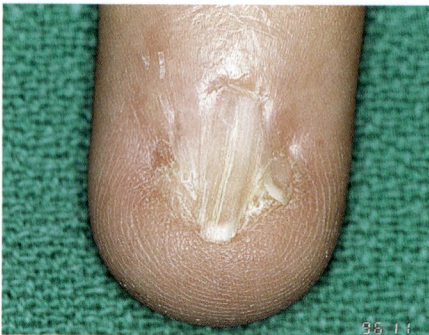

Figure 3.129 Nail lesions of lichen planus.

Figure 3.130 Intraoral lesions: white and red lesions of lichen planus.

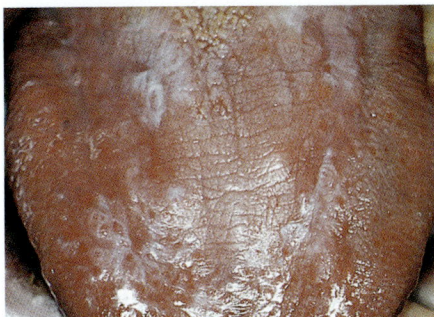

Figure 3.131 Intraoral lesions: white and red lesions of lichen planus.

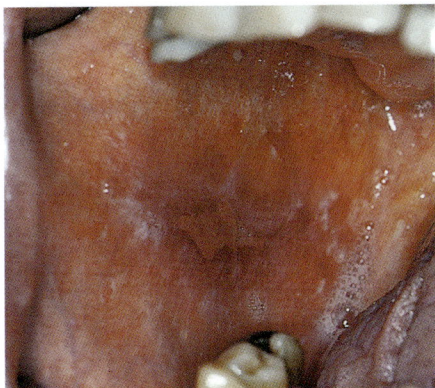

Figure 3.132 Intraoral lesions: white and red lesions of lichen planus.

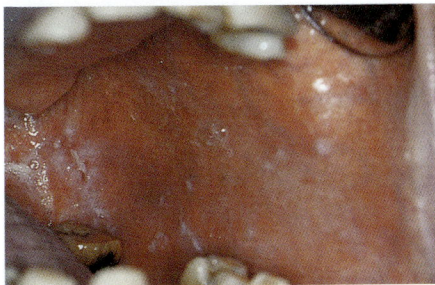

White lesions (continued)

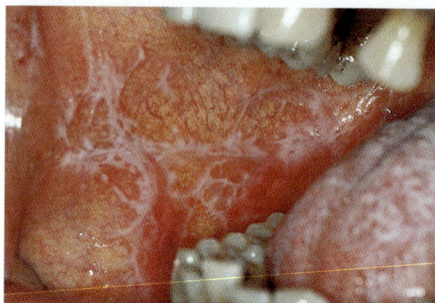

Figure 3.133 Intraoral lesions: white reticular lesions of lichen planus.

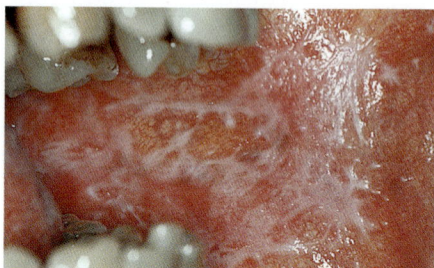

Figure 3.134 Intraoral lesions: white lesions of lichen planus.

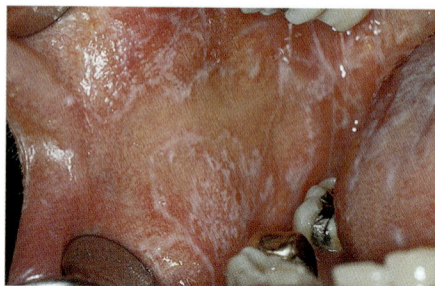

Figure 3.135 Intraoral lesions: white lesions of lichen planus.

- white lesions most commonly; reticular lesions are most often found but papular or plaque-like white lesions also
- red lesions of atrophic LP may cause soreness and also can simulate erythroplasia. LP can cause 'desquamative gingivitis'.
- erosions are irregular, persistent and painful, with a yellowish slough, and are often associated with other LP lesions.

Main oral sites affected: buccal mucosa, sometimes on the tongue or gingivae.

Aetiopathogenesis: usually no aetiological factor is identifiable. A minority are due to drugs (lichenoid lesions, graft-versus-host disease, liver disorders (e.g. HCV infection) or reactions to amalgam or gold.

Gender predominance: female.

Age predominance: middle age or older.

Extraoral possible lesions: skin rash: pruritic, polygonal, purplish papules predominantly on flexor surfaces of wrists, and shins, rarely on the face. Trauma may induce lesions (Koebner phenomenon). Genital lesions (similar to oral). Alopecia or nail deformities are seen occasionally.

Main associated conditions: rarely graft-versus-host disease, liver disorders (e.g. HCV infection), autoimmune disorders.

Differential diagnosis: other causes of white lesions and ulcers, especially DLE and keratoses.

Investigations: drug history; biopsy.

Main diagnostic criteria: clinical supported by histology.

Main treatments: asymptomatic: no treatment. Symptomatic: corticosteroids topically and, rarely, intralesionally or systemically. Other drugs such as retinoids, griseofulvin, ciclosporin or tacrolimus have not proved reliably superior, or may have adverse effects. There is a small malignant potential in LP (1–3% after 10 years).

Linea alba
Common.

Typical orofacial symptoms and signs: symptomless horizontal white raised linea keratosis.

Main oral sites affected: buccal mucosa and often lateral margin of tongue bilaterally.

White lesions (continued)

Aetiopathogenesis: trauma usually in a patient who clenches or grinds the teeth.
Gender predominance: none.
Age predominance: adult.
Extraoral possible lesions: masseteric hypertrophy in some.
Main associated conditions: attrition.
Differential diagnosis: cheek biting, lichen planus, leukoplakia.
Investigations: none.
Main diagnostic criteria: clinical features.
Main treatments: reassurance; relaxation therapy.

Measles
Rarely seen.

Typical orofacial symptoms and signs: Koplik spots – small white spots on oral mucosa during prodrome (Figure 3.136).
Main oral sites affected: buccal mucosa.
Aetiopathogenesis: measles virus.
Gender predominance: none.
Age predominance: children.
Extraoral possible lesions: rash – maculopapular; conjunctivitis, runny nose, cough; fever, malaise and anorexia.
Main associated conditions: none.
Differential diagnosis: thrush, Fordyce spots.
Investigations: none.
Main diagnostic criteria: clinical features; rising antibody titre confirmatory.
Main treatments: symptomatic (see herpes simplex).

Oral submucous faibrosis (OSMF)
Uncommon.

Typical orofacial symptoms and signs: tight vertical bands in buccal mucosa that may progress to severely restricted oral opening (Figure 3.137).
Main oral sites affected: buccal mucosa, sometimes palate or tongue.
Aetiopathogenesis: use of areca nuts (alone as paan, or with betel leaf and sometimes tobacco and spices in betel quid) and thus virtually only a disease of adults from the Indian subcontinent and SE Asia.

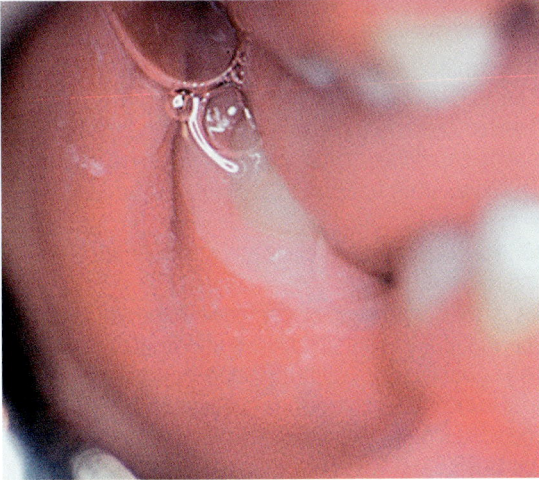

Figure 3.136 Intraoral lesion: white lesions of Koplik spots in measles prodrome.

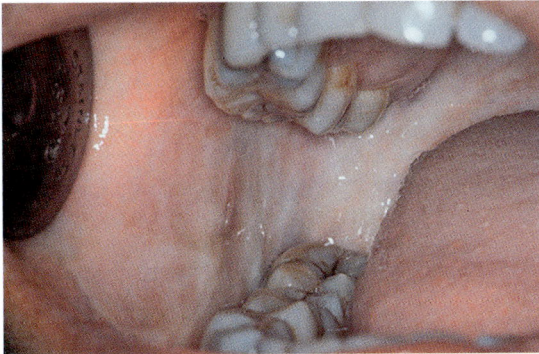

Figure 3.137 Intraoral lesion: oral submucous fibrosis showing pallor, banding and restricted oral opening.

White lesions (continued)

Gender predominance: female.

Age predominance: adult.

Extraoral possible lesions: can affect oesophagus, and can predispose to cancers in liver, mouth, oesophagus, stomach, prostate, cervix and lung.

Main associated conditions: often anaemia is present. Maybe other betel adverse effects.

Differential diagnosis: from scars, lichen planus and scleroderma.

Investigations: biopsy; haematology.

Main diagnostic criteria: clinical features; biopsy; haematology.

Main treatments: stop use of areca nut and chillies and tobacco. Asymptomatic: observe only. Symptomatic with restricted opening: exercises, expansion appliances to increase oral opening, intralesional corticosteroids, surgery. Possibly penicillamine or interferon. Malignant potential – carcinoma possibly in up to 25%.

White sponge naevus

Rare genetic condition.

Typical orofacial symptoms and signs: asymptomatic, diffuse, bilateral white lesions with shaggy or spongy, wrinkled surface (Figure 3.138).

Main oral sites affected: buccal mucosa, but sometimes tongue, floor of mouth, or elsewhere.

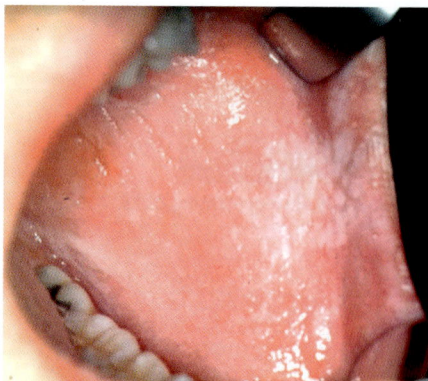

Figure 3.138 Intraoral lesion: white lesions of white sponge naevus (extends beyond occlusal area).

Aetiopathogenesis: autosomal dominant, but family history may be negative.

Gender predominance: none.

Age predominance: from infancy but often recognized later in life.

Extraoral possible lesions: may involve the pharynx, oesophagus, nose, genitals and anus.

Main associated conditions: none.

Differential diagnosis: other white lesions, especially cheek biting.

Investigations: biopsy.

Main diagnostic criteria: clinical features; histology is confirmatory.

Main treatments: reassurance.

Intraoral soft tissue lumps and swellings

Carcinoma (see page 269)

Denture-induced hyperplasia (denture granuloma)

Common.

Typical orofacial symptoms and signs: painless lump that does not enlarge, has a smooth pink surface, and lies parallel with alveolar ridge and may be grooved by denture margins (Figures 3.139, 3.140).

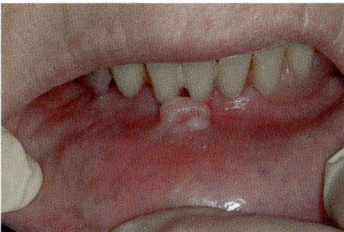

Figure 3.139 Intraoral lesion: swelling of denture-induced hyperplasia (see Figure 3.140).

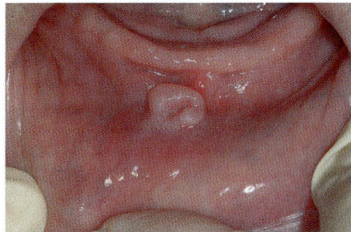

Figure 3.140 Intraoral lesion: swelling of denture-induced hyperplasia.

Intraoral soft tissue lumps and swellings (continued)

Main oral sites affected: anterior lower buccal sulcus.

Aetiopathogenesis: pressure from denture flange causes chronic irritation and hyperplastic response. It is usually related to lower complete denture.

Gender predominance: none.

Age predominance: middle age or older.

Extraoral possible lesions: none.

Main associated conditions: none.

Differential diagnosis: other causes of lumps, especially malignancy.

Investigations: biopsy (excision).

Main diagnostic criteria: usually the diagnosis is clear-cut if the lesion is in relation to denture flange. If ulcerated, it may mimic carcinoma (rarely).

Main treatments: excision biopsy to confirm diagnosis; relieve denture flange to prevent recurrence.

Fibrous nodule or lump ('fibroepithelial polyp')

Common.

Typical orofacial symptoms and signs: pedunculated or broadly sessile, sometimes ulcerated, firm or soft swelling with normal overlying mucosa (Figures 3.141, 3.142). It is termed epulis if on gingival margin.

Main oral sites affected: buccal mucosa, gingiva, palate, tongue.

Aetiopathogenesis: chronic irritation causing fibrous hyperplasia.

Gender predominance: none.

Age predominance: adults.

Extraoral possible lesions: none.

Main associated conditions: none.

Differential diagnosis: papilloma, any other soft tissue tumour.

Investigations: excise for histological confirmation.

Main diagnostic criteria: clinical, confirmed by histology.

Main treatments: excision biopsy.

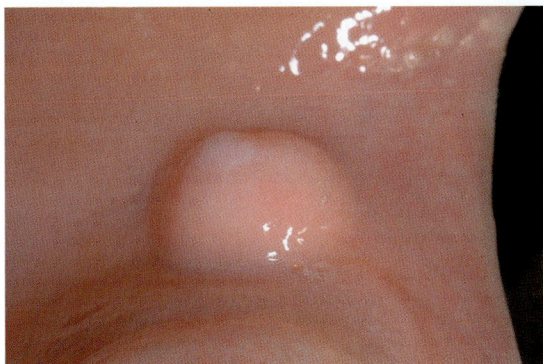

Figure 3.141 Intraoral lesion: swelling of fibrous lump (fibroepithelial polyp): the smooth lesion was firm and has normal overlying mucosa.

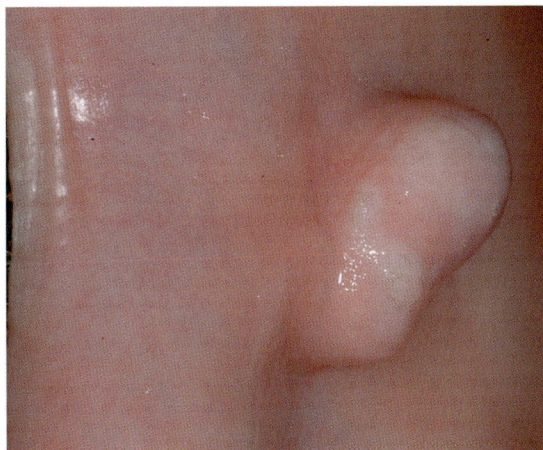

Figure 3.142 Intraoral lesion: swelling of fibrous lump (fibroepithelial polyp).

Intraoral soft tissue lumps and swellings (continued)

Lymphangioma

Rare.

Typical orofacial symptoms and signs: colourless, sometimes finely nodular soft or fluctuant mass (Figure 3.143). Bleeding into lymphatic spaces may cause sudden purplish discoloration. If in tongue and extensive, it is a rare cause of macroglossia. If in lip, it is a rare cause of macrocheilia.

Main oral sites affected: tongue, lip.

Aetiopathogenesis: hamartoma or benign neoplasm of lymphatic channels.

Gender predominance: none.

Age predominance: none.

Extraoral possible lesions: none.

Main associated conditions: none.

Differential diagnosis: papillomas when small.

Investigations: aspirate, biopsy.

Main diagnostic criteria: clinical and histology.

Main treatments: excise for microscopy.

Human papillomavirus (HPV) infections

HPV most commonly produce papillomas, but are also implicated in various warts including venereal warts (condyloma acuminatum), and rare disorders, e.g. multifocal epithelial hyperplasia (Heck disease).

Typical orofacial symptoms and signs: lesions can be warty papules or more smooth-surfaced, and white or pink in colour (Figures 3.144, 3.145). Variants include:

- *Warts* – rare in mouth – are usually transmitted from skin lesions (verruca vulgaris) and are found predominantly on the lips.
- *Papillomas* are most common; they are papillated asymptomatic, pedunculated, either pink or white if hyperkeratinized.
- *Condyloma acuminatum* (genital warts), transmitted from anogenital lesions, are found on the tongue or palate. A higher prevalence is seen in patients with multiple sexual partners, those with sexually shared diseases or those who are immunocompromised, as in HIV/AIDS.
- *Multifocal epithelial hyperplasia* (Heck disease) is rare, predominantly affects Inuits (Eskimos) and American Indians and causes multiple papules.

Figure 3.143 Intraoral lesion: swelling caused by lymphangioma.

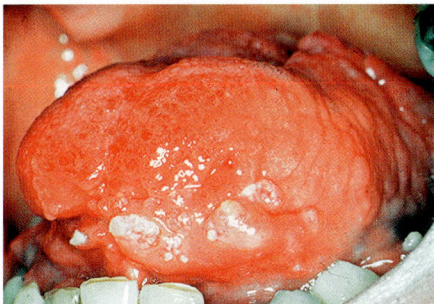

Figure 3.144 Intraoral lesion: papilloma.

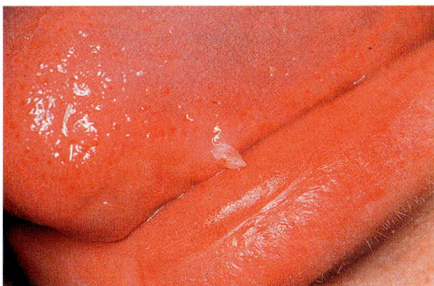

Figure 3.145 Intraoral lesion: papilloma.

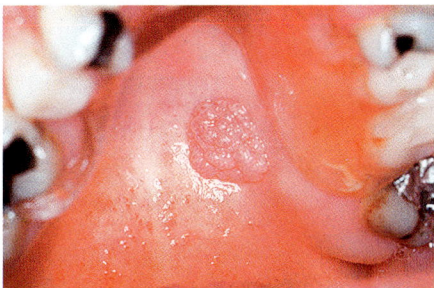

Main oral sites affected: lip, tongue, palate
Aetiopathogenesis: HPV infection.
Gender predominance: none.
Age predominance: wide age range depending on the type.
Extraoral possible lesions: sexually shared infections in some.

Intraoral soft tissue lumps and swellings (continued)

Main associated conditions: papillomas are found also in some rare syndromes (e.g. Cowden multiple hamartoma syndrome).

Differential diagnosis: fibrous hyperplasia, giant cell fibroma, neoplasms.

Investigations: biopsy.

Main diagnostic criteria: clinical and histology.

Main treatments: excision and microscopy; laser; cryosurgery.

Neoplasms (page 269)

See Figures 3.146 and 3.147.

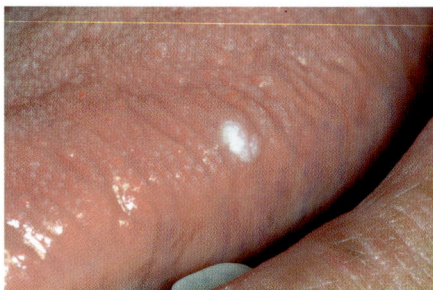

Figure 3.146 Intraoral lesion: white lesion thought to be keratosis but proved to be carcinoma.

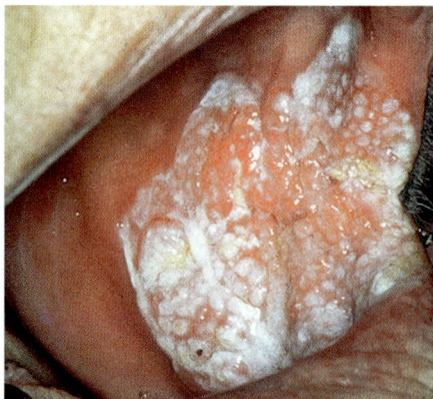

Figure 3.147 Intraoral lesion: white lesion of candidal (speckled) leukoplakia, which contained a carcinoma.

Tongue lesions

Keypoints

- Coloured lesions on the tongue are often red and caused by erythema migrans (geographic tongue), lichen planus, glossitis or candidosis but may indicate erythroplasia or carcinoma.
- Purple or blue lesions on the tongue are usually of vascular origin (e.g. angioma or Kaposi sarcoma).
- Amalgam tattoos may cause grey or black macules seen in the ventrum of tongue, floor of mouth.
- Bleeding from the tongue is mainly from trauma or a vascular lesion such as telangiectasia.
- Soreness of the tongue may be caused by a burn or trauma, mucositis, or red or ulcerated lesions (see Ulceration).
- White lesions on the tongue may be caused by debris (coated tongue), thrush (candidosis), lichen planus or keratosis, carcinoma or, rarely, a congenital cause.
- Ulceration may be due to local causes (especially trauma), aphthae, malignancy, drugs (e.g. nicorandil), or systemic disease (blood, infectious, gastrointestinal, or skin disease). Lichen planus is a fairly common cause of erosions.
- Localized tongue swellings may be congenital (e.g. lingual thyroid, haemangioma, lymphangioma, lingual choristoma); inflammatory (infection, abscess, median rhomboid glossitis, granuloma, foliate papillitis, insect bite); traumatic (e.g. oedema, haematoma); neoplastic (fibrous lump, papilloma, neurofibroma, carcinoma, sarcoma, granular cell tumour [granular cell myoblastoma]); or can be due to a foreign body, cyst, wart or condyloma.
- Diffuse tongue swellings may be congenital (e.g. Down syndrome, cretinism, mucopolysaccharidoses, lymphangioma, haemangioma); inflammatory (infection, insect bite, Ludwig angina); traumatic (oedema, haematoma); angioedema; metabolic (multiple endocrine adenomatosis type 3 [2b]; deposits (glycogen storage disease, I cell disease, mucopolysaccharidoses, amyloidosis); acromegaly; or muscular (Beckwith–Wiedemann syndrome).
- Sore tongue may be associated with obvious localized lesions (any cause of oral erosion, glossitis or ulceration), foliate papillitis, transient

Tongue lesions (continued)

lingual papillitis, geographic tongue, median rhomboid glossitis, deficiency glossitis (anaemias, avitaminosis B), candidosis, or mucositis (chemotherapy, graft-versus-host disease, or post-irradiation).

- Sore tongue may be a complaint with no identifiable physical abnormality in anaemia/sideropenia, depression or cancerophobia, diabetes, glossodynia (burning mouth syndrome), or hypothyroidism.

Ankyloglossia (tongue-tie)

Rare, especially complete or lateral ankyloglossia; partial is more common.

Typical orofacial symptoms and signs: the lingual fraenum anchors the tongue tip, restricting protrusion and lateral movements (Figure 3.148). Breastfeeding may be impaired. Later in life, oral cleansing, sometimes speech, playing a wind instrument, licking an ice-cream cone or even kissing can be impeded. Lingual gingival recession develops in some cases.

Main oral sites affected: tongue only.

Aetiopathogenesis: may be genetic basis. Most cases are partial.

Gender predominance: male.

Age predominance: from birth.

Extraoral possible lesions: none.

Main associated conditions: some rare syndromes such as orofaciodigital, Opitz and Beckwith–Wiedemann syndromes.

Differential diagnosis: from tethering of tongue by scarring in epidermolysis bullosa.

Investigations: assessment of speech or functional nutritional intake disorders.

Main diagnostic criteria: clinical.

Main treatments: surgery or laser fraenectomy if it causes a severe impairment.

Amyloidosis

Rare.

Typical orofacial symptoms and signs: manifestations may include macroglossia or deposits elsewhere, and petechia or blood-filled bullae (secondary purpura due to blood clotting factor X binding to amyloid) (Figure 3.149).

Main oral sites affected: tongue, lip.

Figure 3.148 Tongue lesion: ankyloglossia (tongue-tie).

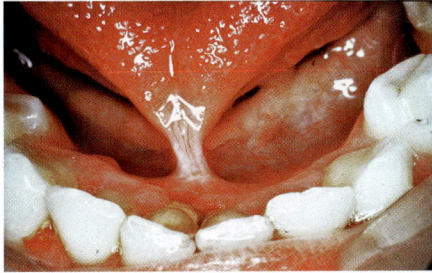

Figure 3.149 Tongue lesion: macroglossia from amyloidosis, also showing purpura.

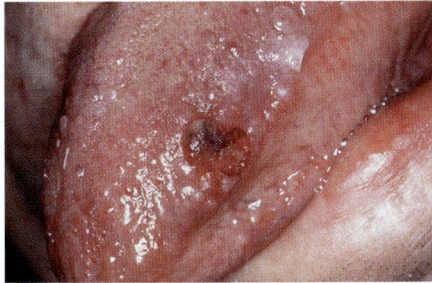

Aetiopathogenesis: amyloid is deposited in tissues of eosinophilic hyaline material, which has a fibrillar structure on ultramicroscopy. Oral amyloidosis is almost exclusively primary, when the deposits are of immunoglobulin light chains (as in myeloma-associated amyloid). Secondary amyloidosis is now seen mainly in rheumatoid arthritis, ulcerative colitis and autoinflammatory disorders, and rarely affects the mouth, and different proteins (AA proteins) are present. Amyloidosis in long-term renal dialysis patients (dialysis-related amyloid) is caused by deposition of β_2-microglobulin.

Gender predominance: none.

Age predominance: adult.

Extraoral possible lesions: cutaneous purpura, including periorbital.

Main associated conditions: concurrent autoimmune, chronic infectious diseases or malignancies, especially multiple myeloma.

Differential diagnosis: from other causes of macroglossia, and from other causes of petechia/bullae, such as localized oral purpura and bleeding tendency.

Tongue lesions (continued)

Investigations: biopsy. Oral deposits may be detected histologically even in the absence of clinically apparent lesions. Blood picture; erythrocyte sedimentation rate and marrow biopsy; serum proteins and electrophoresis; urinalysis (Bence Jones proteinuria); skeletal survey for myeloma.

Main diagnostic criteria: histology and staining with dyes such as Congo red.

Main treatments: chemotherapy with melphalan, corticosteroids or fluoxymesterone. Surgical reduction of the tongue is inadvisable as the tissue is friable, often bleeds excessively and the swelling quickly recurs.

Benign nerve sheath tumor (neurofibroma; neurilemmoma [schwannoma])

Rare.

Typical orofacial symptoms and signs: slowly enlarging painless mass (Figure 3.150).

Main oral sites affected: usually in tongue.

Aetiopathogenesis: benign neoplasm of neurilemmal cells of axonal sheath.

Gender predominance: none.

Age predominance: none.

Extraoral possible lesions: skin café-au-lait hyperpigmentation.

Main associated conditions: multiple neurofibromas can sometimes be found in von Recklinghausen neurofibromatosis. Macroglossia and bone hypertrophy are rarely present. Neurofibromas occasionally undergo sarcomatous change. Mucosal neuromas (plexiform neuromas) may be seen in multiple endocrine neoplasia type III or IIB syndrome (with medullary carcinoma of the thyroid).

Differential diagnosis: from other soft tissue tumours.

Investigations: ultrasound, histopathology; genetic evaluation if multiple findings.

Main diagnostic criteria: ultrasound, advanced imaging histopathology.

Main treatments: excision and microscopic examination; genetic counselling when appropriate.

Black hairy tongue (see page 58)

Carcinoma

Most oral cancer is squamous cell carcinoma. Uncommon but important.

Typical orofacial symptoms and signs: may present as a single persistent ulcer, red or white lesion, lump or fissure or cervical lymphadenopathy. Usually forms a chronic indurated ulcer typically with raised rolled edge and granulating floor (Figures 3.151–3.157). Sometimes manifests with pain. When on gingiva or alveolus it may present with tooth mobility or non-healing extraction socket.

Figure 3.150 Tongue lesion: swellings on tongue, lips and face due to neurofibromatosis.

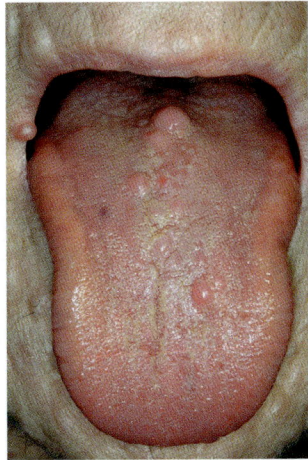

Figure 3.151 Tongue lesion: carcinoma.

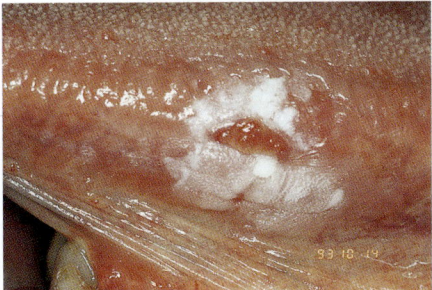

Tongue lesions (continued)

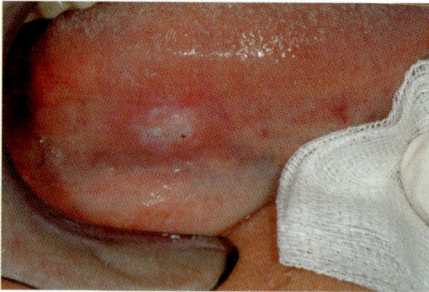

Figure 3.152 White lesion that proved on biopsy to be carcinoma.

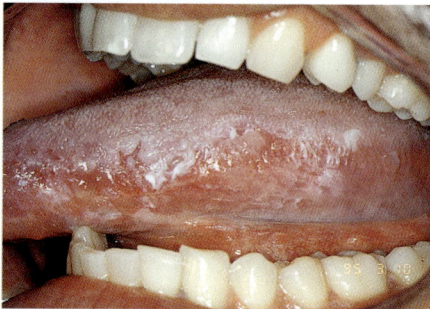

Figure 3.153 White lesion which developed carcinoma as in 3.154.

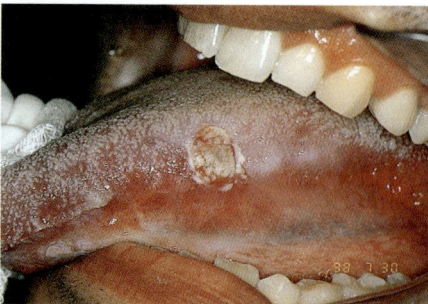

Figure 3.154 Carcinoma.

Figure 3.155 Tongue lesion: red lesion that proved on biopsy to be carcinoma.

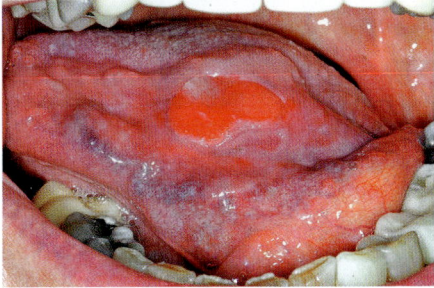

Figure 3.156 Tongue lesion: white lesion that proved to be a carcinoma.

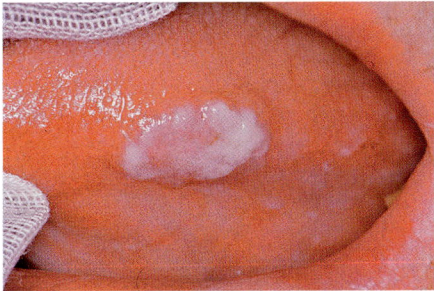

Figure 3.157 Tongue lesion: carcinoma.

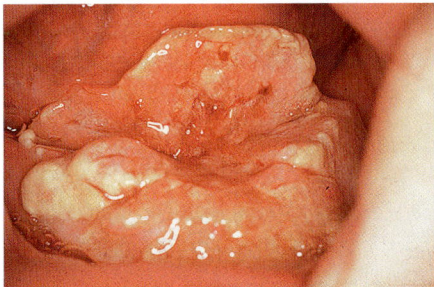

Tongue lesions (continued)

Main oral sites affected: posterolateral margin of tongue.

Aetiopathogenesis: tobacco and/or alcohol or betel use, human papilloma-virus (HPV) and potentially malignant disorders may predispose to carci-noma. Potentially malignant disorders include erythroplakia, dysplastic leukoplakias, candidosis, tertiary syphilis, lichen planus, discoid lupus ery-thematosus, Fanconi anaemia, dyskeratosis congenita, oral submucous fibrosis and Paterson–Kelly syndrome.

Gender predominance: male.

Age predominance: older adults.

Extraoral possible lesions: cervical lymph node or distant metastases; patients must be thoroughly examined and investigated for these and second primary tumours elsewhere in the upper aerodigestive tract.

Main associated conditions: tobacco, alcohol or betel use.

Differential diagnosis: other causes of mouth ulcers, especially major aphthae, traumatic granuloma or, rarely, chronic infections, e.g. tubercu-losis or deep mycosis (e.g. histoplasmosis).

Investigations: biopsy, fibreoptic pharyngolaryngoscopy with autofluores-cence (symptom-directed bronchoscopy/oesophagoscopy); ultrasound-guided fine needle aspiration (USgFNA) biopsy of any neck mass; staging – tumour, node and metastasis (TNM) – supported by MRI (or CT) from skull base to sternoclavicular joints (plus USgFNA and/or FDG-PET if any-thing equivocal). CT of thorax.

Main diagnostic criteria: clinical confirmed by histology.

Main treatments: one or more of the following – frequently using surgery, sometimes also irradiation and, occasionally, chemotherapy or photody-namic therapy (PDT). Morbidity can be high after surgery (aesthetics, impaired speech and swallowing) but higher with radiotherapy (mucositis, hyposalivation, osteoradionecrosis, taste disturbance, trismus).

The prognosis of intraoral carcinoma is poor – about 50% 5-year survival rates – because of the high proportion of late-stage cases at presentation.

Candidal glossitis

Uncommon.

Typical orofacial symptoms and signs: diffuse erythema and soreness (Figure 3.158). There may also be patches of thrush, chapped lips and angular cheilitis.

Main oral sites affected: tongue and vestibule, especially the upper buccal sulcus posteriorly.

Aetiopathogenesis: opportunistic infection with candidal species, particularly *C. albicans*. Predisposing factors include broad-spectrum antimicrobials, particularly tetracycline; hyposalivation; topical corticosteroids (more often thrush); immune defect (more often thrush).

Gender predominance: none.

Age predominance: none.

Extraoral possible lesions: in women, vaginal candidosis.

Main associated conditions: see aetiopathogenesis.

Differential diagnosis: from deficiency glossitis, contact allergy, geographic tongue, lichen planus.

Investigations: cytologic smear for candidal hyphae.

Main diagnostic criteria: clinical.

Main treatments: treat predisposing cause; antifungals.

Figure 3.158 Tongue lesion: depapillation (glossitis) in hyposalivation complicated by candidosis.

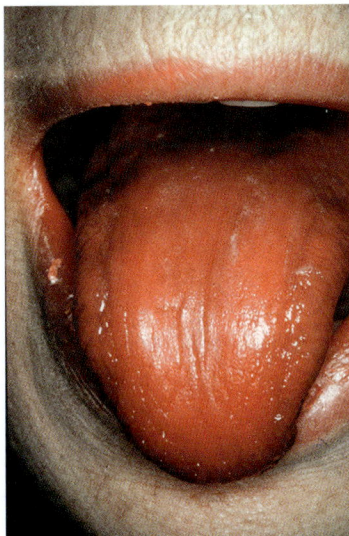

Tongue lesions (continued)

Crenated tongue
Common.

Typical symptoms and signs: shallow impressions of the margins of the tongue due to the neighbouring teeth (Figure 3.159).

Main oral sites affected: lateral borders of tongue.

Aetiopathogenesis: frequent in macroglossia, bruxism and in persons who have the habit of pressing the tongue hard against the teeth.

Gender predominance: none.

Age predominance: none.

Extraoral possible lesions: none.

Main associated conditions: often associated with linea alba and sometimes with tooth attrition.

Differential diagnosis: differentiate from causes of macroglossia.

Investigations: none.

Main diagnostic criteria: history and clinical features.

Main treatments: the condition is of no consequence; reassure.

Deficiency glossitis (see page 134)

Erythema migrans (benign migratory glossitis; geographic tongue)
Common: 1–2% of adults. The cause is genetic and it is associated commonly with a fissured tongue and, rarely, with psoriasis.

Typical orofacial symptoms and signs: often asymptomatic, occasionally sore, especially with acidic foods (e.g. tomatoes). There are irregular, pink or red depapillated macular areas, of variable and varying sizes and shapes (hence 'geographic', as it resembles a map), sometimes surrounded by distinct yellowish slightly raised margins (Figures 3.160–3.164). Red areas change in shape, increase in size, and spread or move to other areas within hours.

Figure 3.159 Tongue lesions: crenated due to stress and clenching.

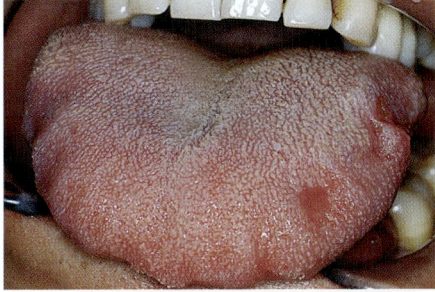

Figure 3.160 Tongue lesions: erythema migrans (geographic tongue).

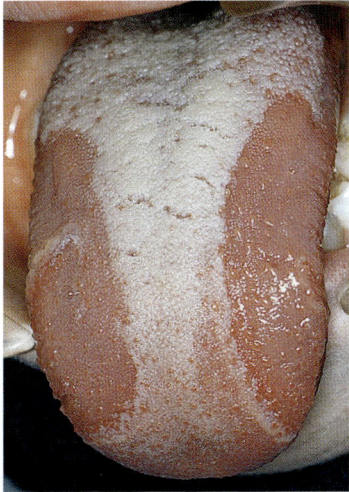

Figure 3.161 Tongue lesions: erythema migrans (geographic tongue).

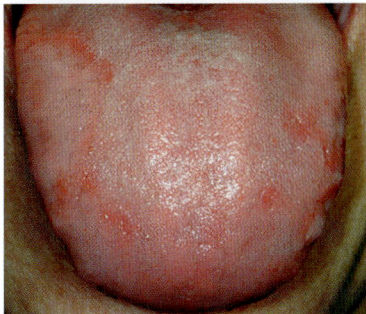

Tongue lesions (continued)

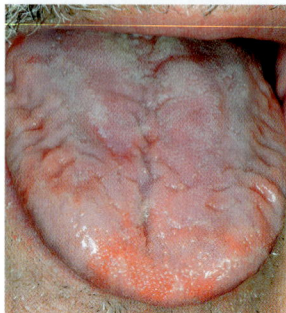

Figure 3.162 Tongue lesions: erythema migrans (geographic tongue).

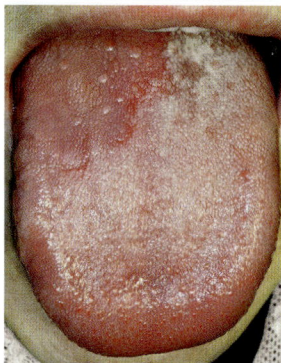

Figure 3.163 Tongue lesions: erythema migrans (geographic tongue).

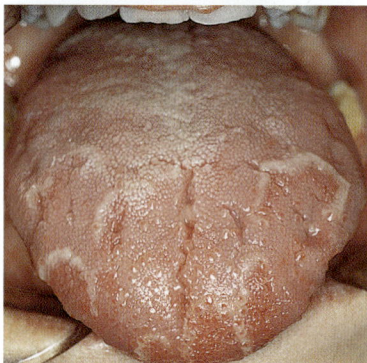

Figure 3.164 Tongue lesions: erythema migrans (geographic tongue).

Main oral sites affected: typically involves the dorsum of the tongue, rarely adjacent oral mucosa (Figure 3.165).

Aetiopathogenesis: genetic. the pathology resembles psoriasis and the lesions are associated with psoriasis in 4%.

Gender predominance: none.

Age predominance: found from infancy.

Extraoral possible lesions: none.

Main associated conditions: the tongue is often also fissured; relatives may have psoriasis.

Differential diagnosis: similar lesions may be seen in psoriasis and Reiter syndrome (reactive arthritis) (transiently). There may also be confusion with lichen planus and lupus erythematosus.

Investigations: history of migrating pattern.

Main diagnostic criteria: clinical.

Main treatments: reassure; benzydamine topically may ease discomfort.

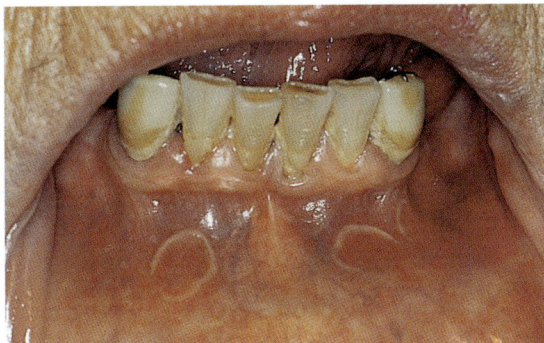

Figure 3.165 Erythema migrans is rarely seen elsewhere.

Tongue lesions (continued)

Fissured (scrotal) tongue
Common.

Typical symptoms and signs: multiple fissures on dorsum only (Figure 3.166). Sometimes the tongue is sore, commonly because of associated erythema migrans.

Main oral sites affected: dorsum of the tongue.

Aetiopathogenesis: hereditary; increases with age.

Gender predominance: none.

Age predominance: none.

Extraoral possible lesions: none.

Main associated conditions: fissured tongue is found in many normal persons, but more often in Down syndrome and in Melkersson–Rosenthal syndrome (fissured tongue, cheilitis granulomatosa, and unilateral facial nerve paralysis).

Differential diagnosis: lobulated tongue of Sjögren syndrome.

Investigations: none, but blood picture if tongue is sore.

Main diagnostic criteria: clinical; the diagnosis is usually clear-cut.

Main treatments: the condition is of no consequence; reassure.

Foliate papillitis
Common.

Typical symptoms and signs: foliate papillae occasionally become inflamed or irritated, with associated enlargement and tenderness, and upon examination these areas are enlarged and somewhat lobular in outline with an intact overlying mucosa (Figure 3.167).

Main oral sites affected: posterolateral margin of the tongue.

Aetiopathogenesis: reactive hyperplasia of lymphoid tissue in deep crypts of foliate papillae.

Gender predominance: none.

Age predominance: none.

Extraoral possible lesions: none.

Main associated conditions: none.

Differential diagnosis: carcinoma.

Investigations: if carcinoma suspected biopsy is mandatory.

Main diagnostic criteria: history and clinical features.

Main treatments: reassure.

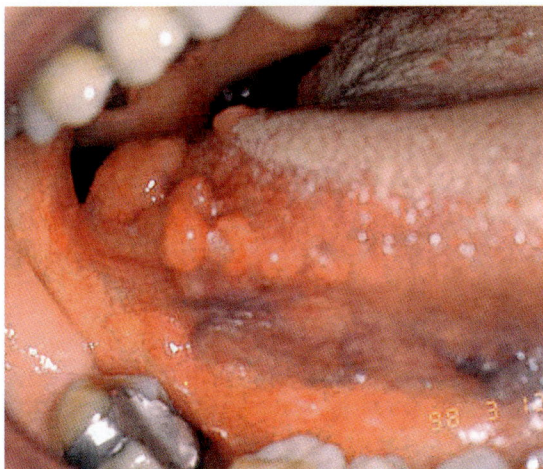

Figure 3.166 Tongue lesion: foliate papillitis.

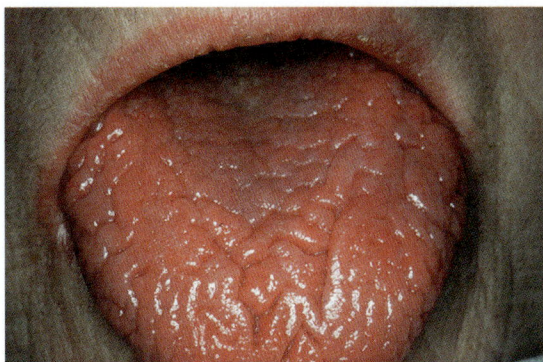

Figure 3.167 Tongue lesion: depapillation and fissuring in hyposalivation.

Tongue lesions (continued)

Macroglossia (see page 114)

Median rhomboid glossitis (central papillary atrophy, posterior lingual papillary atrophy, posterior midline atrophic candidosis)

Uncommon.

Typical orofacial symptoms and signs: rhomboidal (diamond-shaped) red, or nodular and depapillated or white, in midline of dorsum of tongue, just anterior to circumvallate papillae due primarily to the absence of filiform papillae (Figures 3.168, 3.169).

Main oral sites affected: tongue only.

Aetiopathogenesis: acquired, and is sometimes infected with *Candida* species. Smoking may predispose by increasing carriage of *Candida*. Similar lesions may be seen in HIV infection.

Gender predominance: males who smoke.

Age predominance: adults.

Extraoral possible lesions: none.

Main associated conditions: may also be candidosis in the palate ('kissing lesion') and elsewhere ('multifocal candidosis').

Differential diagnosis: from erythema migrans, erythroplasia and carcinoma (see above), rarely lingual thyroid, gumma, tuberculosis, deep mycosis, or granular cell tumour.

Investigations: cytologic smear for *Candida albicans.* Biopsy is rarely required (can show pseudoepitheliomatous hyperplasia). Prior to biopsy, ensure the lesion does not represent a lingual thyroid, as this may be the only thyroid tissue present.

Main diagnostic criteria: clinical.

Main treatments: antifungals if candidal; stop smoking; reassure. Remove if recalcitrant or concerned about carcinoma.

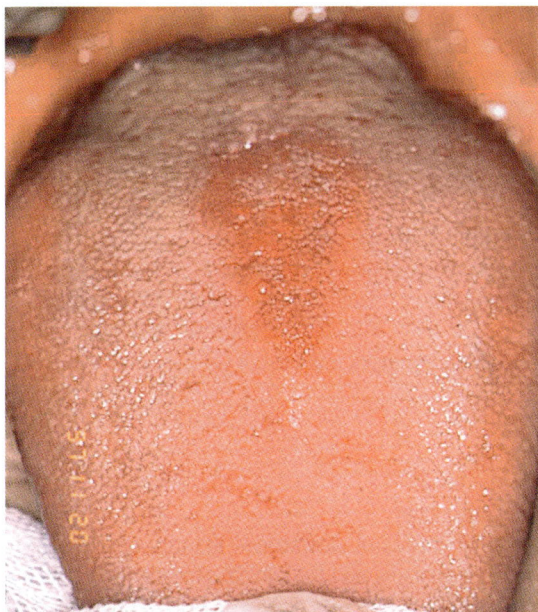

Figure 3.168 Tongue lesion: median rhomboid glossitis (a candidal lesion).

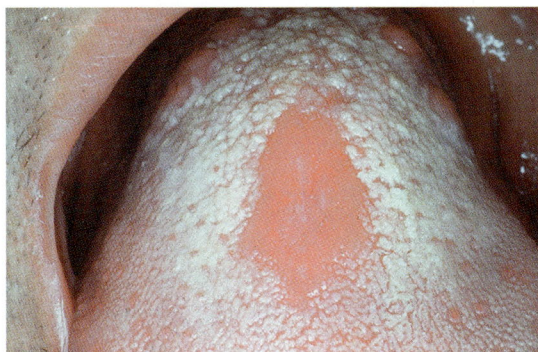

Figure 3.169 Tongue lesion: median rhomboid glossitis.

Tongue lesions (continued)

Traumatic ulcerative granuloma (TUG; also known as traumatic ulcerative granuloma with stromal eosinophilia [TUGSE])
Uncommon.

Typical orofacial symptoms and signs: chronic single ulcer or lump (Figure 3.170).

Main oral sites affected: lateral margin of the tongue.

Aetiopathogenesis: traumatic in origin. Characterized by a diffuse, pseudoinvasive, mixed inflammatory reaction that includes numerous eosinophils and often extends deep into the submucosa and may involve underlying muscle, and can represent a subset of CD30+ lymphoproliferative disorders.

Gender predominance: none.

Age predominance: none.

Extraoral possible lesions: none.

Main associated conditions: none.

Differential diagnosis: other causes of ulceration – the rare appearance of the traumatic ulcerative granuloma and the clinical similarity to carcinoma cause difficulties in diagnosis. Riga–Fede disease is a form of TUGSE that appears rarely; it usually occurs on the anterior ventrum of the tongue in infants who have natal lower incisors due to irritation during suckling.

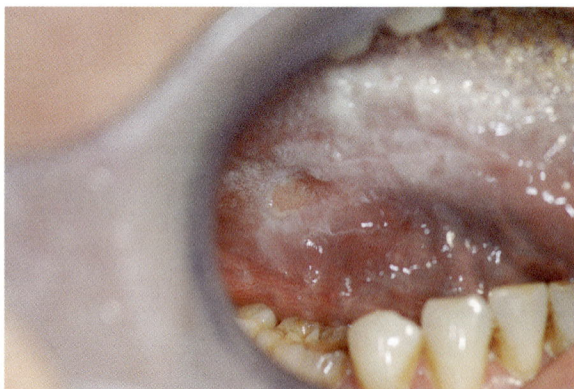

Figure 3.170 Tongue lesion: TUGSE (traumatic ulcerative granuloma with stromal eosinophilia).

Investigations: possible biopsy; determine if a foreign body is present.

Main diagnostic criteria: clinical and histology.

Main treatments: this is a benign persistent lesion, eventually self-healing. Symptomatic care is indicated, with excision if not spontaneously healing in 3 weeks.

Palatal lesions

Keypoints

Cleft palate is a dramatic lesion with multiple implications, but surprisingly few other conditions are found only or mainly in the palate.

- Coloured lesions in the palate are not uncommon. Red lesions may be caused by candidosis, pemphigus, erythroplasia, Kaposi sarcoma or other lesions. Redness restricted to the denture-bearing area of the palate is almost invariably denture-related stomatitis (candidosis), although erythematous candidosis of HIV disease can commonly occur as a red patch of the palate. Brown pigmented lesions in the palate are usually naevi, but Kaposi sarcoma and melanoma have a predilection for this site also and may be brown, black or bluish.
- Bleeding from the palate is rare but may be seen from telangiectasia or in localized oral purpura.
- Soreness in the palate is frequently of local cause such as trauma or from a burn (but see Ulceration).
- White lesions may be seen in the palate, especially in smoker's keratosis, leukoplakia (mainly proliferative verrucous leukoplakia; PVL), candidosis and lupus erythematosus and, on the palatal gingivae mainly, lichen planus.
- Ulceration in the palate is uncommon, and usually due to local causes (e.g. burns, trauma), aphthae, or systemic conditions (e.g. recurrent herpes, pemphigoid, pemphigus and lupus erythematosus) but occasionally due to ulcerated neoplasms such as lymphoma, salivary gland tumours or carcinoma (oral or antral).
- Lumps/swelling is most commonly caused by unerupted teeth or torus palatinus – a common central developmental abnormality. Acquired lumps are often dental abscesses, but fibrous lumps, HPV-associated warts, and neoplasms (particularly carcinomas, salivary neoplasms, Kaposi sarcoma and lymphomas) must be excluded.

Palatal lesions (continued)

Angina bullosa haemorrhagica (ABH; localized oral purpura)
Not uncommon.

Typical orofacial symptoms and signs: blood blisters of rapid onset, with breakdown in a day or two to ulcer (Figure 3.171). No bleeding tendency.
Main oral sites affected: soft palate, posterior buccal mucosa and occasionally the lateral border of the tongue.
Aetiopathogenesis: trauma in most cases; occasionally associated with use of corticosteroid inhalers.
Gender predominance: none.
Age predominance: older.
Extraoral possible lesions: pharyngeal involvement occasionally.
Main associated conditions: none.
Differential diagnosis: thrombocytopenia; pemphigoid; amyloidosis.
Investigations: confirm platelet count, full blood picture and haemostasis normal; biopsy (rarely) to exclude pemphigoid.
Main diagnostic criteria: clinical and blood tests.
Main treatments: reassure; topical analgesics.

Denture-related stomatitis
Common, sometimes termed denture sore mouth, but rarely sore. It is caused mainly by a yeast (*Candida*) that usually lives harmlessly in the mouth and elsewhere and the condition may be precipitated by prolonged wearing of a dental appliance, especially at night, which allows the yeast to grow. It predisposes to sores at the corners of the mouth (angular stomatitis or cheilitis).

Typical orofacial symptoms and signs: diffuse erythema of denture-bearing area only (Figures 3.172–3.176), with occasional petechia or thrush. It is almost always asymptomatic, the only known complications being angular stomatitis and aggravation of palatal papillary hyperplasia.
Main oral sites affected: almost invariably the hard palate alone.
Aetiopathogenesis: usually *C. albicans*. Constant denture-wearing predisposes, but other factors may include poor denture hygiene, and occasionally hyposalivation, high carbohydrate diet and immune defects.
Gender predominance: none.
Age predominance: older patients.
Extraoral possible lesions: may be angular stomatitis.

Figure 3.171 Palatal lesion: collapsed blood blister from localized oral purpura (angina bullosa haemorrhagica).

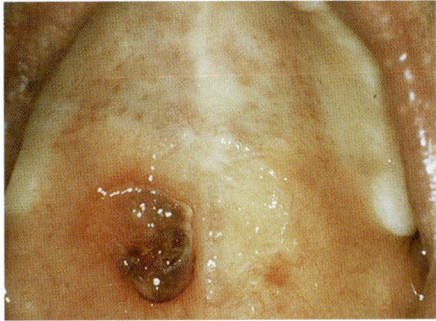

Figure 3.172 Palatal lesion: erythema in denture-related stomatitis (see same patient shown in Figure 3.173).

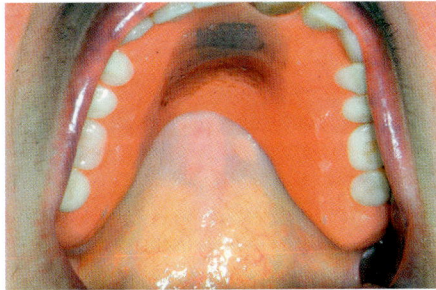

Figure 3.173 Palatal lesion: erythema in denture-related stomatitis (patient as in Figure 3.172).

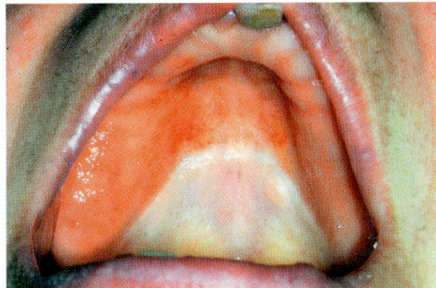

Palatal lesions (continued)

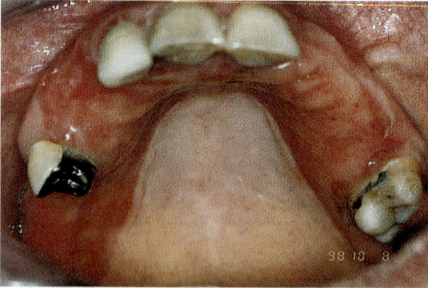

Figure 3.174 Palatal lesion: erythema in denture-related stomatitis.

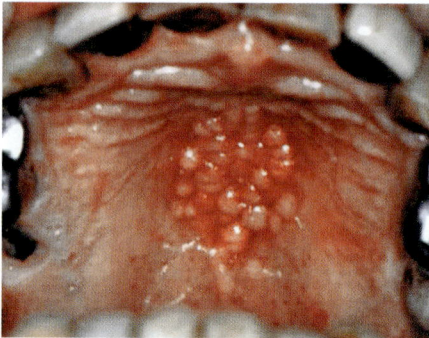

Figure 3.175 Palatal lesion: papillary hyperplasia.

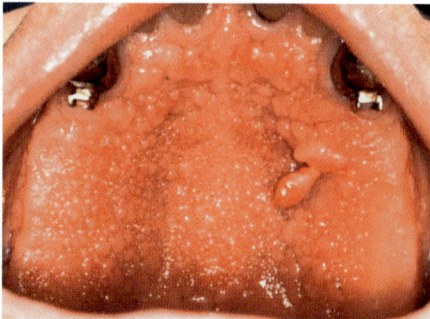

Figure 3.176 Palatal lesion: extensive papillary hyperplasia.

Main associated conditions: edentulous; if dentate, usually narrow V-shaped palate; may have candidal glossitis.

Differential diagnosis: nicotine stomatitis (red form).

Investigations: possibly cytologic smear for hyphae.

Main diagnostic criteria: clear-cut clinically.

Main treatments: leave dentures out at night and for 1 hour immerse in antifungal solution (e.g. hypochlorite, chlorhexidine); topical antifungals; attention to dentures; relining with soft material.

Kaposi sarcoma (KS)

Typical orofacial symptoms and signs: lesions are initially red, purple or brown macules (Figures 3.177, 3.178). Later these become nodular, extend, disseminate and may ulcerate.

Main oral sites affected: palate (over the greater palatine vessels) or gingivae.

Aetiopathogenesis: human herpesvirus-8 (HHV-8), now termed Kaposi sarcoma herpesvirus (KSHV). A malignant neoplasm of endothelial cells, KS is virtually unknown in the mouth except in HIV/AIDS and related syndromes (commonly) or in immunosuppressed organ transplant patients (rarely).

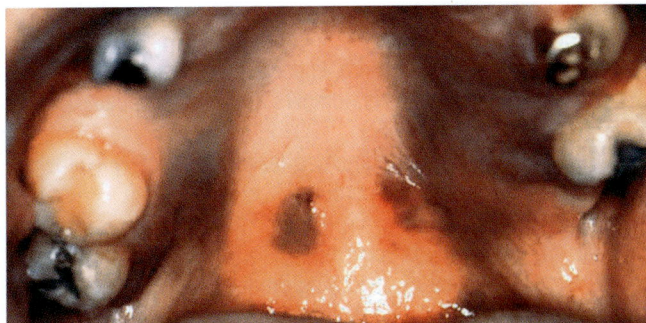

Figure 3.177 Palatal lesion: Kaposi sarcoma – multiple purple-brown macules in typical locations.

Palatal lesions (continued)

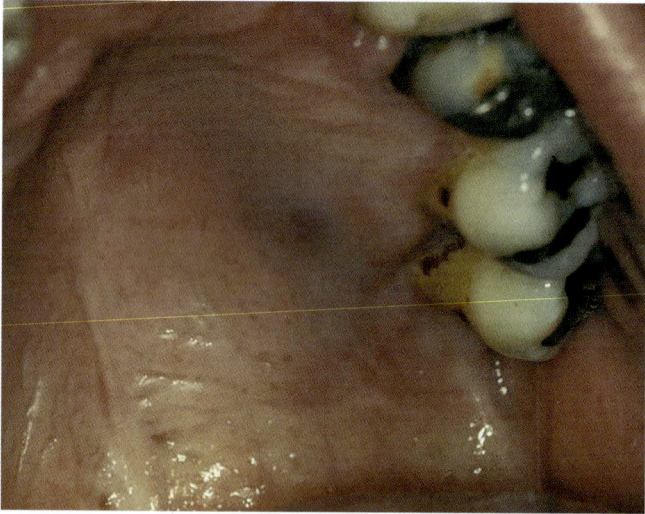

Figure 3.178 Palatal lesion: Kaposi sarcoma – nodular lesion.

Gender predominance: males.

Age predominance: adult.

Extraoral possible lesions: KS elsewhere, especially on the nose.

Main associated conditions: infections, tumours and encephalopathy of HIV/AIDS.

Differential diagnosis: from other pigmented lesions, especially epithelioid angiomatosis, haemangiomas and purpura.

Investigations: biopsy; HIV testing.

Main diagnostic criteria: biopsy is confirmatory.

Main treatments: management of underlying predisposing condition if possible; radiotherapy; vinca alkaloids and other chemotherapy drugs.

Lupus erythematosus (see page 230)

Necrotizing sialometaplasia

A rare non-neoplastic inflammatory condition of the salivary glands that clinically mimics cancer.

Typical orofacial symptoms and signs: single, often painless, persistent ulcer (Figure 3.179); less frequently, pain and numbness. The clinical features may suggest cancer.

Main oral sites affected: soft palate or alveolar ridge.

Aetiopathogenesis: salivary gland ischaemia related to trauma, vascular obstruction or smoking, leading to infarction.

Gender predominance: male.

Age predominance: older.

Extraoral possible lesions: occasionally the condition affects the pharynx, breast or other sites.

Main associated conditions: none usually.

Differential diagnosis: other causes of ulcers, especially squamous cell carcinoma, salivary gland malignancy or lymphoma.

Investigations: biopsy.

Main diagnostic criteria: clinical and histology.

Main treatments: clinical and histopathological features of necrotizing sialometaplasia often simulate those of malignancies such as squamous cell carcinoma or salivary gland malignancy – but it is self-healing.

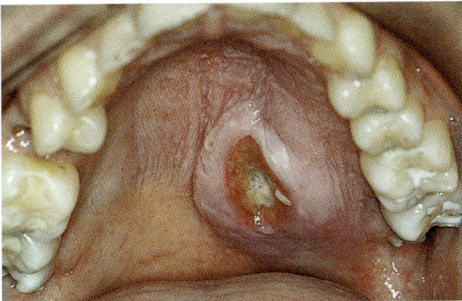

Figure 3.179 Palatal lesion: necrotizing sialometaplasia clinically and histologically can mimic carcinoma.

Palatal lesions (continued)

Smokers' keratosis (stomatitis nicotina; nicotine stomatitis)

Uncommon. This lesion appears to be benign in itself, but carcinoma may develop nearby.

Typical orofacial symptoms and signs: symptomless. Red orifices of swollen minor salivary glands of palate within a widespread white lesion involving most of the hard and often the soft palates give striking appearance of red spots on white background (Figures 3.180, 3.181).

Main oral sites affected: palate.

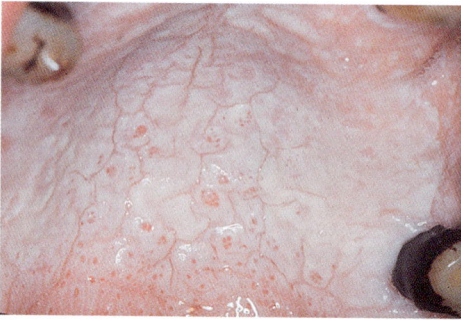

Figure 3.180 Palatal lesion: smokers' keratosis (stomatitis nicotina) and tar-stained teeth from tobacco.

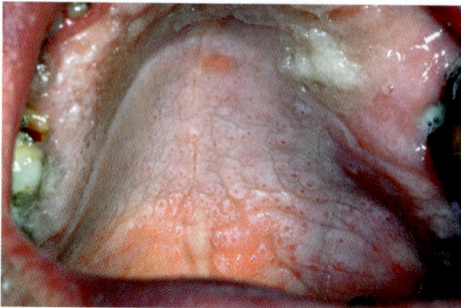

Figure 3.181 Palatal lesion: smokers' keratosis (stomatitis nicotina) and tar-stained teeth from tobacco.

Aetiopathogenesis: pipe smoking is an important cause but heavy cigarette use more common.

Gender predominance: male.

Age predominance: older.

Extraoral possible lesions: may be nicotine-stained fingers.

Main associated conditions: tobacco-associated disorders.

Differential diagnosis: Darier disease, inflammatory papillary hyperplasia, erythroleukoplakia.

Investigations: biopsy.

Main diagnostic criteria: clinical and biopsy.

Main treatments: tobacco cessation.

Oral submucous fibrosis (see page 256).

Gingival lesions

Most gingival and periodontal diseases are inflammatory and related to dental plaque, and others may be aggravated by the effects of plaque accumulation. Dental bacterial plaque is a complex biofilm containing various microorganisms which forms rapidly on teeth, particularly between them, along the gingival margin and in fissures and pits. Plaque is not especially obvious clinically, although teeth covered with plaque lack the lustre of clear teeth. Various dyes (disclosing solutions) can be used to reveal the plaque.

Keypoints

- Coloured lesions of the gingivae are usually red and most are inflammatory and plaque related. Chronic gingivitis is the most common, the redness being restricted to the gingival margins. More diffuse erythema may signify desquamative gingivitis – typically caused by pemphigoid or lichen planus. Red lesions occasionally may be vascular or due to atrophy or malignancy. Brown gingival lesions may be racial, due to tobacco or betel use, or naevi, and grey or black lesions are often due to amalgam tattoos.
- Bleeding from the gingivae is usually due to plaque-induced gingivitis but a bleeding tendency such as leukaemia is occasionally responsible.

Gingival lesions (continued)

- Soreness of the gingiva may be caused by ulceration – in children often due to herpetic stomatitis (Figure 3.182).
- Soreness, if persistent and widespread, is often caused by desquamative gingivitis (Figure 3.183).
- White lesions of the gingivae may be caused by debris (materia alba), thrush (candidosis), lichen planus or keratosis – mainly proliferative verrucous leukoplakia.
- Ulceration of the gingiva is usually traumatic or caused by primary or recurrent herpes simplex infection, or infrequently by necrotizing gingivitis which may be indicative of immunodeficiency, especially acute leukaemia, neutropenias or HIV disease. The gingivae can, however, be affected by most other causes of mouth ulcers.
- Lumps/swelling of the gingivae if localized is usually fibrous epulides or pyogenic granuloma but malignancy (usually lymphoma, carcinoma or myeloma) must be excluded. If generalized, swelling may be congenital, inflammatory, or drug-induced, but occasionally is seen in malignant disease such as leukaemia. Gingival swelling is most characteristic of acute myelomonocytic leukaemia, is most common in adults and is characterized by swelling, petechia, ecchymoses or haemorrhage and ulceration.
- Tooth mobility is usually caused by periodontitis or trauma but an immune defect or malignancy or odontogenic tumour may be underlying. The association between inflammatory periodontal disease and candidate gene polymorphisms is controversial, but interleukin-1 (IL-1), IL-6, IL-10, IL-12, IL-16 and vitamin D receptor may be involved. A range of immunodeficiencies or other defects or lifestyle choices may underlie accelerated or aggressive periodontitis.
- Halitosis (oral malodour) is usually caused by oral or periodontal infections or ulcers.

Acute ulcerative gingivitis (AUG; acute necrotizing ulcerative gingivitis, ANUG)

Uncommon, except in immune defects or where hygiene is lacking.

Typical orofacial symptoms and signs: severe gingival soreness and profuse bleeding, halitosis and a bad taste.

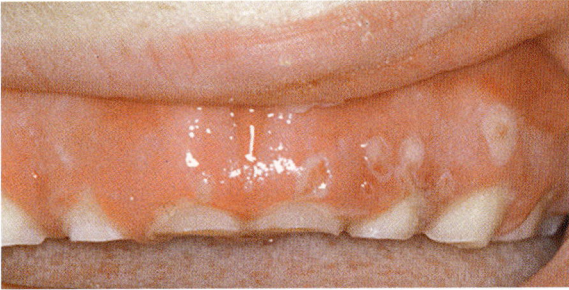

Figure 3.182 Gingival lesions: ulceration in primary herpes simplex stomatitis.

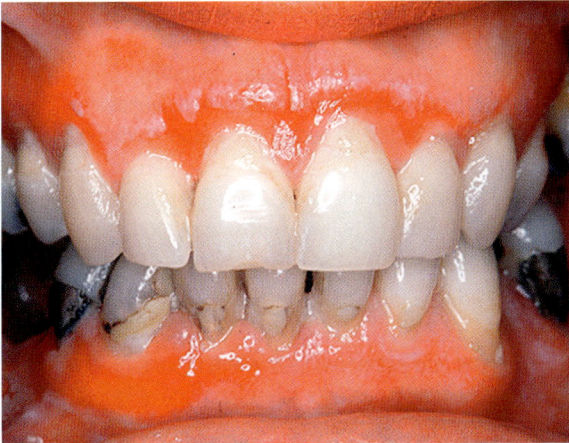

Figure 3.183 Gingival lesions: erosions and desquamation in lichen planus.

Gingival lesions (continued)

Main oral sites affected: ulcers at the tips of interdental papillae, occasionally spreading along gingival margins (Figures 3.184, 3.185).

Aetiopathogenesis: non-contagious anaerobic infection associated with overwhelming proliferation of *Borrelia vincentii* and fusiform bacteria. Predisposing factors include poor oral hygiene, smoking, viral respiratory infections such as EBV, and immune defects such as in HIV/AIDS.

Gender predominance: male.

Age predominance: adolescents and young adults.

Extraoral possible lesions: malaise, fever and/or cervical lymph node enlargement (unlike herpetic stomatitis) are rare. Cancrum oris (noma) is a rare complication, usually seen in debilitated children, when necrosis of the buccal mucosa leads to perforation of the cheek and an orofacial fistula.

Main associated conditions: immune defects.

Differential diagnosis: acute leukaemia or herpetic stomatitis.

Investigations: smear for fusospirochaetal bacteria and leukocytes; blood picture and haematinics; HIV tests and occasionally other immune studies.

Main diagnostic criteria: clear-cut.

Main treatments: amoxicillin or metronidazole (penicillin in pregnant females); oral debridement and hygiene instruction. Peroxide or perborate mouthwashes. Periodontal assessment.

Alveolar ridge keratosis
Common.

Typical orofacial symptoms and signs: painless white lesions on alveolus.

Main oral sites affected: usually posterior alveolar ridge (Figures 3.186, 3.187), often bilateral (bilateral alveolar ridge keratosis, BARK) and typically in retromolar area.

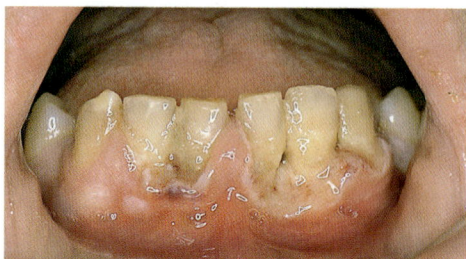

Figure 3.184 Gingival lesions: ulceration in necrotizing ulcerative gingivitis.

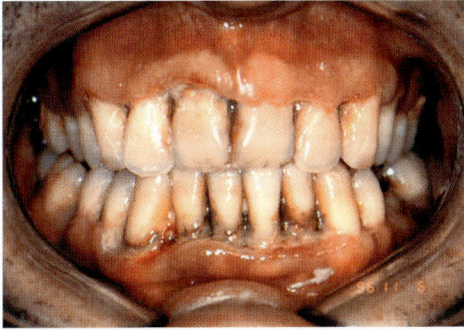

Figure 3.185 Gingival lesions: ulceration in necrotizing ulcerative gingivitis.

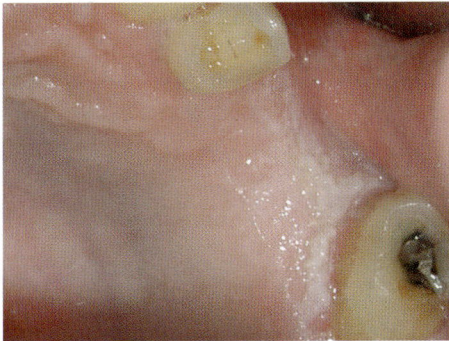

Figure 3.186 Gingival lesion: keratosis from trauma of mastication on alveolar ridge.

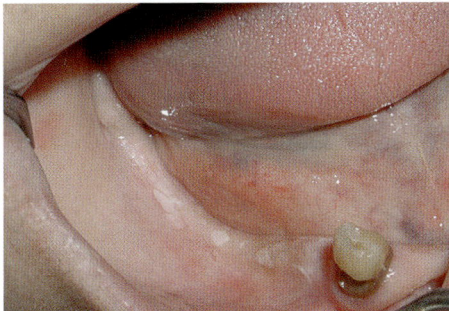

Figure 3.187 Gingival lesion: keratosis from trauma on alveolar ridge.

Gingival lesions (continued)

Aetiopathogenesis: friction from mastication.
Gender predominance: none.
Age predominance: adults.
Extraoral possible lesions: none.
Main associated conditions: none.
Differential diagnosis: leukoplakia.
Investigations: biopsy only if concerned (histology features are similar to those of skin lichen simplex chronicus)
Main diagnostic criteria: clinically obvious.
Main treatments: reassurance.

Chronic marginal gingivitis
Almost universal in adults to some degree.

Typical orofacial symptoms and signs: erythema, oedema and painless swelling of marginal gingivae with bleeding on brushing or eating hard foods (Figure 3.188).
Main oral sites affected: any.
Aetiopathogenesis: dental bacterial plaque.
Gender predominance: none.
Age predominance: adolescents and adults.
Extraoral possible lesions: none.
Main associated conditions: none.
Differential diagnosis: desquamative gingivitis.
Investigations: periodontal probing.
Main diagnostic criteria: clinically obvious.
Main treatments: oral hygiene, including scaling; root-planing etc., if periodontitis-associated.

Drug-induced gingival swelling (drug induced gingival overgrowth: DIGO)
Common.

Typical orofacial symptoms and signs: gingival enlargement characteristically affects the interdental papillae first, which enlarge and are firm, pale and tough, with coarse stippling (Figures 3.189, 3.190).
Aetiopathogenesis: the gene encoding CTLA-4 (cytotoxic T-lymphocyte antigen 4) may influence the gingival swelling, which is a recognized

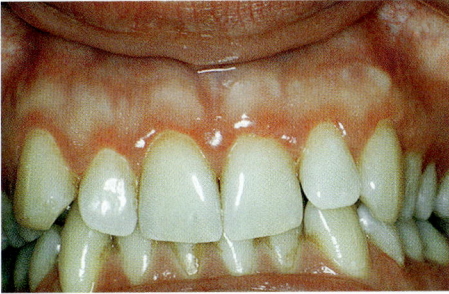

Figure 3.188 Gingival lesion: marginal gingivitis.

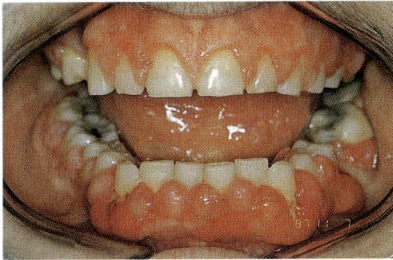

Figure 3.189 Gingival lesion: drug-induced swelling.

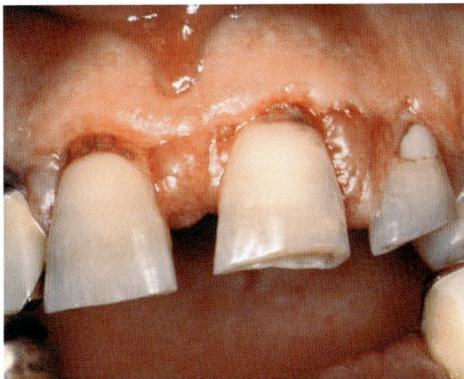

Figure 3.190 Gingival lesion: drug-induced swelling.

Gingival lesions (continued)

adverse effect of phenytoin, calcium channel blockers (dihydropyridines, especially nifedipine) and ciclosporin. The swelling is aggravated by dental bacterial plaque.

Main oral sites affected: any.

Gender predominance: none.

Age predominance: adolescents and adults.

Extraoral possible lesions: possible hirsutism.

Main associated conditions: none.

Differential diagnosis: hereditary gingival fibromatosis.

Investigations: periodontal probing.

Main diagnostic criteria: clinically obvious.

Main treatments: if the drug can be stopped and oral hygiene improved, the lesions may regress. Often, excision of the enlarged tissue may be indicated.

Hereditary gingival fibromatosis (HGF)

Uncommon.

Typical orofacial symptoms and signs: gingival enlargement characteristically affects the interdental papillae first, which enlarge and are firm, pale and tough, with coarse stippling (Figure 3.191). Generalized painless gingival enlargement is obvious especially during the transition from deciduous to permanent dentition. The swelling, if gross, may move or cover the teeth and even bulge out of the mouth. There are occasional associations with supernumerary teeth. Variants include tuberosity enlargements (Figure 3.192).

Aetiopathogenesis: autosomal dominant or recessive. The gene responsible may be *SOS1* on chromosome 2.

Main oral sites affected: any.

Gender predominance: male.

Age predominance: from early childhood.

Extraoral possible lesions: possible hirsutism and, rarely, sensorineural deafness and rare syndromes.

Main associated conditions: none usually.

Differential diagnosis: drug-induced gingival swelling; juvenile hyaline fibromatosis and infantile systemic hyalinosis.

Investigations: periodontal probing.

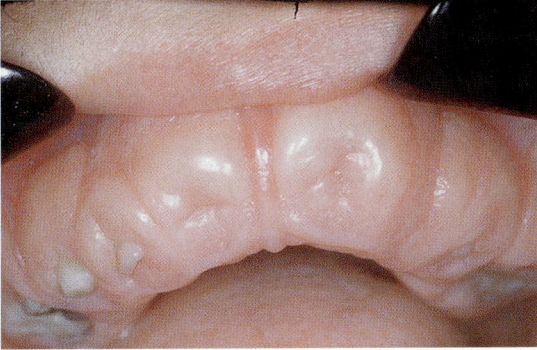

Figure 3.191 Gingival lesion: swelling in hereditary gingival fibromatosis.

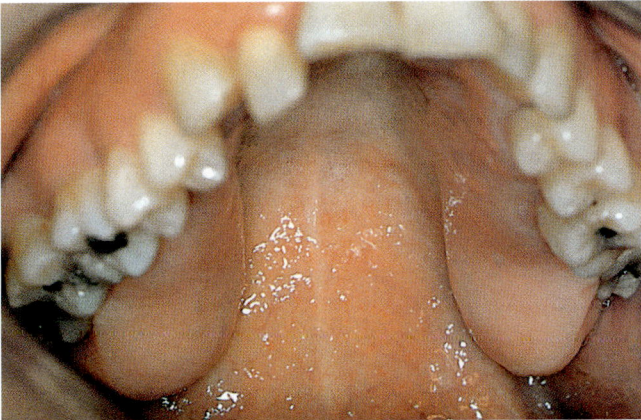

Figure 3.192 Gingival lesions: swelling in a variant of hereditary gingival fibromatosis.

Gingival lesions (continued)

Main diagnostic criteria: clinically obvious. The family history is positive.
Main treatments: often, excision of the enlarged tissue may be indicated.

Pregnancy gingivitis

Common mainly after 2nd month of pregnancy.

Typical orofacial symptoms and signs: erythema, swelling and liability to bleed (Figure 3.193).

Main oral sites affected: gingivae.

Aetiopathogenesis: exacerbation of chronic gingivitis by pregnancy. A proliferative response at the site of a particularly dense plaque accumulation may lead to pregnancy epulis (pyogenic granuloma).

Gender predominance: female.

Age predominance: adolescents and adults.

Extraoral possible lesions: features of pregnancy.

Main associated conditions: pregnancy.

Differential diagnosis: gingivitis, pyogenic granulomas.

Investigations: none.

Main diagnostic criteria: history and clinical.

Main treatments: oral hygiene.

Pregnancy epulis

Common mainly after 2nd month of pregnancy.

Typical orofacial symptoms and signs: soft, red or occasionally firm, swelling of dental papilla (Figure 3.194). It may be asymptomatic unless traumatized by biting or toothbrushing.

Main oral sites affected: gingivae facially and anteriorly.

Aetiopathogenesis: pyogenic granuloma – proliferative response at the site of a particularly dense plaque accumulation.

Gender predominance: female.

Age predominance: adolescents and adults.

Extraoral possible lesions: features of pregnancy.

Main associated conditions: pregnancy.

Differential diagnosis: gingivitis, fibrous epulis, giant cell tumour, Wegener granulomatosis.

Investigations: none usually. Biopsy sometimes; pregnancy test occasionally.

Main diagnostic criteria: history and clinical.

Main treatments: oral hygiene. If asymptomatic, leave alone – may regress after childbirth (parturition). If symptomatic or if patient desires, excision biopsy.

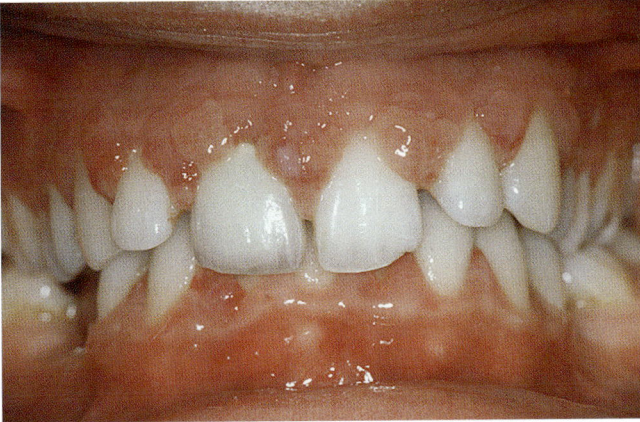

Figure 3.193 Gingival lesion: swelling in pregnancy gingivitis.

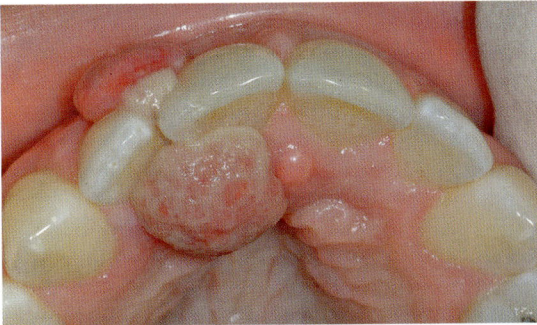

Figure 3.194 Gingival lesion: swelling caused by pyogenic granuloma in pregnancy (pregnancy epulis).

Jaw and musculoskeletal conditions

Keypoints

- Odontogenic infections are a common cause of lesions in the jaws (Figures 3.195, 3.196).
- Other infections such as actinomycosis and osteomyelitis are far less common but almost invariably more serious.
- Jaw cysts and tumours are uncommon and usually of odontogenic origin and some (ameloblastoma and keratocystic odontogenic tumour) are problems since they tend to recur after treatment.
- Diseases of bone such as fibro-osseous lesions are uncommon but can be disfiguring and aggressive.
- Bone necrosis (osteonecrosis) can follow radiotherapy to the jaws, or the use of drugs (bisphosphonates especially).

Actinomycosis

Rare.

Typical orofacial symptoms and signs: chronic purplish swelling eventually discharging pus through sinuses.

Main oral sites affected: below mandibular angle (not arising from the lymph nodes).

Aetiopathogenesis: bacterial infection that may follow jaw fracture or tooth extraction. Caused usually by *Actinomyces* species such as *A. israelii* or *A. gerencseriae*, it can also be caused by *Propionibacterium propionicun*.

Gender predominance: male.

Age predominance: young adult.

Extraoral possible lesions: lung or gastrointestinal.

Main associated conditions: none except possible preceding trauma.

Differential diagnosis: mycobacterial or mycotic infection, or other causes of facial swelling.

Investigations: examination of purulent leakage for 'sulphur granules' (bacterial colonies), culture and sensitivities.

Main diagnostic criteria: history, clinical and microbiology.

Main treatments: prolonged antibacterial therapy, usually with penicillin.

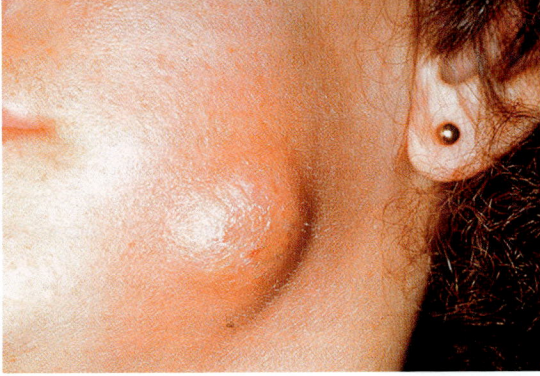

Figure 3.195 Jaw lesions: infection – actinomycosis.

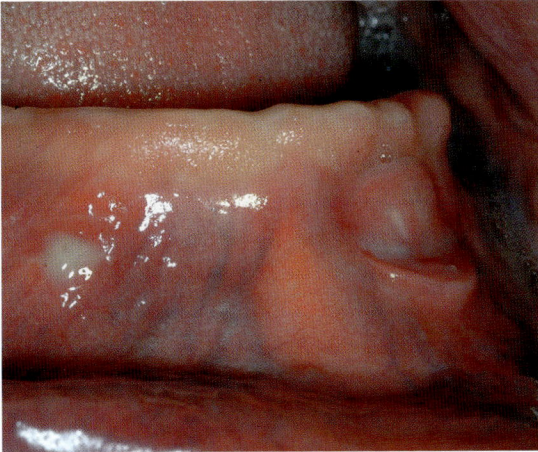

Figure 3.196 Jaw lesions: infected odontogenic cyst.

Jaw and musculoskeletal conditions (continued)

Antral carcinoma

Rare; usually a squamous carcinoma.

Typical orofacial symptoms and signs: may be asymptomatic until carcinoma invades orbit or other structures to cause swelling of cheek or eye area, nasal obstruction or pain. Symptoms depend on main direction of spread.

- Oral invasion: pain and swelling of palate (Figure 3.197), alveolus or sulcus. Teeth may loosen.
- Ocular invasion: ipsilateral epiphora (tears overflowing), diplopia (double vision) or proptosis (eye protrusion).
- Nasal invasion: nasal obstruction or a bloodstained discharge.

Main oral sites affected: may penetrate palate or maxillary vestibule.

Aetiopathogenesis: the only identified predisposing factor appears to be occupational exposure to wood dust.

Gender predominance: male.

Age predominance: older.

Extraoral possible lesions: see above.

Main associated conditions: none.

Differential diagnosis: sinusitis, polyps and salivary gland neoplasms.

Investigations: biopsy, radiographs and MRI.

Main diagnostic criteria: clinical supported by histology and imaging (shows opaque antrum and later destruction of antral wall or floor).

Main treatments: surgery (sometimes with radiotherapy). Prognosis 10–30% 5-year cure rate; better in those with no lymph node involvement.

Fibrous dysplasia

Rare fibro-osseous disorder.

Typical orofacial symptoms and signs: painless unilateral swelling of jaw (Figure 3.198).

Main oral sites affected: posterior maxilla.

Aetiopathogenesis: mutation in the gene encoding G protein.

Gender predominance: none.

Age predominance: from childhood. The polyostotic type is seen mainly in young children and the monostotic type is more common in the twenties.

Extraoral possible lesions: see below.

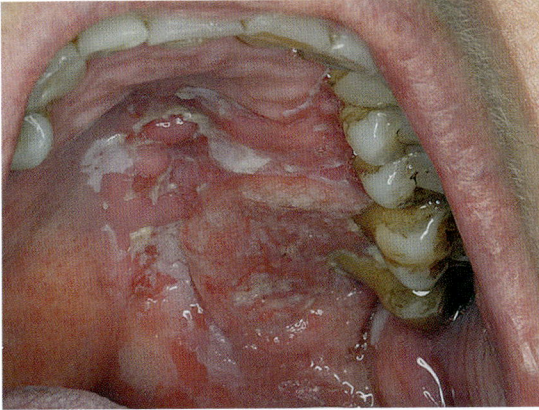

Figure 3.197 Jaw lesions: antral carcinoma.

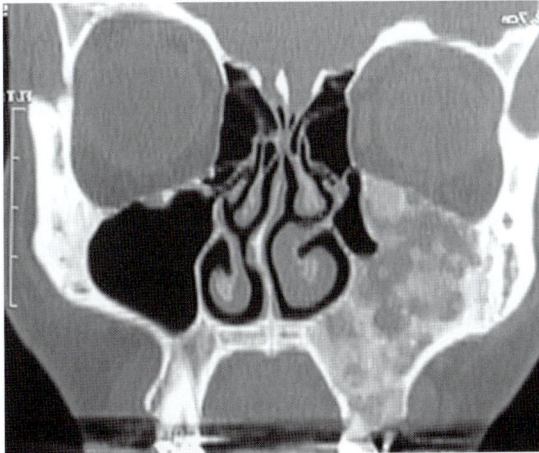

Figure 3.198 Jaw lesions: fibrous dysplasia in one maxilla.

Jaw and musculoskeletal conditions (continued)

Main associated conditions: Albright syndrome is polyostotic fibrous dysplasia with skin hyperpigmentation and endocrinopathy (precocious puberty in females and hyperthyroidism in males).

Differential diagnosis: central ossifying fibroma, diffuse sclerosing osteomyelitis, segmental odontomaxillary dysplasia, Paget disease.

Investigations: radiography; biopsy.

Main diagnostic criteria: CT can best assess the extent; histology.

Main treatments: typically self-limiting and no treatment needed. Bisphosphonates can help and cosmetic surgery may be indicated if there is major deformity or the eye is affected.

Gardner syndrome

This rare condition presents with jaw osteomas, polyposis coli, epidermoid cysts, desmoid tumours and pigmented lesions of fundus of eye.

Langherhans cell histiocytoses (histiocytosis X)

This rare disorder of Langherhans dendritic cells includes:

- Solitary eosinophilic granuloma of bone – localized chronic form.
- Multifocal eosinophilic granuloma (Hand–Schuller–Christian disease) – disseminated chronic form.
- Letterer–Siwe disease – disseminated acute form.

Masseteric hypertrophy

Uncommon.

Typical orofacial symptoms and signs: painless bilateral or unilateral swelling of masseter muscle(s) (Figure 3.199).

Main oral sites affected: masseter.

Aetiopathogenesis: clenching or bruxism.

Gender predominance: none.

Age predominance: adult.

Extraoral possible lesions: see below.

Main associated conditions: linea alba; crenated tongue; tooth attrition.

Differential diagnosis: may clinically simulate the appearance of a parotid mass.

Investigations: cross-sectional imaging.

Main diagnostic criteria: clinical.

Main treatments: typically self-limiting and no treatment needed. Botulinum toxoid can help. Surgery may be indicated if there is a serious cosmetic defect.

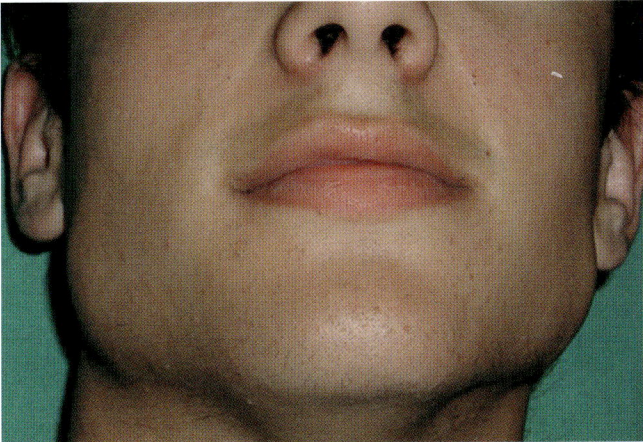

Figure 3.199 Jaw lesions: bilateral masseteric hypertrophy due to clenching and bruxism.

Jaw and musculoskeletal conditions (continued)

Odontogenic cysts and tumours

Uncommon. Cysts can be inflammatory (radicular, residual and paradental) or developmental (several subtypes), and cysts and tumours are classified into specific types by the World Health Organization (1992 and 2005).

Typical orofacial symptoms and signs: often asymptomatic and an incidental finding on imaging (Figures 3.200–3.205). Slow-growing but may eventually cause:

- swelling; initially a smooth bony hard lump with normal overlying mucosa but, as bone wall thins, it may crackle on palpation ('egg shell' crackling), and may resorb bone to show as a bluish fluctuant swelling
- discharge
- pain; if infected or the jaw fractures pathologically.

Main oral sites affected: mandible.

Aetiopathogenesis: odontogenic cysts and tumours arise from odontogenic ectoderm, mesenchyme or a combination (ectomesenchyme) and may be at the site of a tooth germ, or associated with a tooth.

Gender predominance: male.

Age predominance: adult.

Extraoral possible lesions: facial enlargement if large size.

Main associated conditions: keratocystic odontogenic tumour (KCOT, formerly termed odontogenic keratocyst) has a tendency to recur and may be associated with naevoid basal cell carcinoma syndrome (Gorlin syndrome).

Differential diagnosis: central jaw granuloma, early fibro-osseous lesions.

Investigations: imaging; biopsy; occasionally aspiration.

Main diagnostic criteria: clinical, imaging and histology.

Main treatments: surgery; enucleation or marsupialization. Most odontogenic cysts and most tumours have a good prognosis. Ameloblastoma and KCOT are a particular problem since these odontogenic tumours must be excised but tend to recur. Malignant tumours are rare but have a poor prognosis.

Figure 3.200 Jaw lesions: complex odontome.

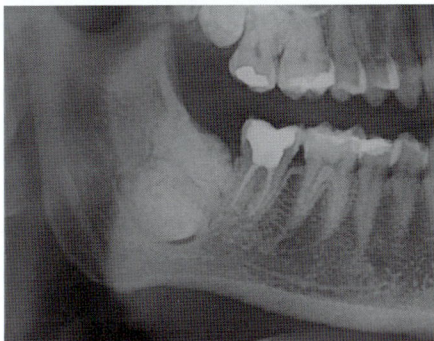

Figure 3.201 Jaw lesions: ameloblastoma, which coincidentally envelops the third molar.

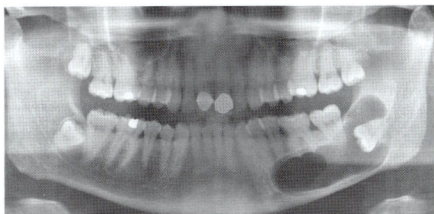

Figure 3.202 Jaw lesions: keratocystic odontogenic tumour.

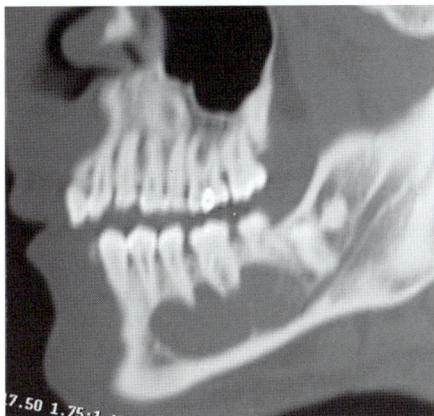

Jaw and musculoskeletal conditions (continued)

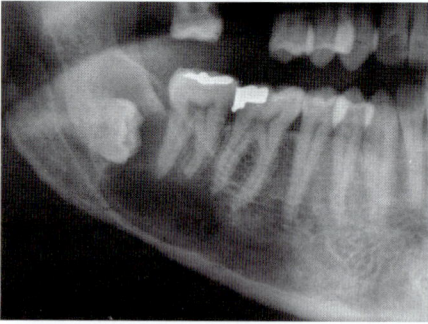

Figure 3.203 Jaw lesions: dentigerous cyst (compare with Figure 3.201).

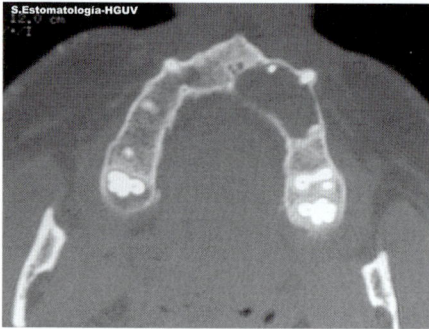

Figure 3.204 Jaw lesions: radicular cyst.

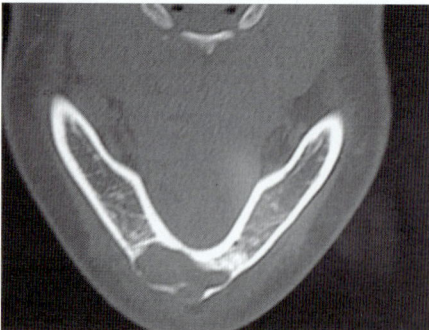

Figure 3.205 Jaw lesions: central giant cell granuloma.

Osteitis (alveolar osteitis or dry socket)

Common.

Typical orofacial symptoms and signs: onset of fairly severe pain 2–4 days after tooth extraction, bad taste and halitosis. The socket contains no clot, the surrounding mucosa is inflamed and the area is tender to palpation.

Main oral sites affected: molar regions.

Aetiopathogenesis: the extraction socket blood clot breaks down from the action of fibrinolysins, and the socket becomes 'dry' with localized osteitis. Most common after traumatic extraction under local anaesthesia in the mandibular molar region. Smoking, oral contraceptive use, immuno-compromising conditions, bone disorders and use of bisphosphonates predispose.

Gender predominance: male.

Age predominance: young adult.

Extraoral possible lesions: none.

Main associated conditions: none.

Differential diagnosis: fracture, osteomyelitis, osteosarcoma, other jaw malignancies.

Investigations: imaging may be indicated to exclude other causes of post-operative pain such as pathology associated with another tooth or a jaw fracture.

Main diagnostic criteria: clinical.

Main treatments: irrigate socket and dress with an obtundent antiseptic preparation. Systemic antimicrobial therapy is rarely warranted.

Osteomyelitis

Rare.

Typical orofacial symptoms and signs: severe pain and tenderness, swelling, labial hypoaesthesia and eventual loss of teeth, discharge of pus and necrotic bone (sequestrate).

Main oral sites affected: mandible.

Aetiopathogenesis: mixed infection (usually bacterial), typically originating from trauma or odontogenic infection. Predisposed by trauma, tobacco, alcohol, anaemia, immune defects and malnutrition.

Gender predominance: male.

Age predominance: young adult.

Jaw and musculoskeletal conditions (continued)

Extraoral possible lesions: sinuses.

Main associated conditions: fever.

Differential diagnosis: dry socket, osteonecrosis, actinomycosis.

Investigations: imaging, pus for Gram staining, aerobic and anaerobic culture and sensitivities, full blood picture, white cell count and erythrocyte sedimentation rate.

Main diagnostic criteria: history and clinical features, raised erythrocyte sedimentation rate and white cell count, and imaging findings once the acute inflammatory reaction leads to bone lysis (osteolysis usually takes 2–3 weeks). MRI has high sensitivity in detecting cancellous marrow abnormalities. Bone scan may be indicated.

Main treatments: aggressive therapy with penicillin, clavulanic acid/amoxicillin, or clindamycin and metronidazole. Analgesia. Later, sequestrectomy may be indicated.

Osteonecrosis

Uncommon jaw osteonecrosis is an important condition that can be caused by exposure to the following (most important is highlighted):

- Bevacizumab
- **Bisphosphonates**
- Bortezomib
- Corticosteroids
- Denosumab
- Heavy metals
- Immunocompromising states
- Irradiation in the head and neck
- Red phosphorus
- Severe herpes zoster or other infections
- Sunitinib
- Thalidomide
- Toxic endodontic materials.

Bisphosphonate-related osteonecrosis of the jaw (BRONJ)

Uncommon.

Typical orofacial symptoms and signs: exposed bone in a non-irradiated mouth, with or without external sinuses, pain and pathological fracture.

Main oral sites affected: mandible.

Aetiopathogenesis: damage to osteoclasts from intravenous bisphosphonates (pamidronate and/or zoledronic acid) and very occasionally from oral bisphosphonates such as alendronic acid. Predisposing factors for BRONJ also include use of other anti-angiogenic agents, advanced age, diabetes and dental trauma. Genetic factors may be a risk factor. Exodontia (tooth extraction) is the main precipitant.

Gender predominance: female.

Age predominance: older adults.

Extraoral possible lesions: may be sinus on face or neck.

Main associated conditions: none.

Differential diagnosis: osteomyelitis and osteoradionecrosis.

Investigations: radiography.

Main diagnostic criteria: clinical supported by imaging (bone has a moth-eaten appearance similar to that seen in osteoradionecrosis).

Main treatments: minimal interference is recommended; antimicrobials and analgesics only. Prevention is crucial. In advanced cases surgical debridement or resection in combination with antibiotic therapy may offer palliation with resolution of acute infection and pain.

Osteoradionecrosis (ORN)

Uncommon.

Typical orofacial symptoms and signs: exposed bone in an irradiated mouth, with or without external sinuses, pain and pathological fracture.

Main oral sites affected: mandible.

Aetiopathogenesis: radiation-induced endarteritis obliterans. Risk of ORN is greatest when radiation dose exceeds 60 Gy, from 10 days before to several years after radiotherapy (particularly at 3–12 months) and in the malnourished or immunoincompetent patient. The initiating event is often exodontia.

Gender predominance: none.

Age predominance: older adult.

Extraoral possible lesions: may be sinus on face or neck.

Main associated conditions: severe salivary gland hypofunction, caries, restricted mouth opening.

Differential diagnosis: osteomyelitis, osteosarcoma, other malignancies of the jaw.

Investigations: radiography.

Jaw and musculoskeletal conditions (continued)

Main diagnostic criteria: history and clinical features, imaging ('moth-eaten' appearance of the jaw).

Main treatments: local cleansing, and antimicrobials, especially tetracycline (which has high bone penetrance) long-term are indicated; hyperbaric oxygen and sequestrectomy may assist. Emphasis on oral disease prevention. In severe cases surgery with jawbone reconstruction is needed.

Paget disease

Uncommon fibro-osseous disease affecting bone and cementum.

Typical orofacial symptoms and signs: progressive jaw swelling often associated with severe bone pain and hypercementosis. Dense bone and hypercementosis make tooth extraction difficult, and there is a liability to haemorrhage and infection.

Main oral sites affected: maxilla.

Aetiopathogenesis: genes involved include the *sequestosome1* gene, with disorganization of osteoclastogenesis (osteoclast formation), disrupted bone remodelling and an anarchic alternation of bone resorption and apposition causing mosaic-like 'reversal lines'. Viruses have been implicated – possibly measles or respiratory syncytial virus.

Gender predominance: male.

Age predominance: older.

Extraoral possible lesions: typically polyostotic (affects several bones) and may affect skull, skull base, sphenoid, orbital and frontal bones, bowing of long bones, pathological fractures, broadening/flattening of chest and spinal deformity. Increased bone vascularity can lead to high-output cardiac failure. The healing after extractions is delayed. Predisposition to osteosarcoma. Constriction of skull foraminae may cause cranial neuropathies.

Main associated conditions: as above.

Differential diagnosis: bone neoplasms.

Investigations: biochemistry (see below), radiography, biopsy.

Main diagnostic criteria: radiography (in early lesions, large irregular areas of relative radiolucency [osteoporosis circumscripta] are seen, but later there is increased radio-opacity, with appearance of 'cotton wool' pattern); normal serum calcium and phosphate but raised serum alkaline phosphatase and urinary hydroxyproline, histology.

Main treatments: bisphosphonates or calcitonin.

Sinusitis

Common.

Typical orofacial symptoms and signs: nasal drainage (rhinorrhea or post-nasal drip), nasal blockage, pain in teeth worse on biting or leaning over, halitosis. There may be tenderness on palpation over the maxillary sinuses, nasal turbinate swelling, erythema and injection; mucus; sinus tenderness; allergic 'shiners' (dark circles around eyes), pharyngeal erythema, otitis, etc.

Aetiopathogenesis: bacterial infection is more likely after:

- allergic (vasomotor) rhinitis and nasal polyps
- viral upper respiratory tract infection (URTI)
- diving or flying
- nasal foreign bodies
- periapical infection of maxillary posterior teeth
- oro-antral fistula
- prolonged endotracheal intubation
- cilia damage (e.g. tobacco smoke exposure.

In acute sinusitis, *Streptococcus pneumoniae, Haemophilus influenzae* and (in children) *Moraxella catarrhalis. Staphylococcus aureus* may occasionally be implicated. In chronic sinusitis, also anaerobes, especially *Porphyromonas* (*Bacteroides*).

Gender predominance: none.

Age predominance: teens and up to 40 years.

Extraoral possible lesions: headache, fever, cough, malaise.

Main associated conditions: otitis.

Differential diagnosis: referred pain, or TMJ pathology.

Investigations: none usually; radiography, nasendoscopy.

Main diagnostic criteria: history, clinical (sinus tenderness and dullness on transillumination), imaging.

Main treatments: analgesics, decongestants (ephedrine), antibiotics for at least 2 weeks in acute sinusitis – amoxicillin (or ampicillin or co-amoxiclav), or a tetracycline such as doxycycline, or clindamycin. Chronic sinusitis responds best to drainage by functional endoscopic sinus surgery (FESS).

Temporomandibular pain-dysfunction syndrome (TMPD; myofascial pain dysfunction [MFD], facial arthromyalgia [FAM], mandibular dysfunction, or mandibular stress syndrome)

A common complaint, it appears to be related to muscle spasm (and subsequent ischaemic pain) arising from stress, joint damage or habits (e.g.

Jaw and musculoskeletal conditions (continued)

tooth clenching or grinding). There are no serious long-term consequences; arthritis does not result and it is not inherited. Various treatments such as rest, exercises, splints, physiotherapy, or drugs may be advocated but the symptoms usually clear spontaneously after some months; hence, it is one of the most controversial areas in dentistry.

Typical orofacial symptoms and signs: triad of temporomandibular joint (TMJ) symptoms – clicking, jaw limitation of opening or locking, and pain (mainly from masticatory muscle spasm).

Main oral sites affected: TMJ area but can spread fairly widely, ipsilaterally (Figure 3.206).

Aetiopathogenesis: trauma and stress appear to predispose through increasing tension in the masticatory muscles.

Gender predominance: female.

Age predominance: teens and up to 40 years.

Extraoral possible lesions: headaches, neck aches and lower back pain.

Main associated conditions: psychogenic disorders.

Differential diagnosis: referred pain, rheumatoid arthritis, osteoarthritis, or other TMJ pathology.

Investigations: none usually; radiography if TMJ pathology suspected.

Main diagnostic criteria: history, clinical (may be crepitus from the TMJ, limited or deviated opening, clicking or popping in the TMJ and/or diffuse tenderness or spasm on palpation of masseter, temporalis, medial or lateral pterygoid muscles).

Main treatments: treatment is indicated if there is pain. Try analgesics; reduce psychological stress (by reassurance), rest TMJ by use of:

- soft diet
- avoidance of trauma, wide-opening and abnormal habits
- warmth, massage and remedial jaw exercises
- non-steroidal anti-inflammatory drugs, topically as a gel, or systemically.

It may sometimes also be helpful to use:

- muscle relaxants (e.g. benzodiazepines)
- hard plastic occlusal splints.

Surgery may be required for the extremely small number with obvious intra-articular pathology.

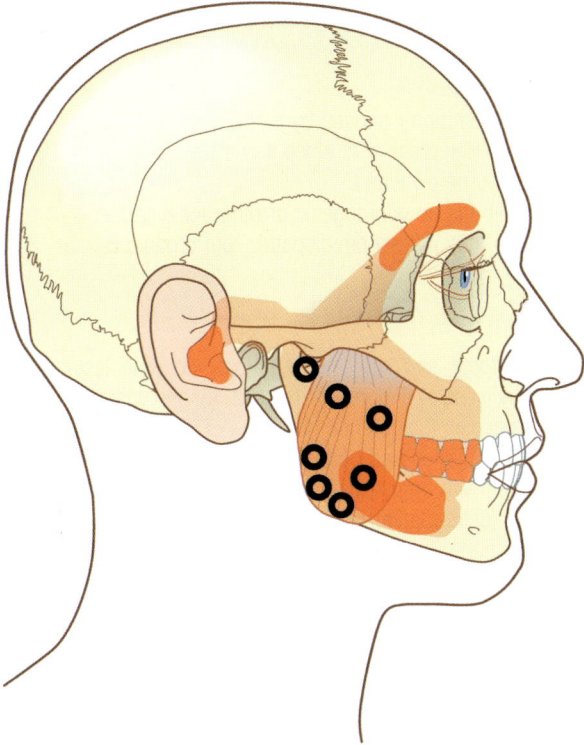

Figure 3.206 Temporomandibular joint lesions: location of pain from TMJ pain-dysfunction.

Neurological and pain disorders

Keypoints

- Facial palsy is most commonly caused by a stroke, or Bell palsy,
- Infections may cause Bell palsy and, since it is a treatable cause, Lyme disease should always be excluded.
- Orofacial pain mostly has an odontogenic or other local cause.
- Idiopathic facial pain may indeed be idiopathic, but organic causes must be excluded.

Bell palsy

Typical orofacial symptoms and signs: lower motor neurone lesion with complete unilateral facial palsy (Figures 3.207, 3.208); and sometimes loss of taste and/or hyperacusis (heightened hearing).

Aetiopathogenesis: inflammation and oedema of the facial nerve, usually in the stylomastoid canal, with demyelination, usually caused by a virus (e.g. HSV, HIV) or bacteria (otitis media; *Borrelia burgdorferi* – Lyme disease).

Gender predominance: none.

Age predominance: young adult.

Extraoral possible lesions: none.

Main associated conditions: rarely pregnancy, diabetes, hypertension, Crohn disease/OFG, sarcoidosis, lymphoma.

Differential diagnosis: stroke, inflammatory, traumatic and neoplastic lesions.

Investigations: neurological; MRI or CT; blood pressure; fasting blood sugar level tests to exclude diabetes; serology to exclude virus infections; serum angiotensin-converting enzyme (SACE) levels to exclude sarcoidosis; serum antinuclear antibodies (ANA) to exclude connective tissue disease; and enzyme-linked immunosorbent assay (ELISA) for *B. burgdorferi* to exclude Lyme disease.

Main diagnostic criteria: clinical.

Main treatments: treat defined causes; systemic corticosteroids.

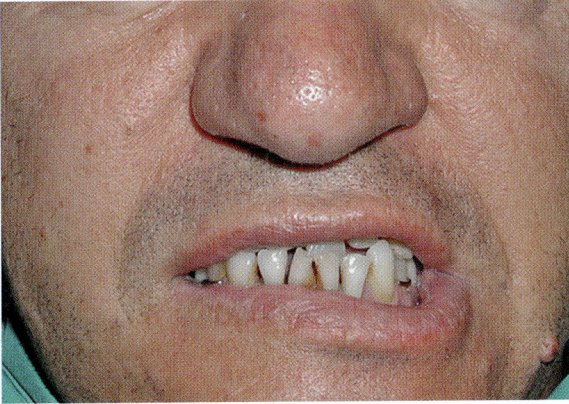

Figure 3.207 Neurological: right sided facial palsy.

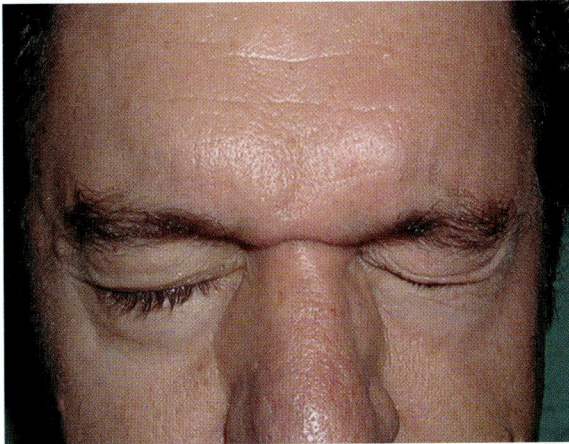

Figure 3.208 Neurological: right sided facial palsy.

Neurological and pain disorders (continued)

Giant cell arteritis (cranial or temporal arteritis)

Rare but may threaten sight and is thus an emergency.

Typical orofacial symptoms and signs: pain on chewing, or headache usually concentrated in the temple – which may be tender to touch (Figure 3.209).

Main oral sites affected: temple; rarely tongue or lip.

Aetiopathogenesis: inflammatory condition that affects medium-sized arteries, in particular the temporal and optic artery.

Gender predominance: female.

Age predominance: older.

Extraoral possible lesions: superficial temporal artery may be dilated and tender.

Main associated conditions: polymyalgia rheumatica.

Differential diagnosis: other causes of headache.

Investigations: erythrocyte sedimentation rate, arterial biopsy, echo Doppler.

Main diagnostic criteria: clinical supported by raised erythrocyte sedimentation rate, and arteritis on biopsy.

Main treatments: can lead to a sudden loss of vision from retinal artery blockage – an emergency necessitating systemic corticosteroid treatment.

Idiopathic facial pain (atypical facial pain)

Common. The cause is not completely known but may the pain may result from increased nerve sensitivity and there may be a background of stress. Atypical odontalgia (chronic continuous alveolar dental pain: CCADP) is generally regarded as a variant.

Typical orofacial symptoms and signs: a dull boring or burning continuous poorly localized pain that does not disturb sleep and is confined initially to a limited area (unrelated to the trigeminal nerve distribution) on one side only, but may spread. Other features are a lack of objective signs, lack of detectable dental/jaw problems and a poor treatment response. Often also multiple other complaints, such as dry mouth and bad taste.

Main oral sites affected: maxilla.

Aetiopathogenesis: no known organic cause – rather, a psychogenic basis.

Gender predominance: female.

Age predominance: older.

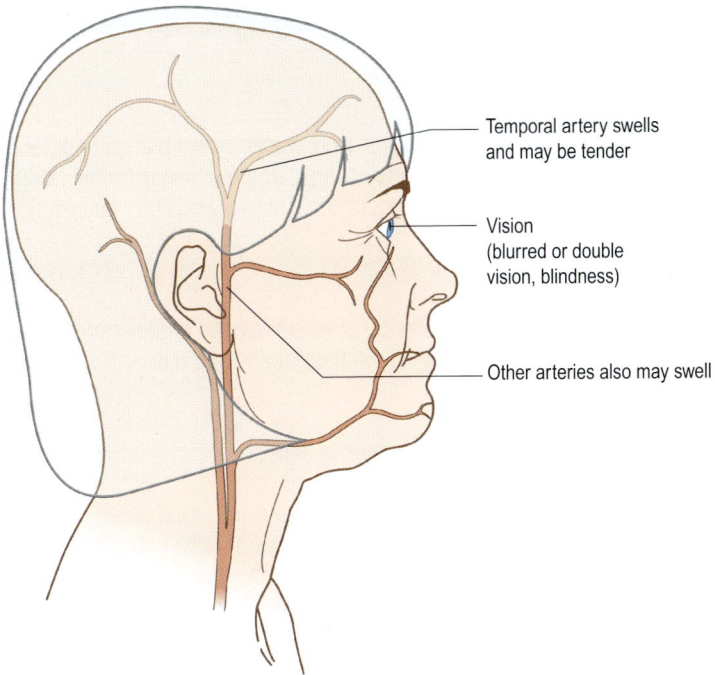

Figure 3.209 Neurological and pain disorders: giant cell arteritis features.

Extraoral possible lesions: headaches, chronic back pain, irritable bowel syndrome and/or dysmenorrhoea.

Main associated conditions: stress, anxiety, a few have hypochondriases, neuroses (often depression) or psychoses.

Differential diagnosis: other causes of orofacial pain including local and neurological causes, and Lyme disease.

Investigations: dental, otolaryngological, and neurological examination, and imaging (tooth/jaw/sinus/skull radiography and MRI/CT scan of the head with particular attention to skull base), serology for *Borrelia burgdorferi*.

Main diagnostic criteria: clinical, with negative investigation results.

Main treatments: cognitive-behavioural therapy (CBT); antidepressant trial, e.g. nortriptyline, may be warranted. There is a high level of utilization of healthcare services with multiple failed consultations and treatment attempts.

Neurological and pain disorders (continued)

Trigeminal neuralgia

Uncommon.

Typical orofacial symptoms and signs: pain is unilateral in branch or division of trigeminal nerve and is severe, sharp 'stabbing' intermittent, lasting seconds only. Often there is a trigger zone. There are no other neurological symptoms or signs.

Main oral sites affected: mandibular division of trigeminal nerve (Figure 3.210).

Aetiopathogenesis: unknown; possibly pressure from an arteriosclerotic posterior inferior cerebellar artery on the trigeminal nerve root.

Gender predominance: female.

Age predominance: older.

Extraoral possible lesions: trigger zones on face.

Main associated conditions: none.

Differential diagnosis: other causes of orofacial pain – local causes (usually dental); neurological disorders (multiple sclerosis or brain tumour); vascular causes (migrainous neuralgia; cranial arteritis); psychological disorders (idiopathic facial pain, oral dysaesthesia) and referred (cardiac) pain very rarely.

Investigations: MRI of trigeminal nerve (Figure 3.211).

Main diagnostic criteria: clinical, and typical beneficial response to the anticonvulsant carbamazepine.

Main treatments: carbamazepine prophylaxis (care in Han Chinese who may be hypersensitive); uncontrolled pain may be treated by injecting glycerol or freezing the peripheral nerve (cryosurgery), or neurosurgery.

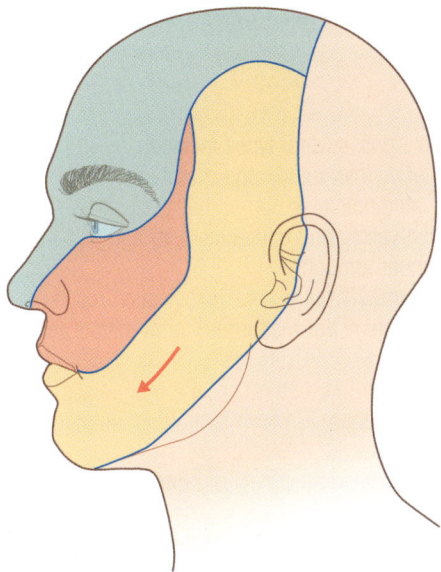

Figure 3.210 Neurological and pain disorders: neuralgia can affect one or occasionally more trigeminal nerve divisions. Arrow: lancinating pain in the mandibular division (the most common site).

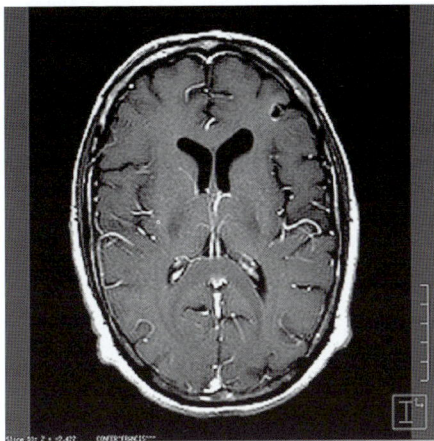

Figure 3.211 Neurological and pain disorders: brain scans may be indicated to exclude a tumour or other pathology.

Teeth-specific disorders

Amelogenesis imperfecta

Uncommon genetic condition.

Typical orofacial symptoms and signs: several types include:

- Hypocalcified type: normal enamel matrix and morphology but incomplete calcification. Morphology is normal but the enamel is opaque, white to brownish-yellow and darkening with age and the teeth are soft and chip under attrition.
- Hypoplastic type: defective matrix but normal calcification results in the enamel being hard and shiny but malformed, often pitted and stained (Figure 3.212).
- Hypomineralized type: defect in the maturation of the enamel's crystal structure. Causes soft enamel, which is mottled, opaque white, yellow and brown (Figure 3.213).

Aetiopathogenesis: genetic defect with wide variety of patterns.

Gender predominance: none.

Age predominance: from infancy.

Extraoral possible lesions: none.

Main associated conditions: none.

Differential diagnosis: fluorosis, tetracycline staining, dentinogenesis imper-fecta, incisor-molar hypomineralization, environmental enamel hypoplasia, oculo-dento-digital dysplasia.

Investigations: imaging.

Main diagnostic criteria: clinical, family history; radiography of teeth.

Main treatments: remineralization of teeth and restorative dental care.

Caries

See dental textbooks.

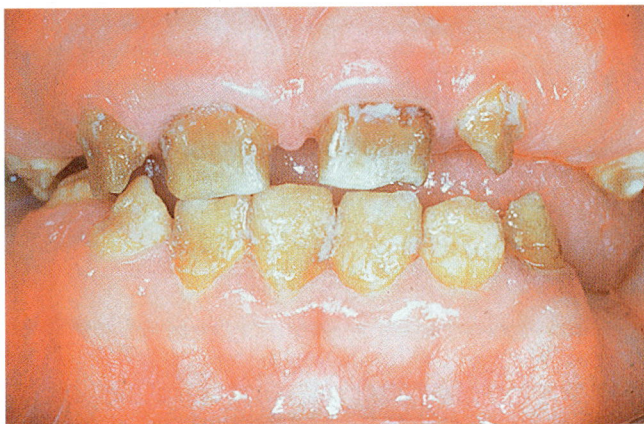

Figure 3.212 Teeth inherited defects – amelogenesis imperfecta (hypoplastic type).

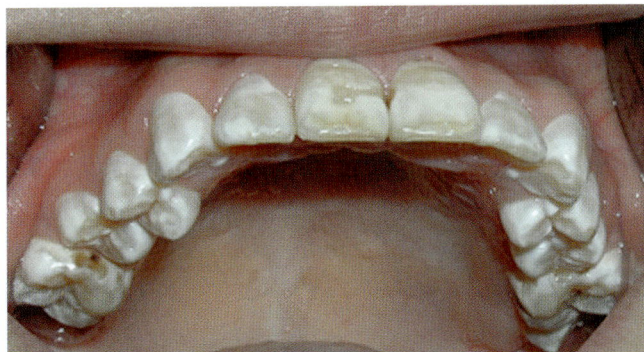

Figure 3.213 Teeth inherited defects – amelogenesis imperfecta (hypocalcified type).

Teeth-specific disorders (continued)

Dentinogenesis imperfecta

Rare.

Typical orofacial symptoms and signs: teeth are abnormally translucent, yellow to blue-grey (Figures 3.214, 3.215). Enamel splits off. Roots are short; pulp is rapidly obliterated by secondary dentine:

- Type I (associated with osteogenesis imperfecta); most severe in deciduous dentition; bone fractures; blue sclera; progressive deafness
- Type II (hereditary opalescent dentine): defect equal in both dentitions
- Type III (brandywine type): associated with occasional shell teeth.

Aetiopathogenesis: usually autosomal dominant inheritance.

Gender predominance: none.

Age predominance: from birth.

Extraoral possible lesions: Type I is associated with osteogenesis imperfecta.

Main associated conditions: as above.

Differential diagnosis: amelogenesis imperfecta, tetracycline staining and dentine dysplasia.

Investigations: imaging.

Main diagnostic criteria: family history; radiography of teeth/bones.

Main treatments: restorative dental care.

Fluorosis

Uncommon in UK/USA. Particularly common in parts of Middle East, India and Africa.

Typical orofacial symptoms and signs: many teeth affected:

- mildest form: white flecks or spotting or diffuse cloudiness
- more severe: yellow-brown or darker patches
- most severe: yellow-brown or darker patches, sometimes with pitting (Figure 3.216).

Aetiopathogenesis: enamel defects caused by high levels of fluoride in drinking water.

Gender predominance: none.

Age predominance: from time of tooth appearance.

Extraoral possible lesions: none.

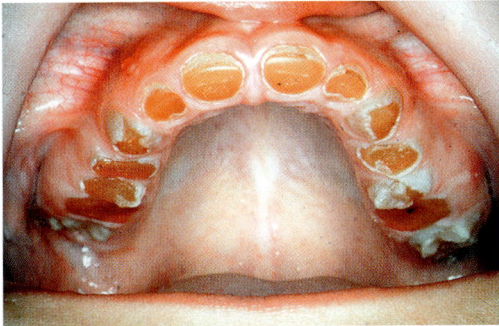

Figure 3.214 Teeth inherited defects: dentinogenesis imperfecta – typical discoloration and attrition.

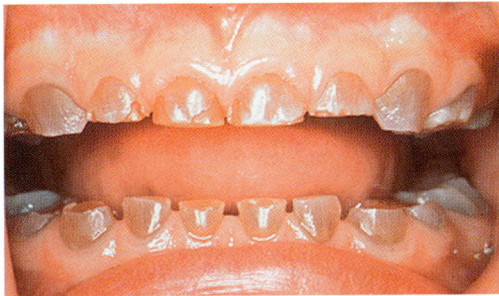

Figure 3.215 Teeth inherited defects: dentinogenesis imperfecta – typical discoloration and attrition.

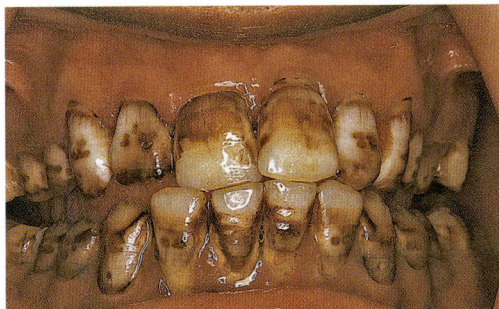

Figure 3.216 Teeth acquired defects: severe fluorosis in a person born in Africa in a very high fluoride area.

Teeth-specific disorders (continued)

Main associated conditions: none.
Differential diagnosis: amelogenesis imperfecta and tetracycline staining.
Investigations: data about fluoride content of drinking water.
Main diagnostic criteria: clinical.
Main treatments: veneers or crowns.

Tetracycline staining

Should be rare but is still not uncommon.

Typical orofacial symptoms and signs: yellow, brown or greyish tooth hyperpigmentation, especially cervically (Figure 3.217). Teeth may also be hypoplastic.
Main oral sites affected: anterior teeth.
Aetiopathogenesis: tetracyclines given to children or before birth to their pregnant or nursing mothers.
Gender predominance: none.
Age predominance: from time of tooth appearance.
Extraoral possible lesions: none.
Main associated conditions: none.
Differential diagnosis: dentinogenesis imperfecta and amelogenesis imperfecta.
Investigations: history of exposure to tetracycline. Teeth fluoresce in ultraviolet light if tetracycline deposition is severe.
Main diagnostic criteria: clinical.
Main treatments: bleaching, veneers or crowns.

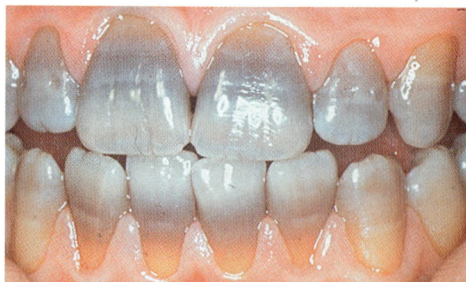

Figure 3.217 Teeth acquired defects: tetracycline staining – multiple coloured bands from repeated therapy.

4

Iatrogenic conditions

An increasing number of therapeutic procedures important in modern medicine and surgery can produce iatrogenic (doctor-induced) unwanted orofacial complications (Tables 4.1–4.6).

Immunosuppressive therapy

Immunosuppressive therapy is designed to suppress T lymphocyte function, and leads to immunoincompetence and liability to infections, especially with viruses (Figures 4.1–4.3), fungi (Figure 4.4) and mycobacteria (Table 4.1).

Such infections may spread rapidly; may be opportunistic; and may be clinically silent or atypical.

Table 4.1 Orofacial complications of immunosuppression

Viral infections	Herpesviruses (HSV, VZV, CMV, EBV, KSHV) and human papillomaviruses (HPV)
Fungal infections	Usually with *Candida* species but also deep mycoses (e.g. zygomycosis, histoplasmosis)
Bacterial infections	Especially with tuberculosis and other mycobacterial infections
Virally related malignant disease	Kaposi sarcoma, lymphomas, carcinomas

Immunosuppressive therapy (continued)

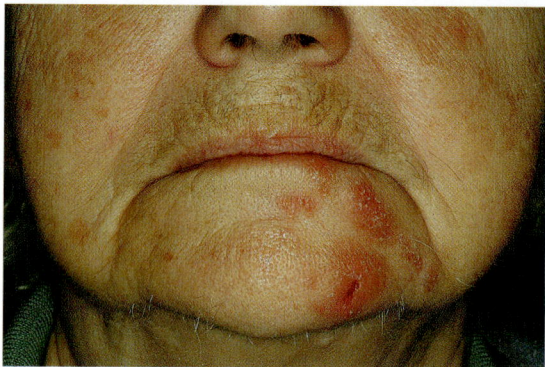

Figure 4.1 Herpes zoster (shingles) of the mandibular division of the trigeminal nerve.

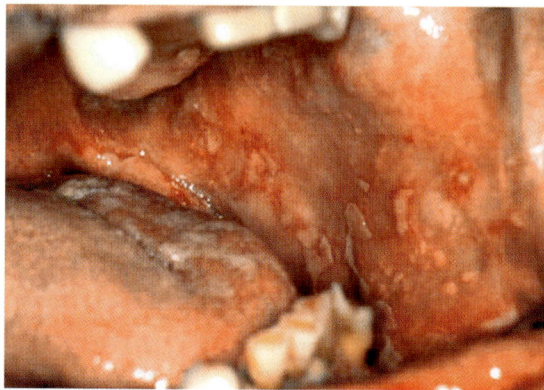

Figure 4.2 Herpes zoster (shingles) of the mandibular division of the trigeminal nerve.

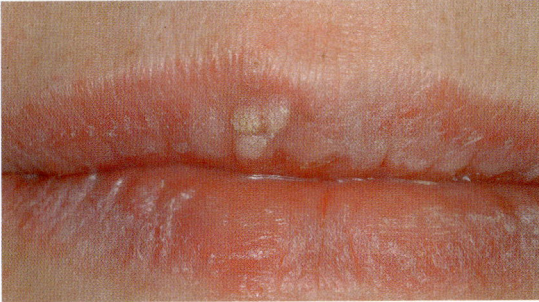

Figure 4.3 Wart (human papillomavirus infection).

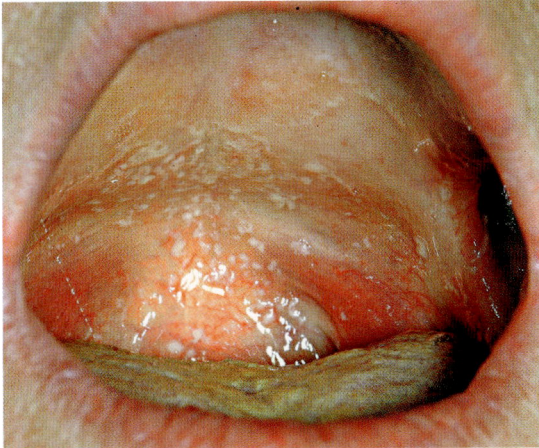

Figure 4.4 Candidosis can complicate systemic or local immunosuppression (from steroid inhalers, as here).

Radiotherapy

Radiation therapy is widely used, especially to control malignant neoplasms, and if involving the mouth and salivary glands invariably produces complications (Table 4.2). These complications may be minimized by using:

- minimal radiation doses and fields
- IMRT (intensity-modulated radio therapy) or IGRT (image-guided radiotherapy)
- mucosa-sparing blocks
- amifostine (a free radical scavenger) before therapy.

Table 4.2 Orofacial complications of radiotherapy

Condition	Causes	Comments
Mucositis	After external beam radiotherapy involving the maxillofacial tissues	Dose-dependent diffuse erythema and ulceration after 10–15 days (Figure 4.5)
Hyposalivation	Damage to salivary glands	(Figure 4.6) Can lead to dysphagia, disturbed taste, candidosis, sialadenitis and radiation caries
Osteoradionecrosis		Pain, jaw necrosis and infection
Trismus	Inflammation and scarring	Distinguish from tumour spread
Taste loss	Damage to taste buds	Temporary
Telangiectasia		Late
Jaw and tooth hypoplasia	Abnormal development	Children treated for neuroblastoma are at particularly high risk
Facial palsy	Carotid artery damage	Cerebrovascular event (stroke)

Figure 4.5 Mucositis can produce widespread erosions and ulcers.

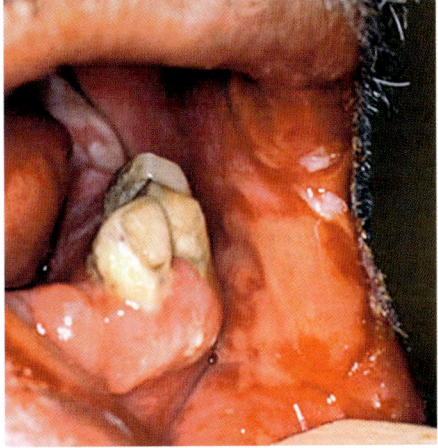

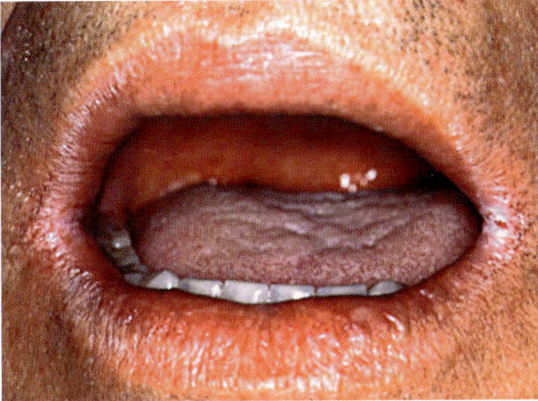

Figure 4.6 Radiation-induced hyposalivation is invariable after radiation involving major salivary glands.

Chemotherapy

Chemotherapy is widely used, especially to treat lymphoproliferative conditions and malignant neoplasms. There can be several complications (Table 4.3). Mucositis is an almost invariable complication and may also be a predictor of gastrointestinal toxicity and of hepatic veno-occlusive disease. It is caused by cisplatin, etoposide, fluorouracil and melphalan, mucositis is especially seen with chemo-radiotherapy regimens, involving:

- cisplatin and fluorouracil
- cisplatin, epirubicin, bleomycin
- carboplatin.

Table 4.3 Orofacial complications of chemotherapy

Condition	Causes	Comments
Mucositis	Cytotoxic drugs impair the mucosal barrier and immunity	Pain appears within 3–7 days, mucosa reddens and thins, may slough and become eroded and ulcerated and sometimes bleeds. Erosions/ulcers often become covered by a yellowish white fibrin clot termed a pseudomembrane
Taste sensation changed	poor oral hygiene, gastric reflux, infections, drugs	Often temporary

Organ transplantation

Transplant recipients are treated with immunosuppressive therapy designed to suppress T lymphocyte function, and they therefore have an increased risk of infections and some malignant neoplasms (Table 4.4).

Table 4.4 Orofacial complications of organ transplantation

Viral infections	Herpesviruses (HSV, VZV, CMV, EBV, KSHV) and human papillomaviruses (HPV),
Fungal infections	Usually with *Candida* species but also deep mycoses (e.g. zygomycosis, histoplasmosis)
Bacterial infections	Especially with tuberculosis and other mycobacterial infections. Bacterial sepsis is the most common cause of deaths occurring during the first post-transplantation months
Virally related malignant disease	Kaposi sarcoma, lymphomas, carcinomas, post-transplant lymphoproliferative disease

Haematopoietic stem cell transplantation

Haematopoietic stem cell transplantation (HSCT or bone marrow transplant) is increasingly used to treat haematological conditions, neoplasms and some genetic defects. Patients are first profoundly immunosuppressed to minimize graft rejection by 'conditioning', often using cyclophosphamide, plus total body irradiation (TBI), or busulphan and are thus very susceptible to infections. Patients must be isolated and may require transfusions of granulocytes, platelets, red cells, granulocyte colony stimulating factors and antimicrobials until the donor bone marrow is functioning. HSCT may be complicated by mucositis, infections, neoplasms, bleeding, or graft-versus-host disease (GvHD) (Table 4.5).

Table 4.5 Orofacial complications of haematopoietic stem cell transplantation

Condition	Causes	Comments
Mucositis	Cytotoxic drugs impair the mucosal barrier and immunity	Pain appears within 3–7 days, mucosa reddens and thins, may slough and become eroded and ulcerated and sometimes bleeds. Erosions/ulcers often become covered by a yellowish white fibrin clot termed a pseudomembrane
Bleeding	Bone marrow damage	Bleeding from gingivae and into tissues
Infections	Viral	Herpesviruses (HSV, VZV, CMV, EBV, KSHV) and human papillomaviruses (HPV)
	Fungal	Usually with *Candida* species, but also deep mycoses (e.g. zygomycosis, histoplasmosis)
	Bacterial	Especially with tuberculosis and other mycobacterial infections. Bacterial sepsis is the most common cause of deaths occurring during the first post-transplantation months
	Virally related malignant disease	Kaposi sarcoma, lymphomas, carcinomas, post-transplant lymphoproliferative disease
Graft-versus-host disease (GvHD)	Donor lymphocytes attack recipient, causing this potentially lethal disorder	Mucositis, lichenoid reactions (Figure 4.7) or hyposalivation
Drug effects	Ciclosporin Tacrolimus	Gingival swelling, predisposition to neoplasms

Figure 4.7 Chronic graft-versus-host disease is common after haematopoietic stem cell transplantation (bone marrow transplants).

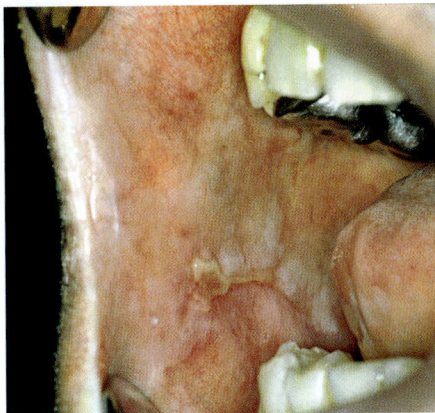

Drugs

Drugs may give rise to a range of orofacial symptoms and signs (Table 4.6) by a wide range of mechanisms – often unknown.

Other iatrogenic conditions

A range of dental operative procedures may cause iatrogenic disease, which are discussed in textbooks of operative dentistry, prosthodontics and oral surgery. These may range from complications of restorative procedures – such as amalgam tattoos (Figure 4.20), or lichenoid lesions (Figure 4.21); dental abscess formation (Figure 4.22); denture-related hyperplasia (Figure 4.23) and stomatitis (Figures 4.24, 4.25); and complications of exodontia such as dry socket and oroantral fistula (Figure 4.26).

Table 4.6 Orofacial adverse effects from drugs

Lesions	Main drugs implicated
Abnormal facial movements (dyskinesias)	Metoclopramide Phenothiazines
Angioedema	Aldesleukin (human recombinant IL-2) Angiotensin-converting enzyme (ACE) inhibitors Interferon (IFN)-alpha Many others
Burning sensation	ACE inhibitors Protease inhibitors Proton pump inhibitors
Candidosis	Any drug that causes hyposalivation Broad-spectrum antimicrobials Cytotoxic drugs Immunosuppressants
Dental hypoplasia	Cytotoxic drugs
Dry mouth	Antihistamines Antihypertensives Calcium channel blockers Lithium Phenothiazines Tolterodine Tricyclic antidepressants
Erythema multiforme	NSAIDs Barbiturates Sulphonamides Very many others
Gingival swelling	Calcium channel blockers such as nifedipine Phenytoin Ciclosporin Tacrolimus (Figures 4.8–4.10)

Table 4.6 Orofacial adverse effects from drugs—cont'd

Lesions	Main drugs implicated
Halitosis	Amphetamines Amyl nitrites Aztreonam Cytotoxic drugs Disulfiram Melatonin Mycophenolate Nicotine Nitrates Phenothiazines Solvent misuse
Herpesvirus infections	Cytotoxic drugs Immunosuppressants
Hyperpigmentation	ACTH Amlodipine Antimalarials (Figure 4.11) Betel Busulfan Capecitabine Hydroxyurea Ketoconazole Minocycline (Figure 4.12) Palifermin Peginterferon and ribavirin Tobacco Zidovudine
Human papillomaviruses (HPV)	Immunosuppressive agents
Lichenoid lesions	A range of drugs, especially NSAIDS (Figure 4.13)
Maxillofacial developmental defects	Alcohol Anticonvulsants Cytotoxic drugs

Continued

Table 4.6 Orofacial adverse effects from drugs—cont'd

Lesions	Main drugs implicated
Mucositis	Cytotoxic agents
Osteonecrosis of the jaws	Bevacizumab Bisphosphonates (Figures 4.14, 4.15) Denosumab Sunitinib
Pain	Doxorubicin Vinca alkaloids
Pemphigoid	Furosemide
Pemphigus	ACE inhibitors Aspirin Captopril Enalapril Fosinopril Levodopa Nifedipine NSAIDs Penicillamine Penicillin (benzyl) Propranolol Ramipril Rifampicin Thiols
Potentially malignant disorders and oral carcinoma	Alcohol Betel Immunosuppressants Khat Tobacco
Sensory changes	Articaine Capsaicin Carmustine Labetalol Prilocaine Sulthiame

Table 4.6 Orofacial adverse effects from drugs—cont'd

Lesions	Main drugs implicated
Sialorrhoea	Aripiprazole Benzodiazepines Cevimeline Cholinesterase inhibitors Clozapine Neuroleptics Pilocarpine Quetiapine
Sialosis	Alcohol Anti-thyroid drugs Methyl dopa Valproic acid Sympathomimetic agents such as isoprenaline
Taste disturbance	ACE inhibitors (e.g. captopril, eprosartan) Amiloride Antidepressants Any chemotherapeutic Any drug causing dry mouth Bisphosphonates Chlorhexidine Clarithromycin H_1-antihistamines (e.g. azelastine and emedastine) Lithium Metformin Metronidazole Omeprazole Penicillamine Pesticides (organochloride compounds and carbamates) Subutramine Terbinafine Tetracyclines Zopiclone

Continued

Table 4.6 Orofacial adverse effects from drugs—cont'd

Lesions	Main drugs implicated
Tics	Anticonvulsants Antiparkinsonian drugs Caffeine Methylphenidate
Tooth discoloration	Extrinsic – chlorhexidine, some antibiotics, tobacco and iron preparations (Figures 4.16, 4.17) Intrinsic – tetracyclines
Tooth root anomalies	Cytotoxic drugs Phenytoin
Ulcers	Alendronate Carbimazole Cytotoxic drugs (Figure 4.18) Deferiprone Nicorandil (Figure 4.19) NSAIDs Sirolimus Tacrolimus

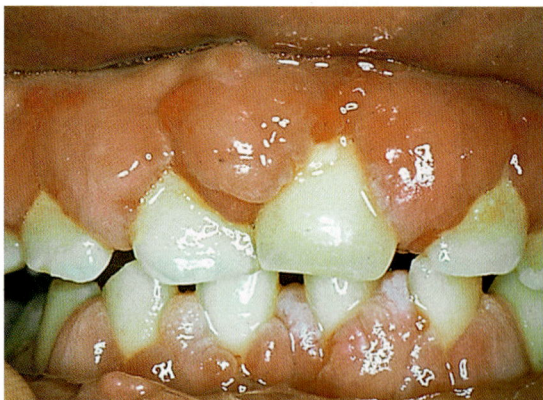

Figure 4.8 Drug-induced gingival swelling (phenytoin) typically originates from interdental papillae.

Figure 4.9
Drug-induced gingival swelling (nifedipine).

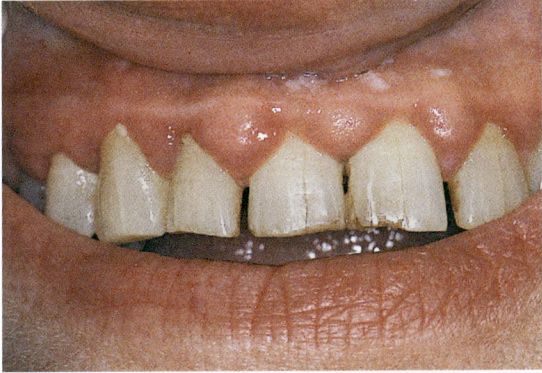

Figure 4.10
Drug-induced gingival swelling (diltiazem and ciclosporin): common after organ transplantation because of anti-rejection therapy.

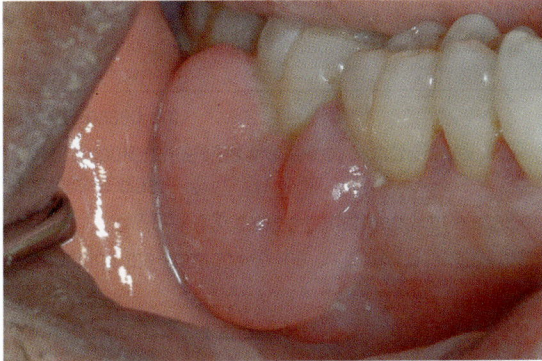

Figure 4.11 Drug-induced palatal pigmentation (hydroxychloroquine).

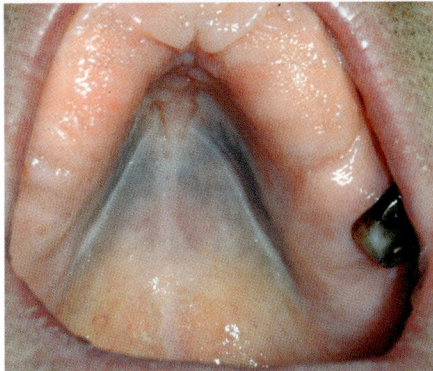

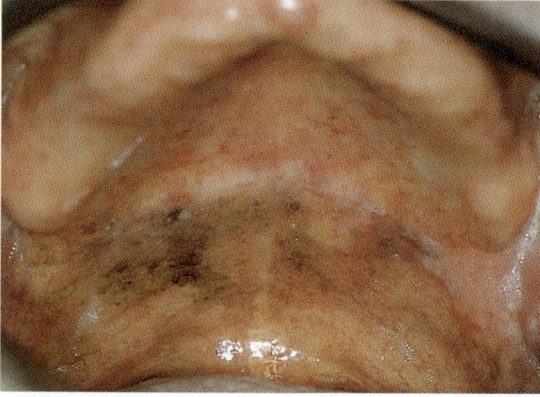

Figure 4.12 Drug-induced palatal pigmentation (minocycline).

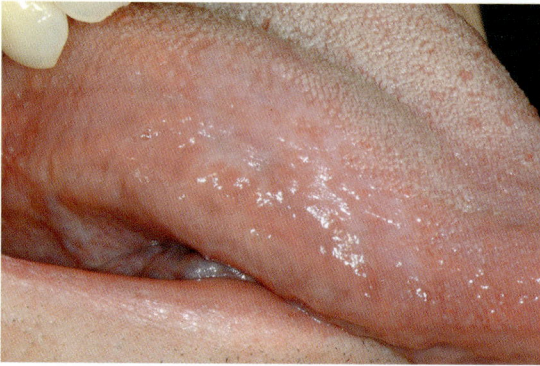

Figure 4.13 Drug-induced lichenoid lesions.

Figure 4.14
Bisphosphonate
related
osteonecrosis
(most common
after intravenous
bisphosphonates
used in cancer
patients).

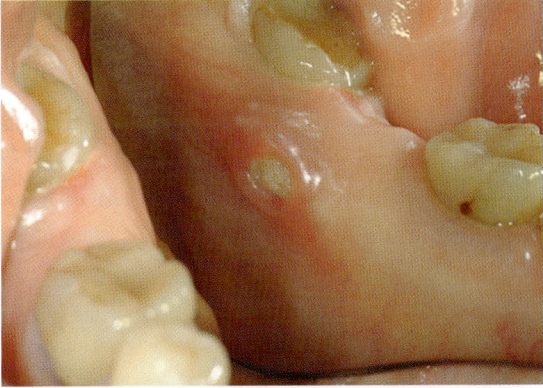

Figure 4.15
Bisphosphonate-
related
osteonecrosis.

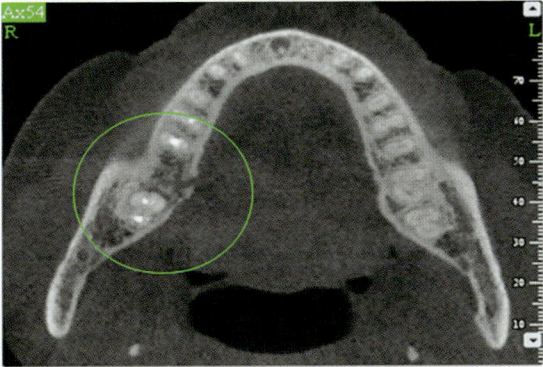

Figure 4.16
Tooth staining
(chlorhexidine).

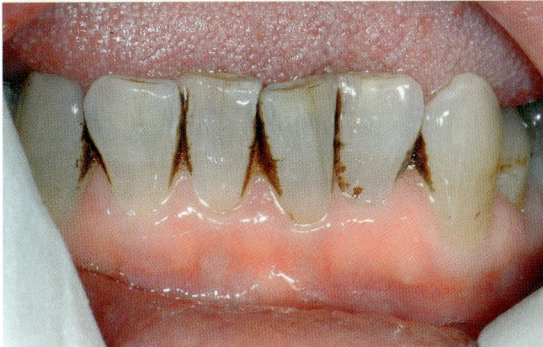

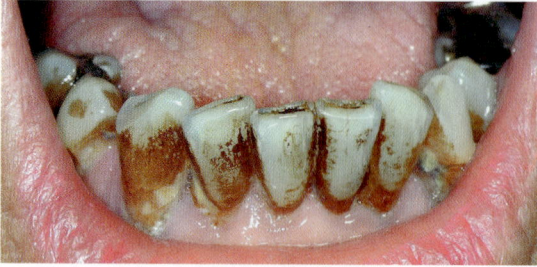

Figure 4.17
Tooth staining (chlorhexidine, smoking and poor oral hygiene).

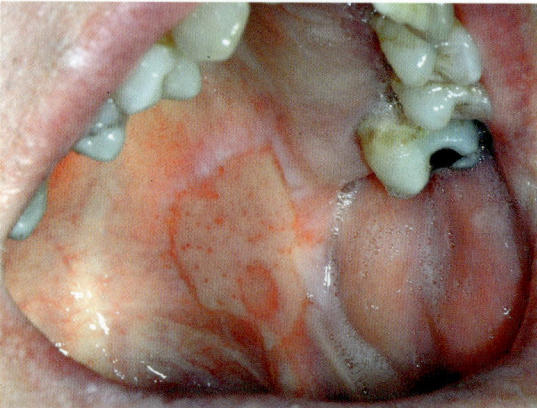

Figure 4.18
Drug-induced ulceration (methotrexate).

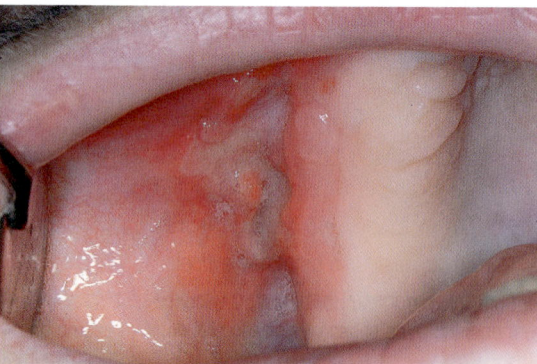

Figure 4.19
Drug-induced ulceration (nicorandil, a potassium channel activator, which can also cause anal ulceration).

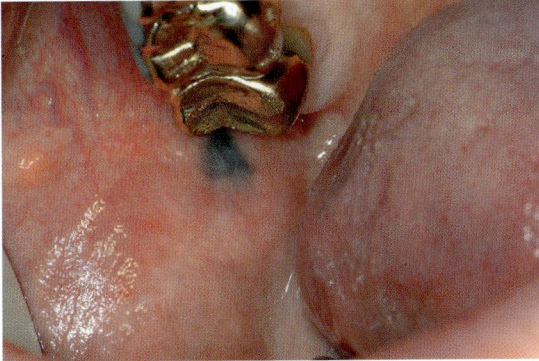

Figure 4.20 Amalgam tattoo.

Figure 4.21 Amalgam related lichenoid reaction.

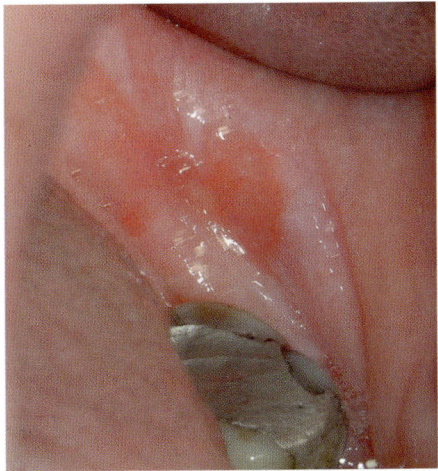

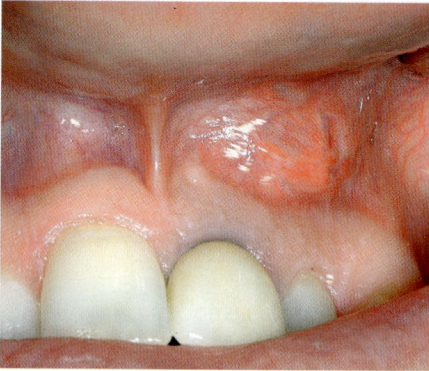

Figure 4.22 Iatrogenic dental abscess related to the crowned incisor.

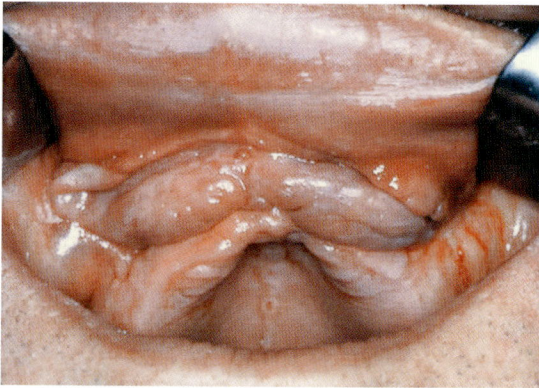

Figure 4.23 Denture-related hyperplasia.

Figure 4.24
Denture-related
stomatitis.

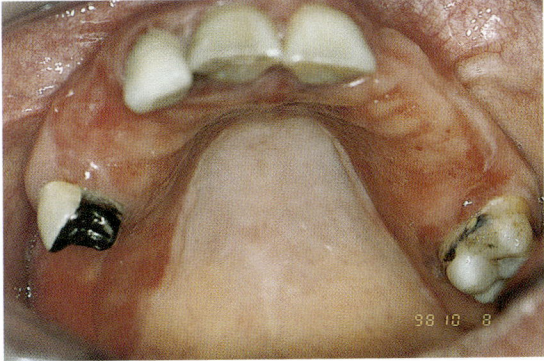

Figure 4.25
Denture-related
stomatitis.

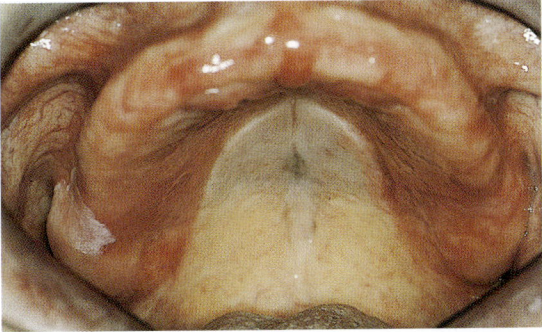

Figure 4.26
Traumatic
oroantral fistula,
after the
maxillary
tuberosity
fractured and
was removed.

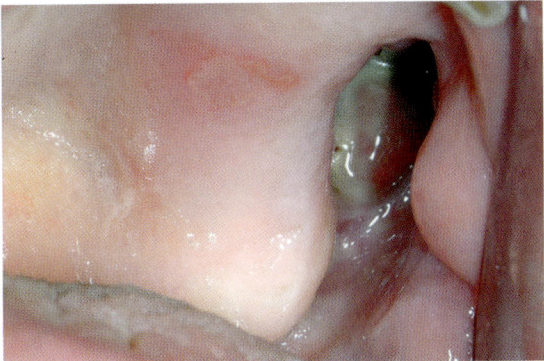

5

Immune defects and haematological defects and malignancies

Human immunodeficiency virus (HIV) disease

HIV is a retrovirus transmitted sexually, via blood, or to the neonate, which has produced a global pandemic, especially affecting people in the developing world. There can be a range of orofacial complications seen in HIV disease (Figure 5.1), and in the acquired immune deficiency syndrome (AIDS) – defined as a CD4 T lymphocyte count of less than 200 cells per microlitre (μl) of blood (Table 5.1).

Orofacial lesions in HIV disease have been classified as follows:

- Group I: Lesions strongly associated with HIV infection
  - Candidosis
    - erythematous Figures 5.2–5.5)
    - hyperplastic
    - thrush
  - Hairy leukoplakia (EBV) (Figures 5.6 & 5.7)
  - HIV-gingivitis (linear gingival erythema) (Figure 5.8)
  - Necrotizing ulcerative gingivitis (Figure 5.9)
  - HIV-periodontitis
  - Kaposi sarcoma
  - Non-Hodgkin lymphoma
- Group II: Lesions less commonly associated with HIV infection
  - Atypical ulceration (oropharyngeal)
  - Salivary gland diseases (Figure 5.10)

Human immunodeficiency virus (HIV) disease (continued)

Table 5.1 Orofacial complications in HIV/AIDS

Viral infection	Herpesviruses (Figure 5.1), and HPV mainly EBV is a herpesvirus that can cause hairy leukoplakia (Figures 5.6, 5.7) which mainly affects margins of the tongue and is a predictor of progression to full-blown AIDS. EBV may cause lymphoma
Fungal infections	Candidosis (Figures 5.2–5.5)
Bacterial infection	Necrotizing ulcerative gingivitis/ periodontitis (Figures 5.8, 5.9)
Virally-related neoplasms	Kaposi sarcoma, lymphoma

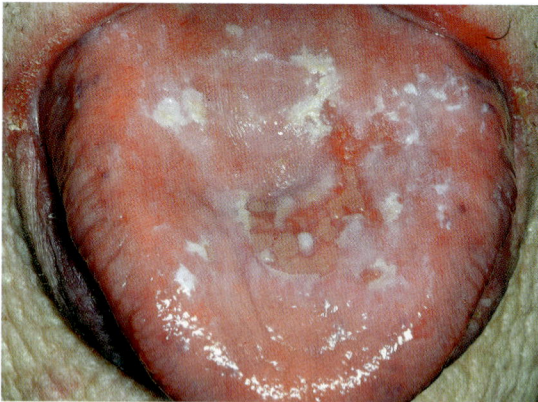

Figure 5.1 HIV disease: chronic candidosis, and herpes simplex ulceration.

Figure 5.2 HIV disease: erythematous candidosis in the classic 'thumbprint' distribution.

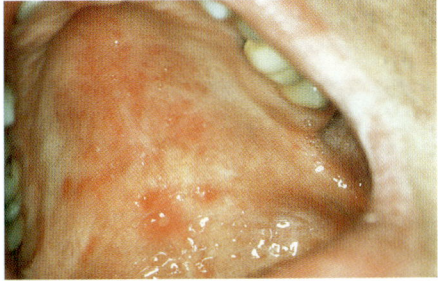

Figure 5.3 HIV disease: erythematous candidosis.

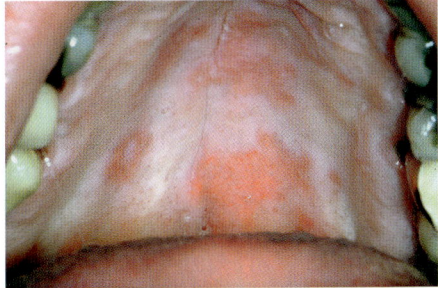

Figure 5.4 HIV disease: erythematous candidosis.

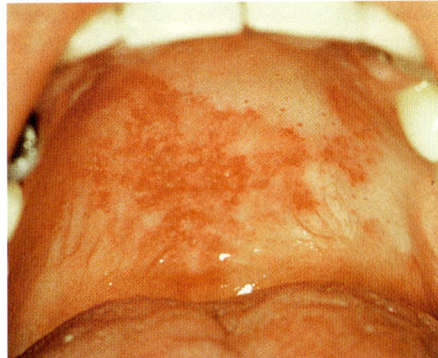

Human immunodeficiency virus (HIV) disease (continued)

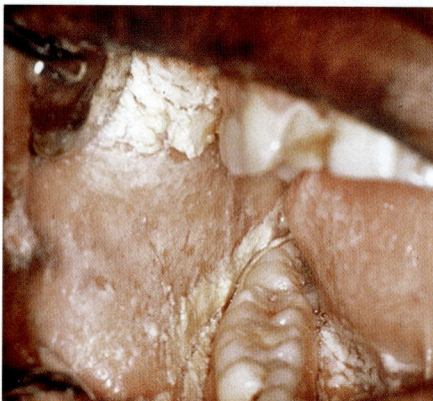

Figure 5.5 HIV disease: white candidosis (pseudomembranous candidosis).

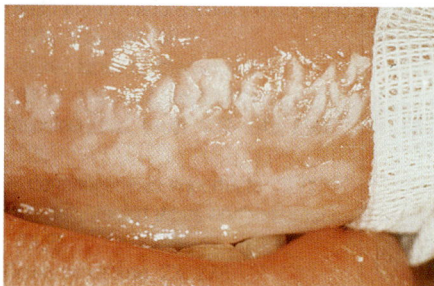

Figure 5.6 HIV disease: hairy leukoplakia related to Epstein–Barr virus (EBV) infection.

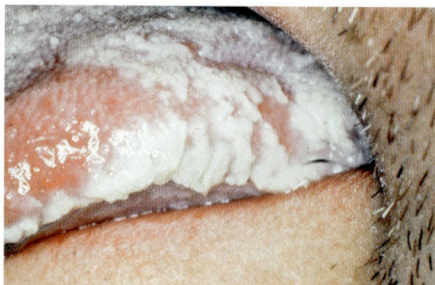

Figure 5.7 HIV disease: hairy leukoplakia appears corrugated rather than hairy and can be seen in any immunocompromised patients.

Figure 5.8 HIV disease: 'linear' gingivitis (linear gingival erythema).

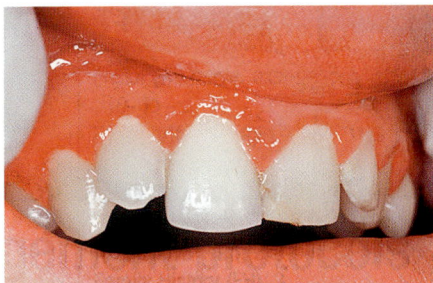

Figure 5.9 HIV disease: necrotizing ulcerative gingivitis.

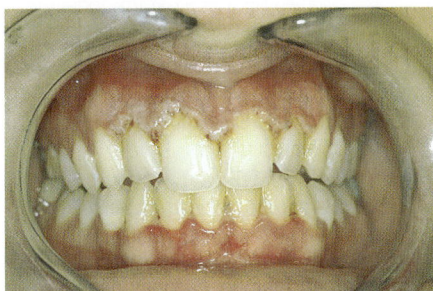

Figure 5.10 HIV disease: salivary gland disease (may be caused by BK virus) can cause swelling and hyposalivation.

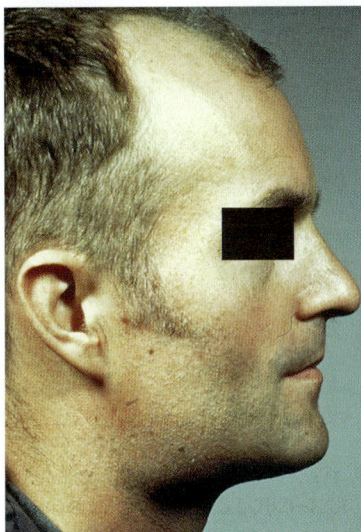

Human immunodeficiency virus (HIV) disease (continued)

    a dry mouth
    b unilateral or bilateral swelling of major salivary glands
       (Figure 5.10)

- Viral infections (other than EBV)
    a cytomegalovirus
    b herpes simplex virus
    c human papillomavirus (warty-like lesions) (see page 262):
       condyloma acuminatum, focal epithelial hyperplasia and verruca
       vulgaris
    d varicella-zoster virus: herpes zoster (see page 216) and varicella.

- Group III: lesions possibly associated with HIV infection. These are a miscellany of rare diseases.

Leukopenia and neutropenia

Leukopenia and neutropenia are haematological defects that may result from viral infections (especially HIV infection), drugs, irradiation, or can be idiopathic.

    Genetic (*ELANE*–related neutropenia) includes congenital neutropenias and cyclic neutropenia. Patients suffer fever, respiratory and cutaneous infections, lymphadenopathy and often orofacial lesions (Table 5.2).

Table 5.2 Orofacial complications of leukopenia

Infections	Mucosal (Figure 5.11) cutaneous, periodontal, antral, or postoperative
Ulcers	Characteristically persistent ulcers lacking an inflammatory halo (Figures 5.12, 5.13)
Lymphadenopathy	Cervical or general

Figure 5.11 Leukopenia: skin infections, as here, if with oral and respiratory infections suggest an immune defect.

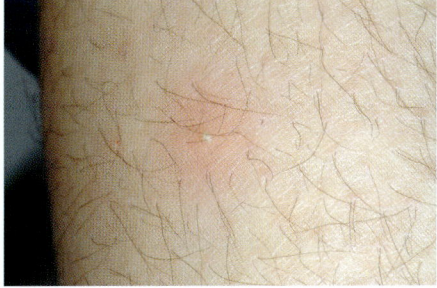

Figure 5.12 Leukopenia: oral ulceration lacks an inflammatory halo.

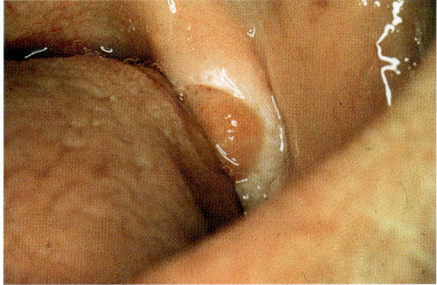

Figure 5.13 Leukopenia: gingival margin ulceration in the patient shown in Figure 5.11.

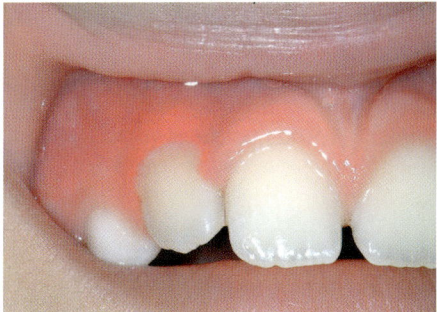

Leukaemias

Malignant neoplasms arising from lymphoid or myeloid cells affect the mouth in many ways (Table 5.3).

Table 5.3 Orofacial complications of leukaemias

Anaemia	Pallor
Infections	Mucosal, cutaneous (Figure 5.14), periodontal, antral, or postoperative
Ulcers	Characteristically persistent ulcers lacking an inflammatory halo (Figures 5.15–5.17)
Bleeding	Gingival bleeding and oral purpura (Figures 5.18, 5.19)
Gingival swelling	Caused by leukaemic deposits mainly in acute myeloid leukaemia
Labial or chin anaesthesia, facial palsy, radiographic changes	Caused by leukaemic deposits. Discrete radiolucencies in the lower third molar region, destruction of lamina dura and widening of the periodontal space or teeth which may appear to be 'floating in air'
Lymphadenopathy	Generalized, with hepatosplenomegaly

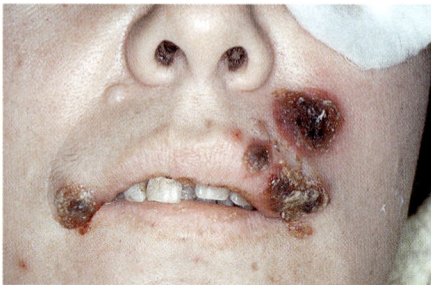

Figure 5.14 Leukaemia: leukaemic deposits in a child with acute leukaemia mimic herpes labialis (which is also common in people with immune defects or malignant disease).

Figure 5.15 Leukaemia: atypical ulceration, together with necrotizing ulcerative gingivitis.

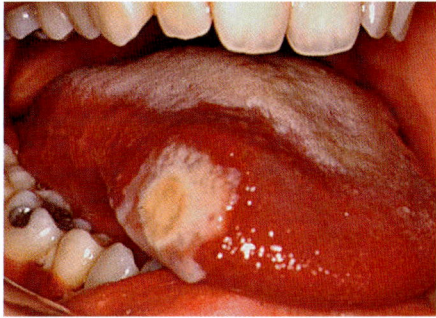

Figure 5.16 Leukaemia: atypical ulceration, together with necrotizing ulcerative gingivitis.

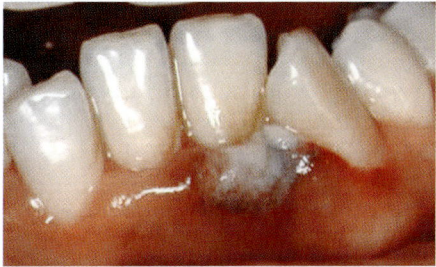

Figure 5.17 Leukaemia: atypical ulceration, covered by fibrin clot.

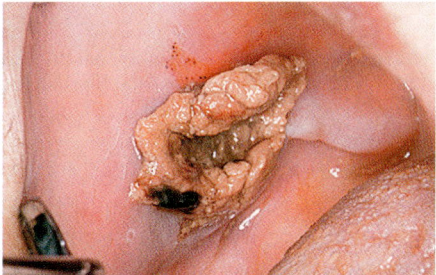

Leukaemias (continued)

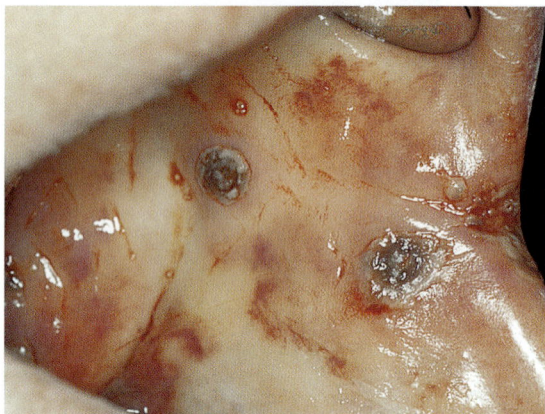

Figure 5.18 Leukaemia: atypical ulceration, together with purpura.

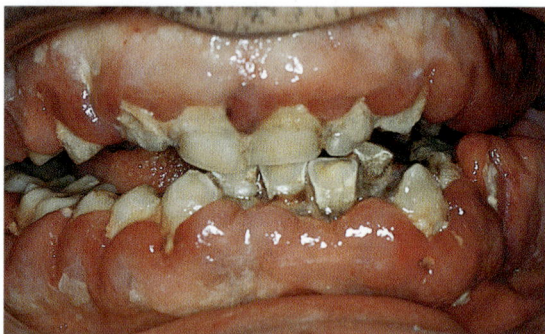

Figure 5.19 Leukaemia: gingival swelling, purpura, haemorrhage and ulceration.

Lymphomas

Malignant neoplasms arising from lymphocytes, lymphomas affecting the oral cavity are mainly B cell lymphomas, and can present in a number of ways (Table 5.4).

Table 5.4 Orofacial complications of lymphomas

Gingival or facial swelling	Caused mainly by non-Hodgkin lymphoma (Figure 5.20)
Ulceration	Characteristically persistent ulceration (Figure 5.21)
Tooth loosening	Or non-healing extraction socket
Lymphadenopathy	Cervical or general

Figure 5.20 Lymphoma presenting as a swelling in a typical site. Non-Hodgkins lymphomas are most common on the gingiva or fauces.

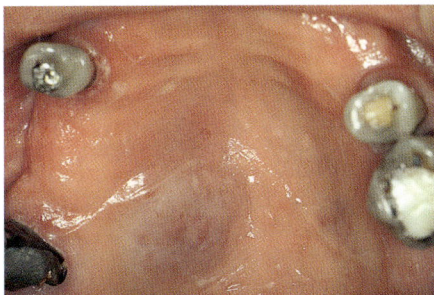

Figure 5.21 Lymphoma presenting as atypical ulceration; any solitary ulcer persisting 3 or more weeks should be biopsied.

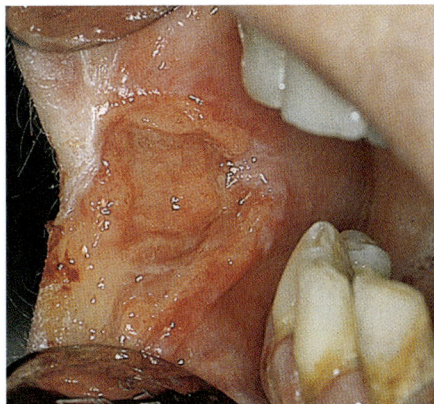

6

Diagnosis

A careful history will often lead to a provisional diagnosis but a careful full clinical examination is always indicated, not least because an unsuspected lesion may be present in addition to the patient's main complaint. The clinician is often then in a position to formulate the diagnosis, or at least a list of differential diagnoses. In the latter case, the diagnosis is provisional, and investigations or another opinion (e.g. specialist referral) may be necessary to reach a firm diagnosis.

Bearing in mind the fact that the whole orofacial tissues and cervical nodes must be examined in every patient, this chapter details diagnosis of disorders in the various sub-sites.

Diagnosis of mucosal disorders

Mucosal disorders are diagnosed mainly from history and examination findings. All mucosae should be examined, in order to detect early lesions. Begin away from the focus of complaint or known lesions. Labial, buccal, floor of the mouth, ventrum of tongue, dorsal surface of tongue, hard and soft palate mucosae, gingivae and teeth should be examined in sequence, recording lesions on a diagram.

Mucosal lesions are not always readily seen and, among attempts to help improve visualisation, are:

- toluidine blue (vital) staining
- chemiluminescent illumination
- fluorescence spectroscopy and imaging.

These are discussed in Chapter 7.

Investigations that may be diagnostically helpful can include biopsy examination, blood tests and microbiological investigations. Informed consent and confidentiality is required for all investigations.

Biopsy is the removal of tissue for diagnosis by histopathological and often immunological examination. **Indications for biopsy** include mucosal lesions that:

- have malignant or potentially malignant features
- are enlarging
- persist > 3 weeks
- are of uncertain aetiology
- fail to respond to treatment
- cause concern.

Blood tests, microbiology tests and other investigations are discussed in Chapter 7. Testing for infections can be a very sensitive issue, especially in the case of human immunodeficiency virus (HIV) and other sexually shared infections and tuberculosis. HIV testing in particular remains voluntary and confidential, and patients must be counselled properly beforehand.

Diagnosis of salivary disease

Salivary disorders are diagnosed mainly from history and examination findings. The salivary glands should be examined by inspecting:

- symmetry
- evidence of enlargement glands
- ducts for salivary flow

and by palpating the parotid glands in front of the ears, to detect pain, or swelling, and the submandibular glands by bimanual palpation between fingers inside the mouth and extraorally.

It is also important to examine the eyes for dryness, redness or discharge, and the oral mucosa; note particularly angular cheilitis, dryness and lingual depapillation or erythema.

Investigations required may include:

- plasma viscosity or erythrocyte sedimentation rate (ESR) or C reactive protein (CRP)
- antibodies

- antinuclear antibodies for lupus erythematosus or rheumatoid arthritis
- rheumatoid factor for rheumatoid arthritis
- SS-A (Ro) and SS-B (La) antibodies for Sjögren syndrome (and allied autoantibodies, e.g. anti-mitochondrial antibodies for primary biliary cirrhosis)
- mumps, HIV, HCV or other viral antibodies
- imaging using:
  - ultrasound
  - orthopantomogram and reverse orthopantomogram
  - oblique lateral views
  - lateral skull views
  - occlusal views
- CT scan
- MRI (which avoids irradiating the patient)
- biopsy: fine needle aspiration biopsy under ultrasound guidance is commonly used.

Diagnosis of jaw disorders

Jaw disorders are diagnosed mainly from history and examination findings. It is especially important to consider the rest of the skeleton, as some jaw disorders are only part of a wider problem.

Investigations required may include:

- full blood picture
- plasma viscosity or erythrocyte sedimentation rate or C-reactive protein
- blood biochemistry – typical features in metabolic disorders such as hyperparathyroidism, fibro-osseous disorders, sarcoidosis:
  - calcium
  - phosphate
  - alkaline phosphatase
  - parathyroid hormone levels
  - serum angiotensin-converting enzyme (SACE)
- serum antibodies
  - antinuclear antibodies – for lupus erythematosus or rheumatoid arthritis
  - rheumatoid factor – for rheumatoid arthritis
  - extractable nuclear antibodies, including SS-A and SS-B antibodies – for Sjögren syndrome

- imaging
  - orthopantomogram
  - oblique lateral views
  - three-dimensional information may be gained from:
    - a tomography in both the coronal and sagittal planes
    - b cone beam CT and T1 and T2 weighting
  - radionuclide scanning
  - MRI – avoids irradiating the patient but is best for soft tissue lesions
- biopsy.

Diagnosis of dental disorders

Disorders affecting teeth are diagnosed mainly from history and examination as discussed in dental texts. All findings should be charted using one of various systems of tooth notations.

Investigations required may include:

- pulp vitality testing
- imaging
  - plain radiography
    - a periapical radiographs
    - b bitewings
    - c oblique lateral views
  - tomographic views
    - a dental pan-oral tomographic views
    - b other tomographic views
  - three-dimensional information from:
    - a tomography in both the coronal and sagittal planes
  - CT scan.

Diagnosis of pain and neurological disorders

Pain

In patients with orofacial pain, it is crucial to exclude local causes, such as odontogenic, by carefully examining the teeth, jaws and joints, mucosae and salivary glands. The cranial nerves should also be examined by inspecting:

- facial symmetry and movement
- fasciculation or deviation of tongue from the centre when protracted

- ocular movements
- hearing testing
- trigeminal nerve functions; those that should be tested include:
  - corneal reflex (this tests Vth and VIIth cranial nerves); puffing air or touching the cornea gently with sterile cotton wool should produce a blink
  - skin sensation, by using:
    a light touch (a puff of air or cotton wool)
    b pin point (sterile needle)
    c temperature
    d vibration
    e two-point discrimination
  - motor function by testing the jaw jerk, and palpating:
    a masseters during clenching
    b temporalis during clenching
    c pterygoids during jaw protrusion
  - taste sensation. Gustometry uses stimuli on a cotton bud, including: citric acid or hydrochloric acid (sour taste), caffeine or quinine hydrochloride (bitter), sodium chloride (salty taste), saccharose (sweet), monosodium glutamate (umami taste).

Investigations required may include:

- imaging
  - jaw/skull radiography
  - CT
  - MRI, which avoids irradiating the patient, has almost completely replaced CT as the modality of choice for investigating trigeminal neuropathy, though CT still plays a role in the assessment of skull base foramina and facial skeleton
  - ultrasound
- biopsy
- urinalysis
- blood tests
  - plasma viscosity or erythrocyte sedimentation rate or C-reactive protein
  - full blood count
  - SACE
  - random glucose

- antibodies
  - a antinuclear antibodies for lupus erythematosus or rheumatoid arthritis
  - b rheumatoid factor (RF) for rheumatoid arthritis
  - c SS-A (Ro) and SS-B (La) antibodies for Sjögren syndrome
  - d RNP antibodies for mixed connective tissue disease
  - e viral antibodies.

Suspected neurological disorders

Neurological disorders may be serious in consequence and thus a neurological opinion may be required in patients with facial palsy, facial sensory loss, or some patients with pain.

It is also important to consider drug use (including recreational drugs and alcohol) and the possibility of related systemic disorders, especially:

- infections (e.g. Lyme disease and HIV)
- cardiovascular disorders (some facial pain may be referred from cardiac or other lesions in the chest)
- respiratory disorders (e.g. sarcoidosis or neoplasms)
- connective tissue disorders, such as lupus erythematosus
- endocrine gland disorders (e.g. diabetes)
- mental health disorders
- nutrition (e.g. eating disorders such as bulimia).

It may be important to:

- check the vital signs (pulse, respiration, temperature, blood pressure)
- look for abnormal posture or gait (e.g. broad based in cerebellar disorders, shuffling in Parkinsonism, swinging leg in stroke)
- assess level of consciousness (Glasgow Coma Scale) and, if necessary, mental state
- assess speech
  - dysarthria (oropharyngeal, neurological or muscular pathology)
  - dysphonia (respiratory pathology) or
  - dysphasia (damage in the brain language areas)
- check for neck stiffness (meningeal inflammation)
- look for tremor (anxiety, drugs, coffee, alcohol or drug withdrawal, CVA, hyperthyroidism, Parkinsonism), tics (partially controlled repetitive movements), maxillofacial dyskinesias (involuntary tic-like movements involving the lips and the tongue – a long term side-effect of

antipsychotics), etc., fasciculations (involuntary twitches of groups of muscle fibres (e.g. in motor neurone disease), dystonia (e.g. torticollis), myoclonus (sudden jerky muscle movements), wasting (motor neurone disease or myopathy)
- test cranial nerves
- If there is any suspicion of a neuropathy there should be a general neurological examination.

7

Investigations

Informed consent and confidentiality are required for all investigations, and the advantages should clearly outweigh any dangers or disadvantages.

Blood tests

Blood tests can help determine disease states, but should be requested only when clinically indicated. There is always a danger of needlestick injury. Furthermore, abnormal 'blood results' do not always mean disease and false-positive results are possible. Serum is used for assaying antibodies, which can help diagnose infections and autoimmune disorders, and for assaying most biochemical substances (e.g. 'liver enzymes').

Microbiological tests

Microbiological diagnosis is based on either demonstration of the microorganism or its components (antigens or nucleic acids) directly in samples or tissues, which are best used as results are speedily obtained. The demonstration in the serum of a specific antibody response can be helpful.

Salivary flow determination

Unless the baseline salivary flow rate for an individual patient is known, it is impossible to be certain if there has been a reduction in salivary flow, since the salivary flow rate varies widely from person to person. Salivary flow rates also vary over time and so estimates should be taken on several occasions.

Normal and reference values are shown in Table 7.1.

Table 7.1 Whole saliva flow rates* (ml/min)

	Normal	Hyposalivation
Unstimulated (resting)	0.3–0.4 ml/min	<0.1 ml/min
Stimulated	1–2 ml/min	<0.5 ml/min

*Unstimulated salivary flow rate (USFR) measurement of whole saliva uses a simple draining test for 5 minutes at rest: a rate less or equal to 0.1 ml/min suggests hyposalivation.

Biopsy

Before beginning, it is important to decide whether an excisional or incisional biopsy is indicated.

Excisional biopsy

Excisional biopsy (Figures 7.1–7.4) is used for small superficial lesions (max 1 cm). If a malignant tumour is suspected, even if small, an excisional biopsy must be done by a specialist.

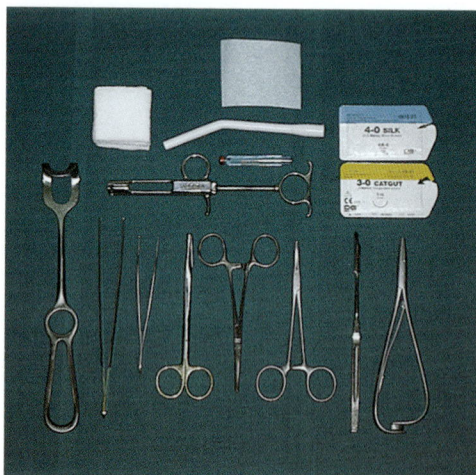

Figure 7.1 Instrumentation for excisional biopsy. Shown are: retractor, aspirator, surgical blade No. 15, surgical forceps, scissors, sutures (catgut or silk 3 or 4), two needle holders, LA (local anaesthetic) syringe and anaesthetic, blotting paper.

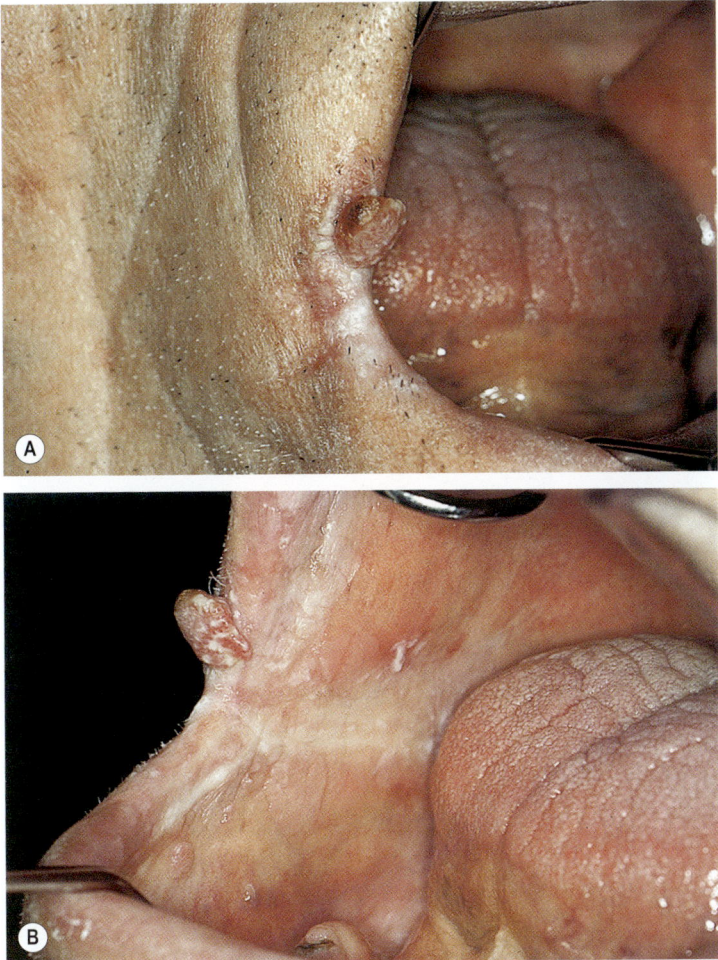

Figure 7.2 (A, B) Excisional biopsy must be used for small superficial lesions (max 1 cm).

Biopsy (continued)

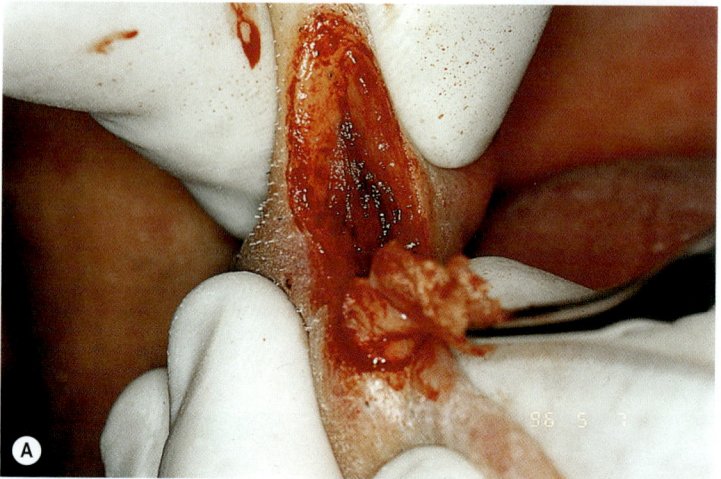

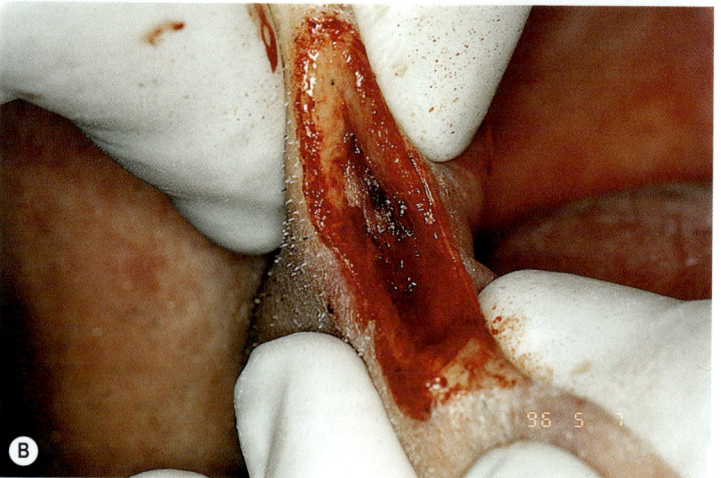

Figure 7.3 (A, B) Remove the tissue completely.

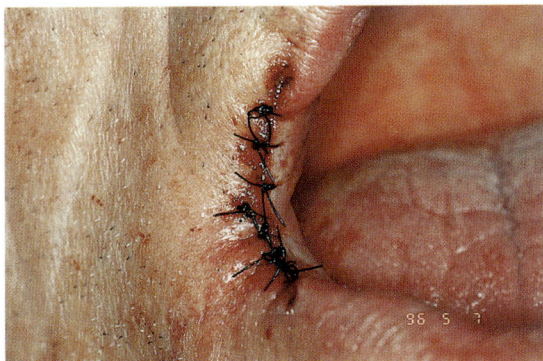

Figure 7.4 Finally, after achieving haemostasis, suture.

Incisional biopsy

Choose the area to biopsy based on:

- appraisal of the clinical appearance (red areas rather than white)
- vital staining with toluidine blue.

An incisional biopsy (Figures 7.5–7.13) can be performed with a scalpel, or dermatology punch.

Steps of incisional biopsy preceded by vital staining, if used
The procedure is shown in Figures 7.14 and 7.15.

Oral lichen planus biopsy (Figures 7.16, 7.17)
For oral lichen planus, the choice of biopsy must consider the following:

- The sample should contain one or more papule or, alternatively, part of striae or plaques.
- The best site is the buccal mucosa; try to avoid, if possible (unless there is the possibility of malignant change), white plaques on the dorsum of the tongue, erosions and ulcers and red atrophic areas, because they are often difficult to interpret histologically.
- The specimen must be sufficiently large and deep.

Note: In cases where the histopathological diagnosis is doubtful it can be useful to carry out direct immunofluorescence, which may show linear deposits of fibrin in the basement membrane zone in lichen planus.

Biopsy (continued)

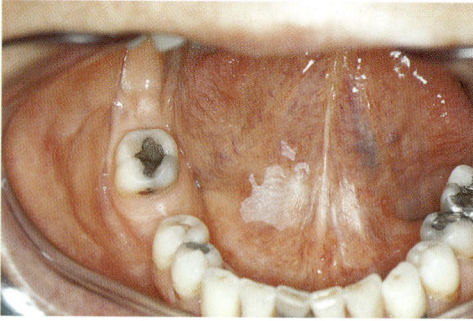

Figure 7.5 Simple incisional biopsy. This is indicated in homogeneous lesions, such as white papules or plaques.

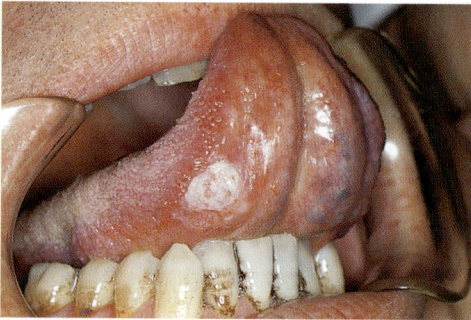

Figure 7.6 A simple incisional biopsy can be made not only in homogeneous lesions but also in red or erosive areas.

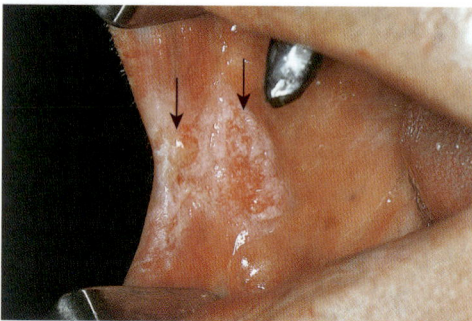

Figure 7.7 A mapping incisional biopsy consists of taking several specimens from different areas. It is usually carried out in non-homogeneous lesions.

Figure 7.8 The incisional biopsy may be preceded by vital staining with toluidine blue (see above). It consists in biopsying several stained areas (royal blue ones). It is carried out in non-homogeneous lesions with extensive red areas.

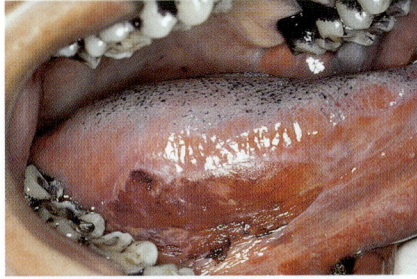

Figure 7.9 Instrumentation for incisional biopsy. Shown are: LA syringe and anaesthetic, scalpel with surgical blade No. 15, surgical forceps, blotting paper.

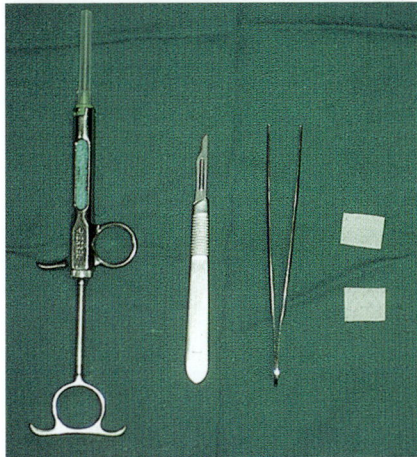

Figure 7.10 Fixative for biopsy specimen. Typically this is 10% formalin in a sufficiently large watertight container with self-adhesive label on which immediately to write the name of the patient (and hospital number). The volume of formalin must be at least three times that one of the pieces of tissue to fix. For immunostaining, the tissue is not put in formalin but in OCS or Michel solution, or frozen in liquid nitrogen.

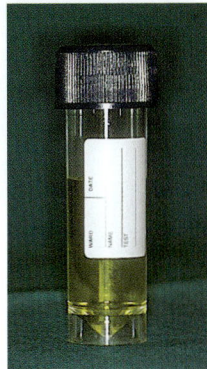

Biopsy (continued)

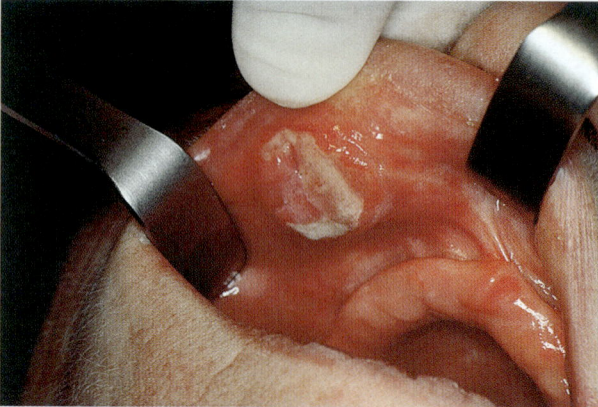

Figure 7.11 Considerations before starting. Examine the lesion carefully and decide (i) which type of incisional biopsy you need, (ii) which area(s) should be biopsied and (iii) whether it is useful to undertake vital staining. *The choices are based on the clinical appearances of the lesion.*

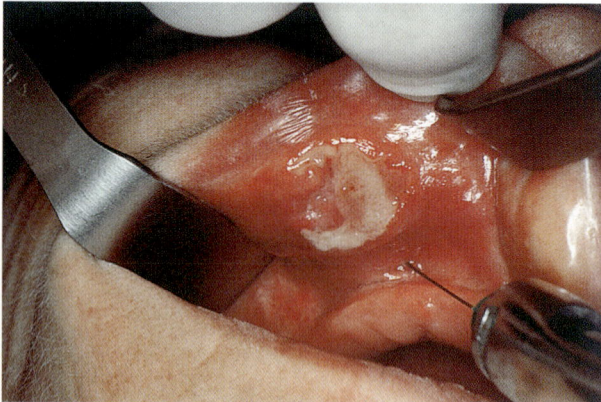

Figure 7.12 Anaesthesia. Do not inject the LA directly into the lesion or with strong pressure, since it is possible to cause pain, damage the tissue and create artefacts.

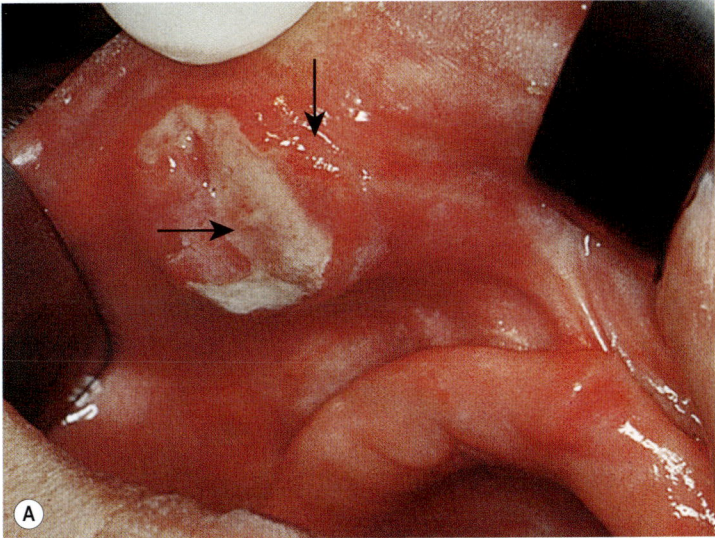

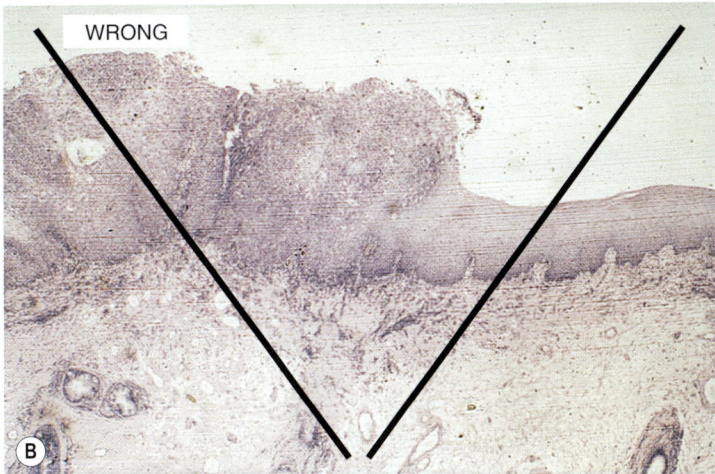

Figure 7.13 (A–E) The sample: never sample a necrotic zone (A). Do not excise a wedge since this samples little of the basal layers (B).

Biopsy (continued)

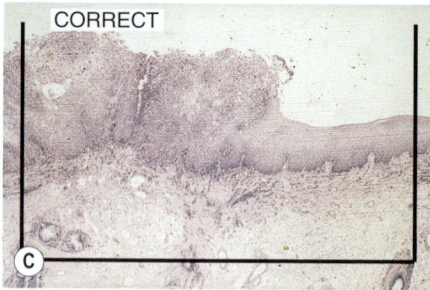

Figure 7.13, cont'd The biopsy must be sufficiently deep to include the epithelium–connective tissue interface (C). The biopsy should be at least 4–5 mm diameter. Take care not to damage the biopsy with forceps; for more delicate lesions (e.g. bullous diseases) use anatomical forceps (D) or a suture. Place the specimen blotting paper with the epithelium upwards to allow orientation by the pathologist (E). Put the sample immediately into the fixative.

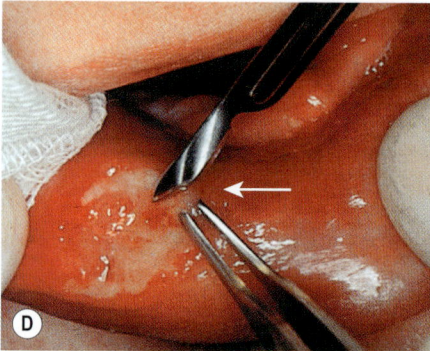

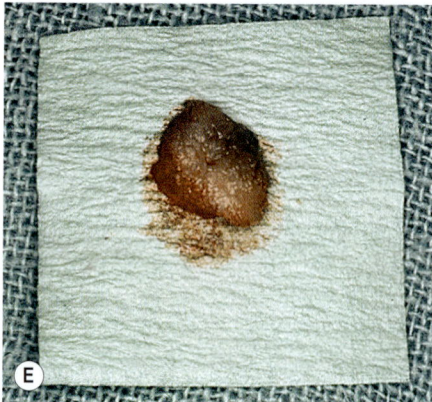

Figure 7.14 (A, B) Vital
staining is used when
lesions are non-
homogeneous, or mixed
red and white lesions, or
where there is an
extensive red component.

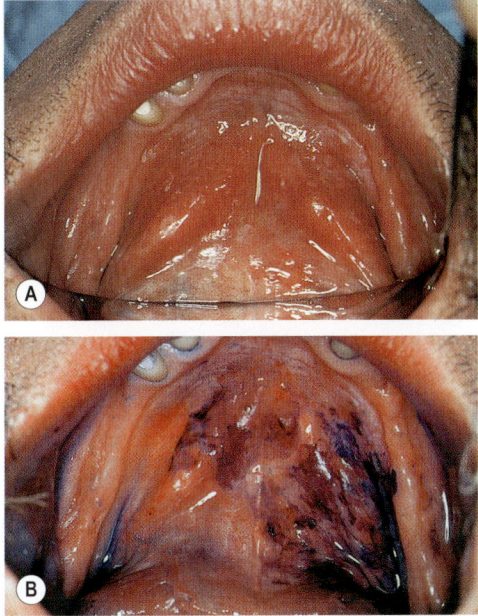

Figure 7.15 The sample taken
should include both areas that are
stained and not.

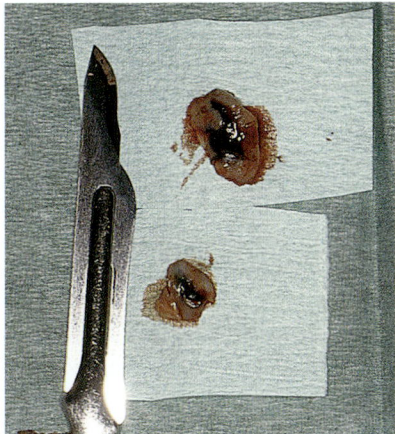

Biopsy (continued)

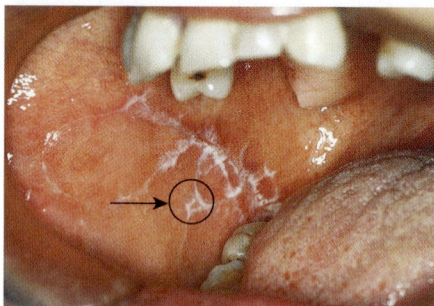

Figure 7.16 Striae are good areas to biopsy to establish the diagnosis of oral lichen planus.

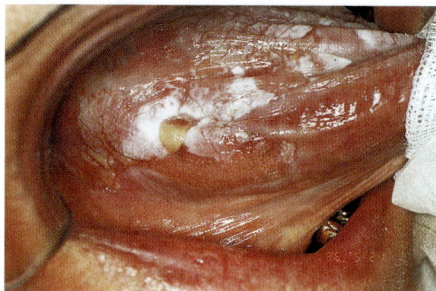

Figure 7.17 Remember that oral lichen planus can be a potentially malignant condition. Therefore carefully evaluate the lesions to decide which areas to biopsy and if there is any reason to suspect early oral cancer, proceed with precaution and refer the patient to a specialist.

Direct immunofluorescence

For oral mucosal diseases which may have an autoimmune or immune pathogenesis (mainly bullous diseases), direct immunofluorescence (DIF) analysis is sometimes fundamental to establishing the diagnosis. For DIF a large biopsy is necessary so that sufficient material is available for half of the specimen to be conserved NOT in formalin. Use Michel solution, OCT or PBS (phosphate buffered saline) and process for DIF; the other half of the sample is fixed in formalin and processed routinely and embedded in paraffin for conventional histology (Figure 7.18).

For lichen planus or lupus erythematosus the criteria to follow are those above. For **bullous diseases** the sample:

- must be taken in areas where epithelium is present (no erosions or ulcers)
- must be handled gently to avoid any epithelium–connective tissue split during removal of the specimen (a scalpel rather than punch is best used)
- must be taken perilesionally

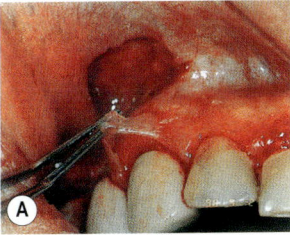

Biopsy of desquamative gingivitis, avoiding the areas in which the epithelium is too easily detached

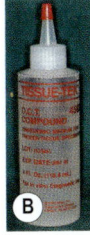

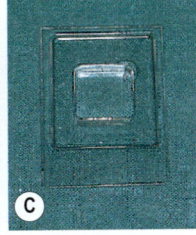

The OCT must be poured in its container without creating bubbles; the fragment must be carefully laid on the bottom with the epithelium upwards

Part of the sample is preserved in one of these two types and carried immediately to a laboratory

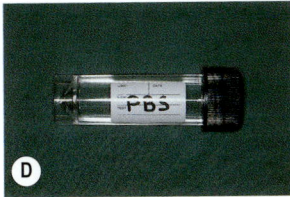

One half of the specimen is preserved in PBS

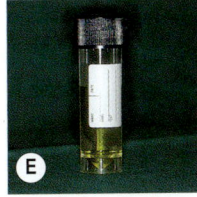

The other half is fixed in formalin for traditional histology

Figure 7.18 (A–E) Direct immunofluorescence procedure.

Imaging

Because of the adverse effects of ionizing radiation and the cumulative effect of radiation hazard, clinicians requesting examination or investigation using X-rays must satisfy themselves that each investigation is necessary and that the benefit outweighs the risk.

Ultrasound and magnetic resonance imaging avoid radiation hazards.

Computed axial tomography (CT or CAT)

This imaging technique shows the bone and teeth white, can be useful in diagnosis of lesions involving hard tissue, but gives a fairly high radiation exposure. Cone beam CT (CBCT) is becoming widely utilized for imaging bone/dental pathology of the jaws and has the advantage of a lower radiation dose to the patient than conventional CT.

Dental panoramic tomography (DPT; or orthopantomography [OPTG])

This imaging technique gives a good overview of the dentition, maxillary sinuses, mandibular ramus and temporomandibular joints, but is subject to considerable and unpredictable geometric distortion, is greatly affected by positioning errors and has relatively low spatial resolution compared with intraoral radiographs.

Intraoral radiography

Intraoral radiography includes periapical, bitewing and occlusal projections and allows detection of small carious lesions and periapical radiolucencies not always detectable with DPT.

Magnetic resonance imaging (MRI)

MRI gives good images of soft tissues and is the modality of choice to aid in the diagnosis and management of:

- trigeminal neuralgia
- idiopathic facial pain.

The disadvantages of MRI are that it is:

- liable to produce image artefacts where metal objects are present (dental restorations, orthodontic appliances, metallic foreign bodies, joint prostheses, implants, etc.)

- contraindicated in
  - implanted electric devices (e.g. heart pacemakers, cardiac defibrillators)
  - ferromagnetic intracranial vascular clips
  - prosthetic cardiac valves containing metal
  - obesity
  - claustrophobia.

Ultrasound scanning (US)

Ultrasound scanning is non-invasive and the first-line imaging modality to use in diagnosis of soft tissue swellings (e.g. lymph nodes, thyroid or salivary glands) and in assisting fine needle aspiration biopsy (ultrasound-guided FNA or FNAB).

Adjunctive screening tests

Saliva pH test

This may help assess caries risk but not the advertised assessment of susceptibility to cancer, heart disease, osteoporosis, arthritis, and many other degenerative diseases.

Breath analyser

This may help assess oral malodour, but only measures a limited range of gases in the breath.

Visualization aids

It is likely that very small and very early lesions could be overlooked by visual examination of the mouth. The search is on for techniques to detect carcinoma at a very early stage – but the very earliest stages are surely at the microscopic or submicroscopic levels. A number of clinical aids have been developed in attempts to be:

- adjuncts to visual examination
- helpful to identify sites for biopsy.

These are discussed in Chapter 1.

However, all current aids suffer from low specificity and/or sensitivity (see Table 7.2)

Table 7.2 Commercial visualization devices

	Sensitivity %	Specificity %
Brush biopsy	71.4–100	32–100
ViziLite	100	0–14.2
VELscope	98–100	94–100

8

Management protocols for patients with oral diseases treated in primary care settings

This chapter tabulates the typical management in primary dental care of patients with the more common complaints.

Condition	Typical main clinical features	Investigations that may be indicated for diagnosis in addition to history and examination
Aphthous stomatitis	Recurrent oral ulcers only	Full blood picture. Exclude underlying systemic disease (e.g. ESR for autoinflammatory disease; transglutaminase for coeliac disease; haematinic assays for deficiencies)
Allergic reactions	Swelling, erythema or erosions	Allergy testing
Burning mouth syndrome	Glossodynia	Full blood picture, haematirics, glucose, thyroid function, electrolytes
Candidosis (including angular stomatitis and denture-related stomatitis)	White or red persistent lesions	Consider smear, or biopsy. Consider immune defect
Chapped lips	Dry, flaking lips	May be dry mouth
Dental infections and pain	Pain usually aggravated by pressure or heat	Vitality test Radiology
Dry mouth	Dryness Caries Candidosis Sialadenitis	Full blood picture Exclude underlying systemic disease (e.g. glucose for diabetes; SSA and SSB antibodies for Sjögren syndrome)

Therapeutic protocols	High levels of available evidence for treatment*
Vitamin B$_{12}$, aqueous chlorhexidine, corticosteroids topically (e.g. hydrocortisone, betamethasone), amlexanox or, only in adults, topical tetracycline (doxycycline)	Yes (for all)
Avoid precipitant. Consider antihistamines (e.g. loratidine)	Yes
Reassurance, CBT. GMPs or specialists may use tricyclic antidepressants or SSRIs	Yes
Antifungals, leave out dental appliances, allowing the mouth to heal. Disinfect the appliance (as per additional instructions). Use antifungal creams or gels (e.g. miconazole) or tablets (e.g. nystatin or fluconazole), regularly for up to 4 weeks	Yes
Topical petrolatum gel or bland creams	No
Restorative dentistry	Yes
Preventative dental care Mouth wetting agents Sialogogues	

Condition	Typical main clinical features	Investigations that may be indicated for diagnosis in addition to history and examination
Erythema migrans	Desquamating patches on tongue	–
Halitosis	Oral malodour	Oral/ENT examination and radiography
Herpetic infection	Oral ulcers, gingivitis, fever	Sometimes PCR or immunostain
Hyposalivation	Dry mouth. May be dry eyes, or a connective tissue disease	Assess salivary flow rate. Exclude drugs, diabetes, Sjögren syndrome (serology – SS-A (Ro) and SS-B (La) antibodies), HCV and HIV. Ultrasound. Consider labial gland biopsy, sialography, MRI or scintiscan
Idiopathic facial pain	Persistent dull ache typically in maxilla in an older female	Imaging to exclude organic disease
Keratosis	Flat, raised or warty white lesion	Biopsy
Leukoplakia	Flat, raised or warty white or white and red lesion (erythroleukoplakia)	Biopsy

Therapeutic protocols	High levels of available evidence for treatment*
Reassurance ± benzydamine	No
Treat underlying cause	No
Symptomatic – aciclovir suspension or tablets	Yes
Preventive dentistry. Mouth wetting agents (artificial salivas, of which there are several available) and artificial tears; salivary stimulants (sialogogues) – such as sugar-free chewing gum, or systemic pilocarpine or cevimeline	Yes
Reassurance, CBT. GMPs or specialists may use SSRIs or tricyclics	Yes (for CBT and tricyclics)
Stop tobacco, betel or alcohol use. Excise if dysplastic	No
Stop tobacco, betel or alcohol use. Excise	No

Condition	Typical main clinical features	Investigations that may be indicated for diagnosis in addition to history and examination
Lichen planus	Mucosal white or other lesions. Polygonal purple pruritic papules on skin. May be genital or skin adnexal involvement	Biopsy – immunofluorescence may be useful
Necrotizing ulcerative gingivitis	Interdental papillary ulceration and bleeding, halitosis, pain	Smear may help Consider immune defect
Pemphigoid	Blisters, mainly in mouth occasionally on conjunctivae, genitals or skin. Scarring	Biopsy – immunostaining
TMJ pain-dysfunction	TMJ pain, click, limitation of movement	Occasionally imaging, rarely arthroscopy

Therapeutic protocols	High levels of available evidence for treatment*
Corticosteroids (e.g. betamethasone or clobetasol propionate) topically. Aloe vera gel may be tried. Stop tobacco or any causal drug use	Yes (for steroids and aloe vera)
Antimicrobials: penicillin or metronidazole. Oral hygiene improvement. Mechanical debridement. Consider excluding HIV	Yes
Topical corticosteroids (e.g. betamethasone or clobetasol propionate). Specialists may use dapsone, systemic steroids or other immunosuppressives	Yes
Reassurance, occlusal splint, anxiolytics or muscle relaxants (e.g. benzodiazepines such as diazepam or temazepam)	No

*Some of the evidence is controversial.

Abbreviations: CBT, cognitive-behavioural therapy; GMP, general medical practitioner; HCV, hepatitis C virus; PCR, polymerase chain reaction; SSRI, selective serotonin re-uptake inhibitor; HIV, human immunodeficiency virus.

In UK, registered dentists are legally entitled to prescribe from the entirety of the *British National Formulary* (BNF) and *BNF for Children* (BNFC), but within the National Health Service (NHS) dental prescribing is restricted to those drugs contained within the List of Dental Preparations in the *Dental Practitioners Formulary* (DPF).

9

Referral for specialist advice

Clinicians should endeavour to recognize the early signs of serious disease and to direct the patient to the appropriate specialist for a second opinion, including results of any relevant investigations.

Patients who may benefit from specialist referral include those where there is:

- a possibly complex or serious diagnosis (e.g. cancer, pemphigus, HIV/AIDS Behçet disease, Crohn disease)
- a doubtful diagnosis
- extraoral involvement or possible systemic disease
- investigations required, but not possible, or appropriate to carry out, in primary care
- a situation where therapy may not be straightforward and may require complex agents
- a situation where drug use needs to be monitored with laboratory or other testing
- a patient who needs repeated access to an informed opinion, outside normal working hours.

Essential details of a referral letter include the following:

- *Name and contact details of the patient*, including age, address and day-time telephone number.
- *Name and contact details of the referring and other clinicians* (name, address, telephone, fax and e-mail)
- *History of present complaint* with brief details and description of the nature and site of lesion(s)

- *Urgency of referral*
- *Social history*
- *Medical history*
- *Special requirements*, e.g. for interpreter, sign language expert or special transport.

Shared clinical care

Table 9.1 Responsibilities of parties involved in shared clinical care (shared care implies good communication between all parties)

Specialist	General practitioner (GP)	Patient
Write to GP suggesting shared care	Tell Specialist, with reasons, if they cannot share care	Comply with recommended care
Provide GP with care guidelines	Prescribe certain treatment agents	Ensure understanding of care regimen
Provide GP with contact details	Provide patient with suitable written information	Ensure attendance of monitoring
Report adverse treatment effects	Undertake monitoring of patient health	Report to and seek advice from GP on any concerns
Prescribe certain treatment agents	Refer to Specialist if treatment fails	Understand that care may be curtailed if patient fails to comply with above
	Report to and seek advice from Specialist on any concerns	
	Report adverse reactions to Specialist, and stop treatment in cases of severe reactions	

10

Further information

Glossary of eponymous diseases and syndromes

Addison disease
Autoimmune hypoadrenocorticism.

Albers–Schönberg disease
Osteopetrosis.

Albright syndrome (McCune-Albright syndrome)
Polyostotic fibrous dysplasia, skin pigmentation and endocrinopathy (usually precocious puberty in girls).

Apert syndrome
Congenital craniosynostosis and syndactyly.

Ascher syndrome
Congenital double lip with blepharoclasia and thyroid goitre.

Beckwith–Wiedemann syndrome
Congenital gigantism, omphalocoele or umbilical hernia.

Behçet disease (Adamantiades syndrome)
Oral ulcers, genital ulceration and uveitis.

Bell palsy
Lower motor neurone facial palsy, caused by inflammation in the stylomastoid canal.

Block–Sulzberger disease (incontinentia pigmenti)
Congenital hyperpigmented skin lesions, skeletal defects, learning disability and hypodontia.

Bloom syndrome
Congenital telangiectasia, depigmentation, short stature.

Bourneville disease (epiloia, tuberous sclerosis)
Nail fibromas (subungual fibromas), hamartomas in the brain, kidneys and heart, and skin nodules in the nasolabial fold (adenoma sebaceum).

Burkitt lymphoma
Lymphoma caused by Epstein–Barr virus, most common in sub-Saharan Africa, often affecting the jaws.

Cannon disease
Congenital white sponge naevus.

Carabelli cusp
Congenital additional palatal cusp on upper molars.

Chediak–Higashi syndrome
Congenital defective neutrophil function, susceptibility to infection, skin pigmentation.

Chondroectodermal dysplasia (Ellis–van Creveld syndrome)
Autosomal recessive; polydactyly and chrondrodysplasia.

Cowden syndrome
Congenital multiple hamartoma syndrome, with oral papillomatosis and risk of breast and thyroid cancer.

Cri-du-chat syndrome
Short arm of chromosome 5 deletion, resulting in microcephaly, hypertelorism and laryngeal hypoplasia causing a characteristic shrill cry.

Crohn disease
Granulomatous disorder that affects mainly the ileum or any part of the gastrointestinal tract, including mouth.

Crouzon syndrome
Autosomal dominant premature fusion of cranial sutures, mid-face hypoplasia and proptosis.

Cushing syndrome
Hyperadrenocorticism.

Darier disease
Inherited skin disorder with follicular hyperkeratosis, and white oral papules.

Di George syndrome
Congenital immunodeficiency with cardiac defects and hypoparathyroidism due to third branchial arch defect.

Down syndrome (trisomy 21)
The commonest recognizable congenital chromosomal anomaly. Patients have learning disability, are of short stature with brachycephaly, mid-face retrusion and upward sloping palpebral fissures (mongoloid slant).

Eagle syndrome
An elongated styloid process associated with dysphagia and pain on chewing, and on turning the head towards the affected side.

Ehlers–Danlos syndrome
A group of congenital disorders of collagen characterized by hyperflexibility of joints, hyperextensible skin and bleeding and bruising.

Ellis–van Creveld syndrome (chondroectodermal dysplasia)
Congenital polydactyly, dwarfism, ectodermal dysplasia. Hypodontia and hypoplastic teeth. Multiple fraenae.

Epstein–Barr virus
A herpesvirus that has been implicated in infectious mononucleosis, hairy leukoplakia, nasopharyngeal carcinoma and some lymphomas.

Fabry disease (angiokeratoma corporis diffusum universale)
X-linked recessive error of glycosphingolipid metabolism with punctate skin angiokeratomas on scrotum, hypertension, fever, renal disease and risk of myocardial infarction.

Fallot tetralogy
Pulmonary stenosis, over-riding aorta, ventricular septal defect and right ventricular hypertrophy.

Fanconi anaemia
Congenital anaemia, abnormal radii, risk of oral carcinoma and leukaemia.

Felty syndrome
Rheumatoid arthritis and neutropenia.

Fordyce disease
Congenital ectopic sebaceous glands.

Frey syndrome
Gustatory sweating and flushing of skin after trauma due to crossover of sympathetic and parasympathetic innervation to the salivary gland and skin.

Gardner syndrome
Autosomal dominant syndrome of intestinal polyposis, multiple osteomas and fibromas and pigmented lesions of fundus of eye.

Gilles de la Tourette syndrome
Coprolalia (utterance of obscenities).

Goldenhar syndrome
A variant of congenital hemifacial microsomia, with microtia (small ears), macrostomia, agenesis of mandibular ramus and condyle, vertebral abnormalities and epibulbar dermoid cysts.

Goltz syndrome (focal dermal hypoplasia)
An inherited condition that involves many body systems but takes its name from patchy skin abnormalities.

Gorlin–Goltz syndrome (multiple basal cell naevi syndrome)
Multiple basal cell carcinomas, keratocystic odontogenic tumours, vertebral and rib anomalies.

Graves disease
Hyperthyroidism with ophthalmopathy and exophthalmos.

Guillain–Barré syndrome
Acute demyelination.

Hailey–Hailey disease
Autosomal dominant benign familial pemphigus presenting in second or third decade with skin and oral blisters and vegetations.

Hallermann–Streiff syndrome
Congenital cranial anomalies, micro-ophthalmia, cataracts, mandibular hypoplasia and abnormal TMJ.

Hand–Schüller–Christian disease
Langerhans histiocytosis causing skull lesions, exophthalmos and diabetes insipidis.

Heck disease
Multifocal epithelial hyperplasia associated with human papillomavirus infection.

Heerordt syndrome
Sarcoidosis with lachrymal and salivary swelling, uveitis and fever (uveoparotid fever).

Henoch–Schönlein purpura
Allergic purpura, which may cause oral petechiae.

Hodgkin disease
Lymphoma.

Horner syndrome
Unilateral:
    ptosis (drooping of the upper eyelid)
    anhydrosis (loss of sweating) of the ipsilateral face
    miosis (pupil constriction)
enophthalmos (retruded eyeball) sometimes.

Hunterian chancre
Syphilitic primary chancre.

Hurler syndrome
Congenital mucopolysaccharidosis causing growth failure, learning disability, large head, frontal bossing, hypertelorism, coarse face (gargoylism) and mandibular radiolucencies.

Hutchinson teeth
Screwdriver-shaped incisor teeth in congenital syphilis

Kaposi sarcoma
Sarcomatous lesion caused by human herpesvirus-8 (KSHV; Kaposi sarcoma herpesvirus), seen mainly in AIDS.

Kartagener syndrome
Congenital dextrocardia, immunodeficiency and sinusitis.

Kawasaki disease (mucocutaneous lymph node syndrome)
Idiopathic disorder with fever, lymphadenopathy, desquamation of hand and feet, cheilitis and cardiac lesions.

Kelly syndrome
Atrophy of edentulous anterior maxilla caused by retained mandibular anterior teeth.

Kikuchi–Fujimoto disease
A self-limited lymphadenopathy that can be confused histologically and clinically with lymphoma or systemic lupus erythematosus.

Klippel-Feil anomaly
Congenital association of cervical vertebrae fusion, short neck, low-lying posterior hairline, syringomyelia and other neurological anomalies and sometimes unilateral renal agenesis and cardiac anomalies.

Kuttner disease
Chronic sialadenitis in IgG_4 disease.

Laband syndrome
Hereditary gingival fibromatosis with skeletal anomalies and large digits.

Langerhans cell histiocytoses (histiocytosis X)
Langerhans cell histiocytoses includes:
   solitary eosinophilic granuloma of bone;
   multifocal eosinophilic granuloma (Hand–Schüller–Christian disease);
   Letterer–Siwe disease.

Laugier–Hunziker syndrome
Acquired, benign hyperpigmented macules of the lips and buccal mucosa and nails.

Laurence–Moon–Biedl syndrome
Congenital retinitis pigmentosa, obesity, polydactyly, learning disability and blindness.

Lesch–Nyhan syndrome
Congenital purine metabolism defect causing learning disability, choreoathetoid cerebral palsy and self-multilation.

Letterer–Siwe disease
Rapidly progressive disseminated form of Langerhans histiocytosis which can be fatal because of pancytopenia and multisystem disease.

Lyme disease
Infection with deer tick-borne *Borrelia burgdorferii* causing rashes, fever, arthopathy and facial palsy (first reported in the town of Lyme, Connecticut, USA).

Maffucci syndrome
Multiple enchondromas, haemangiomas, and risk of malignant chondrosarcomas.

Mantoux test
Skin test for delayed-type hypersensitivity reaction to bacille Calmette-Guérin (BCG; for tuberculosis).

Marcus Gunn syndrome
Jaw-winking syndrome (eyelid winks during chewing), with ptosis.

Marfan syndrome
Autosomal dominant tall, thin stature and arachnodactyly (long, thin spider-like hands), lens dislocation, aortic aneurysms and regurgitation, floppy mitral valve, and occasionally cleft and bifid uvula. Joint laxity is common.

Melkersson–Rosenthal syndrome
Facial paralysis, oedema and fissured tongue – probably a variant of orofacial granulomatosis.

Miescher cheilitis
Oligosymptomatic orofacial granulomatosis or Crohn disease clinically affecting the lip alone.

Mikulicz disease
Salivary gland and lacrymal gland swelling often related to IgG4 systemic disease.

Mikulicz ulcer
Minor aphthous ulceration.

Moebius syndrome
Congenital anomaly involving multiple cranial nerves, including the abducens (VI) and facial (VII) nerves, and often associated with limb anomalies.

Moon molars
Hypoplastic molars from congenital syphilis.

Munchausen syndrome
Fabrication of stories aimed at the patient receiving operative intervention.

Nikolsky sign
Blistering or extension of a blister on gentle pressure (e.g. in pemphigus and pemphigoid).

Noonan syndrome
Congenital short stature, webbed neck sometimes with cardiac anomalies, pulmonary stenosis and cherubism.

Osler–Rendu–Weber disease (hereditary haemorrhagic telangiectasia: HHT)
Autosomal dominant disorder. Telangiectases orally and periorally but also in nose, gastrointestinal tract and occasionally on palms.

Paget disease
Acquired idiopathic disorder of bones presenting with progressive jaw swelling, hypercementosis and deformity.

Papillon–Lefèvre syndrome
Congenital defect in cathepsin causing palmoplantar hyperkeratosis and juvenile periodontitis which affects both dentitions, and immunodeficiency.

Parrot nodes
Frontal bossing in congenital syphilis.

Paterson–Kelly syndrome (Plummer–Vinson syndrome)
Association of dysphagia (post cricoid web of candida), microcytic hypochromic anaemia, koilonychia (spoon-shaped nails) and angular cheilitis.

Paul–Bunnell test
Serological test for heterophile antibodies in infectious mononucleosis (glandular fever).

Peutz–Jeghers syndrome
Autosomal dominant condition of circumoral melanosis and intestinal polyposis.

Pierre Robin syndrome
Congenital micrognathia, cleft palate and glossoptosis.

Prader–Willi syndrome
Congenital obesity, hypogonadism, learning disability, diabetes and dental defects.

Ramsay Hunt syndrome
A lower motor neurone facial palsy due to herpes zoster of the geniculate ganglion of the VIIth nerve.

Rapp–Hodgkin syndrome
Ectodermal dysplasia, kinky hair, cleft lip/palate, popliteal pterygium and ectrodactyly.

Raynaud syndrome
Vascular spasm in response to cooling, seen in the digits in connective tissue disorders.

Reiter syndrome
The association of arthritis, urethritis and balanitis, and conjunctivitis.

Rett disease
Congenital bruxism and hand-wringing, often with learning disability.

Riley–Day syndrome
Inherited dysautonomia; sympathetic dysfunction, enlarged salivary glands and sialorrhoea and self-mutilation, seen particularly in Ashkenazi Jews.

Romberg syndrome (hemifacial atrophy)
Progressive atrophy of the soft tissues of half the face, associated with contralateral Jacksonian epilepsy and trigeminal neuralgia.

Sabin–Feldman test
Serological test for toxoplasmosis.

Seckel syndrome
Congenital microcephaly, learning disability, zygomatic and mandibular hypoplasia.

Shprintzen syndrome (velo-cardio-facial syndrome)
A congenital anomaly with cleft palate, heart defect, abnormal face, learning disability, short stature and microcephaly.

Sipple syndrome (multiple endocrine neoplasia type 2a)
Multiple endocrine neoplasia (MEN) type 3 (MEN 3; sometimes called 2b).

Sjögren syndrome (secondary Sjögren syndrome)
Hyposalivation and keratoconjunctivitis sicca, i.e. dry mouth and dry eyes with connective tissue disease.

Smith–Lemli–Opitz syndrome
Congenital short stature, learning disability, syndactyly, urogenital and maxillary anomalies.

Stevens–Johnson syndrome
Severe erythema multiforme.

Still syndrome
Juvenile rheumatoid arthritis.

Sturge–Weber syndrome (encephalotrigeminal angiomatosis)
Congenital angioma of upper face (naevus flammeus), and underlying bone with convulsions, and hemiplegia.

Sutton ulcers
Major aphthae.

Sweet syndrome
Acute neutrophilic dermatosis; red mucosal lesions and aphthae.

Takayasu disease
Pulseless aorta and large arteries.

Thibierge–Weissenbach syndrome
Diffuse cutaneous scleroderma.

Treacher Collins syndrome (mandibulofacial dysostosis)
Autosomal dominant defect in the first branchial arch with downward sloping (antimongoloid slant) palpebral fissures, hypoplastic malar complexes, mandibular retrognathia, deformed pinnas, hypoplastic

sinuses, colobomas in the outer third of the eye, middle and inner ear hypoplasia (deafness).

Tricho-dento-osseous syndrome
Autosomal dominant; kinky hair, amelogenesis imperfecta and brittle nails.

Trotter syndrome
Acquired unilateral deafness, pain in the mandibular (third) division of the trigeminal nerve, ipsilateral palatal immobility and trismus. Due to invasion of the nasopharynx by malignant tumour.

Turner teeth
Hypoplastic tooth due to damage to the developing tooth germ.

Von-Recklinghausen disease
Multiple neurofibromas with skin pigmentation, skeletal abnormalities and central nervous system involvement.

Waardenburg syndrome
Congenital heterochromia iridis (different-coloured eyes), deafness and white forelock, with prognathism.

Waldeyer ring
Lymphoid tissue surrounding the entrance to the oropharynx (tonsils and adenoids).

Warthin tumour
Salivary gland tumour.

Wegener granulomatosis
Idiopathic granulomatous disorder affecting lungs, kidneys and sometimes mouth.

Wiskott–Aldrich syndrome
X-linked recessive immunodeficiency characterized by thrombocytopenic purpura, eczema, recurrent infections and lymphoreticular malignancies.

Glossary of abbreviations

AC	angular cheilitis
ANA	antinuclear antibodies
bid or **bd**	twice a day
BMS	burning mouth syndrome
BNF	*British National Formulary*
BP	blood pressure
BRONJ	bisphosphonate-related osteonecrosis of the jaw
BS	Behçet syndrome
CAT	computerised axial tomography
CBT	cognitive-behavioural therapy
CMV	cytomegalovirus
CNS	central nervous system
CO	complaining of
COPD	chronic obstructive pulmonary disease
CRP	C-reactive protein
CSF	cerebrospinal fluid
CT	computed tomography or chemotherapy
CVA	cerebrovascular accident
CXR	chest X-ray
DIF	direct immunofluorescence
DLE	disseminated lupus erythematosus
DPF	*Dental Practitioners Formulary*
DXR	radiotherapy
EB	epidermolysis bullosa
EBV	Epstein–Barr virus
ECG	electrocardiogram
ELISA	enzyme-linked immunosorbent assay
EM	erythema multiforme
ENT	ears, nose and throat

ESR	erythrocyte sedimentation rate
FBC	full blood count
FBP	full blood picture
FH	family history
FNA	fine needle aspiration
FNAB	fine needle aspiration biopsy
GDP	general dental practitioner
GI	gastrointestinal
GIT	gastrointestinal tract
GMH	general medical history
GMP	general medical practitioner
GORD	gastro-oesophageal reflux disease
GP	general practitioner
GvHD	graft-versus-host disease
HBV	hepatitis B virus
HCV	hepatitis C virus
HHV	human herpesviruses
HIV	human immunodeficiency virus(es)
HL	Hodgkin lymphoma
HPA	hypothalamus–pituitary–adrenal
HPC	history of the present complaint
HPV	human papillomaviruses
HSCT	haematopoietic stem cell transplantation
HSV	herpes simplex virus
IIF	indirect immunofluorescence
KCOT	keratocystic odontogenic tumour
KS	Kaposi sarcoma
KSHV	Kaposi sarcoma herpesvirus
LA	local anaesthesia
LFT	liver function tests
LP	lichen planus

MDR-TB	multidrug resistant tuberculosis
MEN	multiple endocrine neoplasia
mg	milligram
MMP	mucous membrane pemphigoid
MRI	magnetic resonance imaging
MRS	Melkersson–Rosenthal syndrome
MRSA	methicillin-resistant *Staphylococcus aureus*
NHL	non-Hodgkin lymphoma
NSAID	non-steroidal anti-inflammatory drug
OFG	orofacial granulomatosis
ORN	osteoradionecrosis
OTC	over-the-counter
PCR	polymerase chain-reaction
PFAPA	periodic fever, aphthae, pharyngitis, adenitis
PMH	past medical history
POM	prescription-only medicine
PPI	proton pump inhibitor
prn	as necessary
PV	pemphigus vulgaris
qid or **qds**	four times a day
RAS	recurrent aphthous stomatitis
RF	rheumatoid factor
RMH	relevant medical history
SH	social history
SJS	Stevens–Johnson syndrome
SLE	systemic lupus erythematosus
SS	Sjögren syndrome
SSI	sexually shared infections
SSRI	selective serotonin re-uptake inhibitor
STI	sexually transmitted infection
TB	tuberculosis

tid	three times a day
TMJ	temporomandibular joint
TMPD	temporomandibular pain-dysfunction syndrome
TN	trigeminal neuralgia
TNF	tumour necrosis factor
U&E	urea and electrolytes
URTI	upper respiratory tract infection
US	ultrasound
UTI	urinary tract infection
WBC	white blood cell count
WCC	white cell count
VZV	varicella-zoster virus
XDR-TB	extended drug-resistant tuberculosis

Further reading

http://health.nih.gov/
<accessed 15 June 2011>

http://www.emedicine.com
<accessed 15 June 2011>

http://www.mayoclinic.com/health/DiseasesIndex/DiseasesIndex
<accessed 15 June 2011>

http://www.merckmanuals.com/professional/full-symptoms.html
<accessed 15 June 2011>

Index

Page numbers ending in 'b', 'f' and 't' refer to Boxes, Figures and Tables respectively

B

J

P

R

S